Mary Jane Safford, MD
INDOMITABLE MITE

Elizabeth Coachman, MD

Second Edition 2017

© 2017 Elizabeth Coachman, MD

Book Design: Sergio Waksman

ISBN: 978-0-9986366-3-4

Printed in United States

Publisher: Elizabeth Coachman, MD

Brooksville, Florida

TABLE OF CONTENTS

DEDICATION

In memory of Edward and Jane Hoffman

who dragged me, kicking and screaming,

into the vortex of 19th century history

but to whom I'm forever grateful

for the experience

For Mike who always makes me smile

PREFACE

"A mite of a woman with an indomitable soul," is Dr. Anna Howard Shaw's apt description of medical school professor Dr. Mary Jane Safford whose real life experiences rival Forrest Gump's fictional ones.

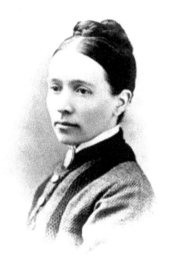

Fearless, with the uncanny ability to appear in right places and times to experience 19th century history, she was among its creators. From the poverty of youth to a European grand tour with a corrupt ex-governor of Illinois, from Civil War nurse to medical school valedictorian to European-trained gynecologic surgeon, from experiencing the Great Chicago fire, Great Boston fire and her own fiery speeches on dress reform and temperance, Mary Safford rose to a fame larger

Mary Jane Safford, undated. Courtesy Cairo Public Library, Cairo, IL.

than life. She wrote and spoke prolifically on travel, progressive reforms, racial equality and medicine. She could address an exclusive women's club as comfortably as she worked among Boston's slum dwellers.

Among her associates were Elizabeth Cady Stanton, Mary Livermore, Clara Barton, Ulysses S. Grant and a host of others; yet somehow Mary Safford slipped through history's cracks and is veritably overlooked. Perhaps it is because she was only four feet four inches tall.

Hopefully, this book will resurrect and revitalize interest in this dynamic woman.

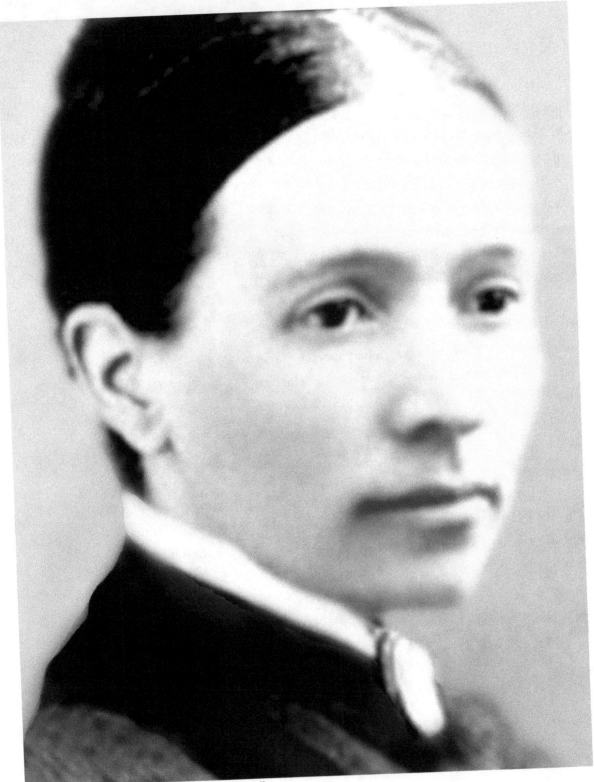

Detail of Mary Jane Safford, undated. Courtesy Cairo Public Library, Cairo, IL.

1 IN THE BEGINNING

Mary Jane Safford's birth year is an enigma. Her 1862 passport application, the only legal documentation of her birth date, states it was December 31, 1837, and says she was 24 years old when, in fact, she was probably 30.[1] Among young scholars' answering roll call in Crete, Illinois,' school for 1837-8 were Mary and her brothers Anson Peasley Keeler Safford (known as A. P. K.), Alfred Boardman Safford, and the oldest Joseph Brewster Safford.[2] An 1837 genealogy book lists all five Safford siblings including eldest Anna and youngest Mary.[3] Unless that book was hot off the press on New Year's Eve or Mary precociously started school before birth, she was born earlier. Engraved on her huge, gray, Vermont granite tombstone in Florida is the incorrect birth year 1834. Safford family photo labels provide the 1831 birth year preferred for this book.[4]

Married in a Morristown, Vermont, civil ceremony Mary's parents Joseph Warren Safford and Diantha Little descended from 17th century English immigrants.[5][6][7] At Mary's birth the family lived in northwestern Vermont's Hyde Park region with beautiful rocky, wooded terrain and an overabundance of ravenous merino sheep that plagued farmers.[8][9] Wool manufacturers were happy, but the ruminants' destructive effects and a national economic panic led to many farmers' departures including that of Joseph Warren Safford. Newly opened water routes Champlain and Erie Canals facilitated the way west. "The West," included northern Illinois, homeland to the Potawatomi Indians who farmed for generations but realized white settlers' intrusion meant a formidable lifestyle change and sought relief from them through a treaty that involved abandoning lands including what became Will County, Illinois.[10][11]

In 1837, Joseph Safford sold almost all his Vermont land and family home for $400.[12] The sales record's wording, "the premises on which I now reside with my family…" implied the Saffords left then, but A.P.K.'s autobiography says the family left for Illinois a year earlier.[13] Whether marauding sheep or a poor economy prompted the Saffords' move is unknown, but conditions must have been extreme for Joseph in his early 60s to uproot his family from land of several generations' home and move to virtually unknown wilderness. The prospect of beginning anew on flat, fertile, black dirt farmland must have been enticing.

Just as birds of a feather flock together, many Vermont friends and relations migrated to northern Illinois in the mid-1830s. Mary's uncle Dr. Wallace Asa Little and family moved as did her Aunt Lydia Little Boardman, cousins William Boardman and Diantha Boardman Wood, and her husband Willard Wood who traveled by water to Detroit then overland to Chicago.[14][15][16][17][18] The trade center's population was growing, but the pioneers bypassed city life to favor open land. They planned continuing west, but spring flooding diverted them about 40 miles south to the Will County area eventually known as Crete.[19] A reference listed Willard Wood and J. W. Safford and three sons among settlers of Will County's Thorn Creek area in 1835-1836 but failed noting Diantha, Mary and her much older sister Anna Safford Gridley who died at age 27 when Mary was only 11.[20][21]

An 1895 interview with then 87-year old Willard Wood described the region as the Saffords found it, "covered with hazel brush, and a few oak trees, or what there was left after fires had swept the prairies."[22] The area was further described as having, "wild and undisturbed beauty," and that, "deer, grouse and quail and many other wild animals made hunting plentiful, but the nights were made weird by the plaintive howling of wolves patrolling the cabins." [23] A. P. K. Safford's autobiographical sketch echoed these primitive conditions:

"The Indians had but recently vacated the country; their trails as they had traveled single file were yet deeply sunk in the alluvial soil. Many of their wigwams were still standing, and the coals were visible where they had cooked their food. Arrow points and implements of war were found on every hand, and the bones of their dead were often unearthed by the plow of the husbandman. Sometimes the grave of one evidently distinguished in his tribe was uncovered as evidenced by the trophies that were buried with him." [24]

Will County commenced in 1836, named for medical Dr. Conrad Will, master of slaves if not their outright owner, and not surprisingly, a politician. [25][26] Despite the Northwest Ordinance of 1787's prohibiting slavery in Illinois, the state's constitution allowed, "leasing of slaves," through a type of indentured servitude for massively labor-intensive salt operations like Dr. Will ran. [27][28] Probably, the Vermonters were unaware of the name's ignominious connotation, as the salt works were in distant southern Illinois. [29]

As of this writing, the Triebold family of Crete, Illinois, owns the property the Saffords developed. A stream runs along the eastern side of the relatively flat land, and corn grows in its rich, black dirt fields. Carol Triebold identified the Saffords' reputed cabin site, but no remnants exist. Saffords' property acquisition details are unknown, but settlers commonly claimed land through squatting on untitled parcels. By building a cabin and fencing a cultivated area, they established a pre-emptive right to purchase the land when the U.S. Government offered it at $1.25/acre. Although Joseph sold the family's Vermont homestead, travel expenses were steep, and he lacked sufficient funds to purchase the Illinois farm outright. A.P. K. reported his parents' poor health, high farm mortgage interest, low returns on their crops and how the family occasionally subsisted on wild onions. [30] It was said of Mary's situation:

"…nearly all her childhood and early life were marked by the struggle with poverty and hardships, which her parents endured as pioneers in the then new country." [31]

Life was tough. The Saffords were among friends and relatives, but Illinois lacked Vermont's established community infrastructure. The exciting opportunity to design and live in a new community came with challenging hardships, but Mary's youth made her blessedly oblivious to poverty's deprivations. It was her normal state of affairs.

A biographer further elaborated:

"Her stories of those days were most thrilling and bore frequent reference to her mother…Her mother was called far and near among the much scattered population in times of sickness, sometimes taking one of her daughters with her, but often leaving the little Mary to take charge of the household in her absence…She was first greatly interested in surgery from an accident which happened to her mother. Mrs. Safford broke her arm, which was clumsily set, and therefore improperly united, and in order to have a perfect and useful arm, she voluntarily broke it, and reset it herself, with lasting success…" [32]

Diantha Safford also had a passion for education and felt schooling was her children's ticket out of difficult pioneer life. [33] Brother A. P. K. studied wherever he could while still farming and later helped establish Arizona Territory's public school system. [34][35] Mary's long and circuitous educational path's description is in following chapters.

In addition to farming, the abolitionist Saffords actively participated in Will County's Underground Railroad to help fugitive slaves attain freedom. An 1876 sketch of Mary Safford's early life illustrated the family's abolitionist work:

"...some of the most striking recollections of Mary's childhood are connected with the underground railroad, of which her father's home formed a station. Many times has she been awakened from sleep by a low tapping at the door, in answer to which her mother would rise and admit the fugitives, giving them food, and, if not too closely pursued, affording them rest and shelter. They always went away with well-filled knapsacks and explicit directions to the next station. On one occasion an old man with his wife and little child came to their door for shelter. They were so much exhausted by fatigue and suffering that it was decided they should stay two or three days, and a hiding-place was made for them in the cellar. Soon after their arrival some men, impelled perhaps by the general principle that an abolitionist's house would bear examination, came to search for them. The only entrance to the cellar, through the house, was by a trap-door. On this door little Mary Safford placed herself and by various childish devices managed to direct the attention of the pursuers, so that after a hasty search of the house, they left without having noticed the door. The mother then spoke to the child in regard to her unusual conduct in their presence and asked the reason of it. 'Why, mother, I was afraid they would see the trap-door if I did not do so,' was the earnest reply. Both parents and brothers were amused by the child's stratagem, which had prevented the discovery of the runaway slaves. Educated amid such scenes and by such parents, we can readily see how a hearty antipathy to oppression in any form became one of the strongest attributes of her nature."[36]

In 1847, Joseph Safford sold a last piece of Vermont property--50 acres for $80, far less per acre than the Illinois property's cost.[37] He was then 72 years old and died a year later.[38] Mary's mother died the following year and lies next to Joseph in Crete.[39] Their deaths' cause is unknown, but old age and pioneer life's tough existence likely contributed. Possibly, they succumbed to Northern Illinois' 1848-49 cholera epidemic.[40] No matter what caused their parents' deaths, 21-year old A. P. K. and 17-year old Mary were alone on the Safford homestead, faced a mountain of debt and lacked adequate farm equipment.[41] Through the help of generous friends and relations the new orphans' dismal lives improved.

2 ANTEBELLUM LIFE

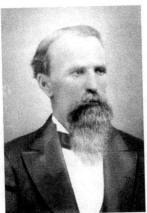

Anson Peasley Keeler (A. P. K.) Safford, early 1850s. Arizona Historical Society AHS25013.

Presumably, Mary kept house while A. P. K. farmed as did nearby married brother Joseph Brewster Safford. Cousin Willard Wood designed the Village of Crete in 1849 and greatly expanded his 1836 log cabin into Wood's Tavern, then Wood's Hotel.[1] Stores opened, and former brother-in-law George Gridley's blacksmith shop prospered. Some might have been content maintaining the status quo with a productive farm, neighboring friends and relations and a developing town. However, the California gold discovery was too tempting for a single male to bypass, and as A. P. K. put it:

"The gold fields of California were then attracting a great deal of attention, and I determined to try my fortunes in the new El Dorado. The thought of parting from me for so long and perilous a trip was painful in the extreme to my young sister; but I reasoned that I could place her in school; that my absence should not extend longer than two years, and then if fortune smiles upon me, we could both obtain an education. After long persuasion, she consented and I commenced at once to make preparation for the journey."[2]

In 1850, while vowing to return to Crete, A. P. K. sold his land to brother Joseph and left with other young male Cretans for California's gold fields. 19-year old Mary moved into Wood's Hotel with Willard's family including seven children, widowed Aunt Lydia Little Boardman and four laborers.[3] It's a wonder any hotel guests found rooms. Mary and A.P.K. next saw each other sixteen years later.[4]

After remaining only a short time to help with those myriad cousins, Mary left for boarding school. Followed by, "Crete, Illinois," her name was among Vermont's Bakersfield North Academy students for the year ending November 1852.[5] Possibly, the Saffords knew of the school previously, as Bakersfield was near Hyde Park. Perhaps Willard Wood who studied law in Vermont knew someone on the school's board of trustees.[6] Later, A. P. K. recounted a Nevada Territory property sale netted him $300.75 of which he, "forwarded $300 to the States for the benefit of my sister."[7] By then she was 20 or 21 years old, but he indicated neither where he sent the money nor his plans for his remaining $0.75. The coeducational Vermont school's course offerings mirrored a modern day rigorous high school curriculum and provided a solid basic education including penmanship taught by Mr. Chase.[8] Mary Safford's later handwriting's appearance suggests he made little impression on her.

While at Bakersfield, Mary lived in Hon. William Campbell Wilson's, "rooms."[9] He was a school trustee and established Bakersfield's law school the prior year.[10] Three of his children attended the academy and lived with Mary and other students, but crowded conditions would not have bothered her, as she lived them in Crete.[11] Although Mary might have considered remaining in Vermont, she chose furthering her education instead:

"After graduating at Bakersfield, Vermont, Miss Safford went to Canada, and entered a French school, in which she remained a year, perfecting herself in the language spoken there. At the end of this time she returned to her brother's home in Illinois, her parents being dead; and soon, after feeling that she must be doing something, she became a

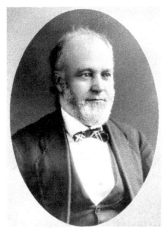

Alfred Boardman Safford, 1850s. Courtesy Cairo, IL, Public Library.

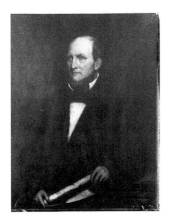

Joel Aldrich Matteson. Abraham Lincoln Presidential Library & Museum (I-2064).

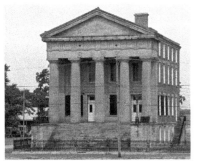

State Bank of Illinois, Shawneetown, IL, as it appeared in 2012. Courtesy Michael R. Coachman.

member of a German family, and spent six months studying their language."[12]

No record exists of her German host family or her matriculation at a Canadian school. However, Montreal was only about 80 miles from Bakersfield, and, logically, an independent, bright young woman might opt for life in a civilized large city.

By the mid-1850s, Mary joined older brother Alfred in Joliet, Illinois, where a few years earlier he studied law briefly with their cousin William Boardman.[13] [14] He was brother-in-law of Joel Aldrich Matteson, another merchant and practiced politician, who became Illinois' governor in 1852.[15] [16] Above his wool store Matteson opened the Merchants' and Drovers' Bank and named Roswell Goodell its cashier.[17] When Matteson became governor he appointed Goodell Secretary of the Illinois Canal Commission, and a subsequent scandal exposed Matteson's part in a false re-issue of over $200,000 in previously redeemed Illinois-Michigan canal scrip.[18] [19] Goodell married Matteson's daughter Mary Jane, and, as well as a potential love match, the union cemented Matteson's political and business relationships with him. Later, the ex-governor named his daughter Olivia's husband John McGinnis, Jr., president of the Matteson's Bank of Quincy, Illinois.[20] [21] Matteson's legendary penchant for nepotism soon involved Alfred and Mary Safford who likely met him through their cousin William.

In 1813, the Bank of Illinois began operations in far southern Shawneetown, and the institution's initial success supported the town's reputation as Illinois' financial capital.[22] The bank soon closed when officers refused loaning Chicago men money while reasoning that the town was, "…too damned far from Shawneetown to ever amount to anything."[23] Current common knowledge said Shawneetown would displace Chicago as Illinois' great metropolis. Ostensibly to promote customer confidence, the officers built an $80,000 stone building fronted by five massive columns reminiscent of a Greek temple. A state act extended the bank's charter, but the institution closed again.[24] In 1854, Governor Matteson sensed a golden opportunity and, by using Alfred Safford as a surrogate, kept a low profile in purchasing the bank.[25] [26] [27] Three years later, with President Roswell Goodell and Cashier Alfred Safford, the institution had the largest capitalization of any Illinois bank at $650,000.[28] [29]

While living in Shawneetown the Saffords may have occupied the bank's upper story, but, wherever they lived, the river, with its inescapable sounds, smells and activity offered easy access to numerous large cities. The town was nine miles below the mouth of the Wabash River and was named for the Shawnee Indians who formerly lived in the vicinity. They wisely decided the locale was an unsuitable village site due to frequent flooding in an area compared to the Nile Delta and even now called, "Egypt."

Also in 1854, in Joel Matteson's hometown of Watertown, New York, 32-year old Alfred Safford married Julia Jane Massey.[30] Living in Shawneetown with Alfred and Julia, Mary sought useful occupation and soon found it:

"They had a school in Shawneetown; but the young men boasted that no teacher had ever yet taught a full term.'

'The earnest mind of Miss Safford, born and educated in New England as she had been, revolted at this state of affairs, and she determined to open a public school herself…Her brother predicted that she would not teach more than two weeks; and almost everyone in the place, who thought of it at all, did so only to laugh at the notion. 'Safford's ragged school' was one of the good jokes in Shawneetown.'

'At the close of the first week fifty scholars were in attendance, and at the end of the term the number had increased to one hundred and fifty. The athletic young men who had been in the habit of throwing fighting teachers out of doors never gave this little woman the slightest trouble…During the first year, a good school-house was built, and thus 'Safford's ragged school' became the pride of Shawneetown…" [31]

The author's reference to, "this little woman," was well founded, as Mary Safford was only 4' 4" tall.[32] Having three older brothers may have prepared her for the Shawneetown boys' challenge, but perhaps her diminutive size and good looks inspired the boys' acting protectively. Mary's winning way with words, humor and natural teaching abilities served her well in this first of the many types of schools where she eventually taught. The name, "Safford Ragged School," might imply ridicule, but in the 19th century, "Ragged Schools," were charitable institutions dedicated to destitute children's free education.[33] The Scottish Ragged School Movement spread, and the poor dirty Shawneetown youths were prime candidates for it. Among her students were the Wilson brothers one of whom became a Major General after graduation with honors from West Point.[34] His brother became U. S. District Attorney for the Southern District of Illinois and subsequently Solicitor of the Treasury. His memory of Mary Safford: "…there is no person whose kindly countenance and advice did so much toward rousing a noble ambition in his mind as that of his teacher…"[35]

Mary's Ragged School teaching ended with an unnamed illness, and her subsequent Shawneetown activities are unknown. She had river access to large cities and a direct stage line to Springfield, but no rail line served Shawneetown. A one-day steamship ride down the Ohio River brought passengers to Illinois' southernmost tip and Cairo, where, since 1855, Illinois Central Railroad trains offered service north to Chicago.[36][37] From Cairo, steamboats traveled as far south as New Orleans.

Shawneetown housed a curious collection of individuals Mary may have known. Among these were Robert Green Ingersoll and John Alexander, "Black Jack," Logan.[38] Ingersoll taught school in Metropolis, Illinois, and had studied law for three months. After admission to the Illinois Bar, Ingersoll first worked for John M. Cunningham at Shawneetown's Federal Land Office before assisting Clerk of the Circuit and County Courts John E. Hall. Sadly, a man with whom Hall had a disagreement ended it in 1856 by shooting him right before Ingersoll in their office.[39] Hall died in Ingersoll's arms. The murderer was Robert Sloo, and his sensational 42-day trial enlisted notable prosecutor John A. Logan.[40] Much to Ingersoll and Logan's disgust, Sloo was acquitted due to, "emotional insanity."[41] Mary Safford undoubtedly knew of Sloo's heinous crime. No correspondence between Mary and Ingersoll exists, but very likely they were acquaintances in Shawneetown and elsewhere, as both worked for Illinois woman suffrage and had early albeit different Civil War involvement.

Across the street from the Shawneetown bank and directly on the Ohio River, was the home of Ingersoll's initial employer Land Registrar John Cunningham.[42] The land office was on the first floor, and the large Cunningham family including eldest daughter Mary occupied the rest.[43] The two Marys, Safford and Cunningham, undoubtedly were acquainted. In the Mexican War John Cunningham served with John Logan who took an interest in pretty 17-year old Mary Cunningham and married her in 1855. Later, he and Mary Safford played significant parts in Illinois' early Civil War activities while Mary Logan wrote about them and eventually about her life as wife of Illinois' U.S. Senator Logan. She referred to Mary Safford as among, "noble souls."[44]

Shawneetown's residents usually accepted the Ohio River's intermittently inundating the town as mere inconvenience, but the catastrophic 1858 flood allowed steamboats to easily navigate the town's streets.[45] As drive-in banking had yet to be invented, the deluge likely encouraged Matteson's moving his bank. In addition, he saw proverbial handwriting on the wall and moved both the bank and the Saffords to the more strategically located Cairo, Illinois, at a most propitious time.[46]

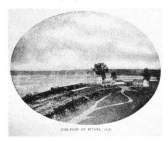

Cairo, IL, 1858, Illinois Central train line along Ohio River levee. A History of the City of Cairo, Illinois, John McMurray Lansden, Chicago, Donnelly & Sons, 1910, p. 72.

The name Cairo can elicit thoughts of an exotic locale with camels' transporting avid travelers to ancient pyramids in a shimmering desert warmed by soft, dry winds. In Illinois the name evokes different images and sounds. First, it is pronounced, "Karo," like the syrup. Second, although the landscape includes the confluence of two mighty rivers, its image differs considerably from that of its African counterpart. Charles Dickens wrote of his 1842 visit:

"At the junction of the two rivers, on ground so flat and low and marshy, that at certain seasons of the year it is inundated to the house-tops, lies a breeding-place of fever, ague, and death;…A dismal swamp, on which the half-built houses rot away:…the hateful Mississippi circling and eddying before it, and turning off upon its southern course a slimy monster hideous to behold; a hotbed of disease, an ugly sepulcher, a grave uncheered by any gleam of promise; a place without one single quality, in earth or air or water, to commend it: such is this dismal Cairo."[47]

Supposedly, Dickens' impressions were the basis for, "New Eden," in his novel Martin Chuzzlewit. Even 20 years later, conditions hadn't improved much, as Anthony Trollope wrote after a February 1862 visit:

"Cairo is the southern terminus of the Illinois Central Railway. There is but one daily arrival there, namely, at half-past four in the morning…Why anybody should ever arrive at Cairo at half-past four A. M., I cannot understand. The departure at any hour is easy of comprehension. The place is situated exactly at the point at which the Ohio and the Mississippi meet, and is I should say—merely guessing on the matter—some ten or twelve feet lower than the winter level of the two rivers. …Who were the founders of Cairo I have never ascertained. They are probably buried fathoms deep in the mud.'

'I tried to walk round the point on the levees, but I found that the mud was so deep and slippery on that which protected the town from the Mississippi that I could not move on it.…On the other, which forms the bank of the Ohio, the railway runs, and here was gathered all the life and movement of the place."[48]

The Saffords moved to this quagmire of existence and den of terraqueous inhabitants in 1858.[49] Cairo's population was around 2000, and its internationally famous muddy streets boasted four shoe stores, seven food stores, five clothing establishments, two doctors, one dentist, one newspaper and fifteen lawyers.[50][51] Perhaps the last were useful to stimulate boardwalk maintenance. Cairo, too, suffered in the 1858 flood when a breached levee uprooted trees and submerged the city.[52] If allowed an option, the Saffords might have picked a different home, but Matteson's plans included Alfred who became cashier of the governor's new City Bank of Cairo.[53] Its building included upper floors' office space where the Saffords lived initially.[54]

While Alfred established the bank and a life for himself and Julia, Mary began teaching school.[55] Beyond that, her activities are unrecorded until the first mustering of troops at Cairo's Camp Defiance in June of 1861. Perhaps in the interim she furthered her education. The coeducational Illinois State University at Normal, Illinois, opened earlier, and, although unlisted among those matriculating, possibly, Mary audited classes.[56] Also, her involvement in scientific and natural history organizations may have begun while she was in Cairo. Among her friends was the handsome geology Professor Joseph H. McChesney, charter faculty member of the exclusively male Old University of Chicago.[57][58]

Today, Cairo's public library has a small climate controlled room with a few Safford family books. One entitled *Life of Our Lord and Savior Jesus Christ* by the Reverend John Fleetwood contains the inscription, "Miss Mary Safford, April 3, 1858." A small volume marked just inside with, "M. J. Safford," is *The Final Memorials of Charles Lamb* said to consist of previously unpublished letters and notes of the British writer's companions. The most elegant of these books is a 3" x 4" x 2" thick, brown leather-bound Bible embossed in gold and inscribed, "Miss M. J. Safford from her brother July 4, 1860." Given Alfred's proximity, the book was more likely from him than from A. P. K. who was in California or Joseph Brewster Safford who continued farming in Crete.[59][60] Whether Mary viewed the Bible from a spiritual, historical or scientific viewpoint is unknown, but the tranquility that allowed her reading time was about to end.

3 WAR ARRIVES

On a small island outside Charleston's harbor and approximately 700 miles from Cairo, Major Robert Anderson received a most polite note:

> "Fort Sumter, S. C. April 12, 1861, 3:20 A. M.
>
> Major Robert Anderson, United States Army, Commanding Fort Sumter:
>
> Sir: By authority of Brigadier General Beauregard, Commanding the Provisional forces of the Confederate States, we have the honor to notify you that he will open the fire of his batteries on Fort Sumter in one hour from this time.
>
> We have the honor to be, very respectfully, your obedient servants,
>
> James Chesnut, Jr. Aid-de-Camp
>
> Stephen D. Lee, Captain, S. C. Army and Aid-de Camp"[1]

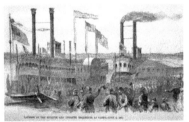

Union troops' arriving in Cairo, IL, 4 Jun 1861. Harper's Weekly, 29 Jun 1861.

Having expressed their respects, the Confederates fulfilled their offer of honorable hostilities with firepower's leading to the Union's retreat. This necessitated Major Anderson's subsequent report to Lincoln's Secretary of War Simon Cameron. In turn, he wrote to Illinois Governor Richard Yates:

"Washington April 15, 1861. His Excellency, Richard Yates: Call made on you by to-night's mail for six regiments of militia for immediate service. Simon Cameron, Secretary of War."

"Washington, April 19, 1861. Governor Yates: As soon as enough of your troops is mustered into service, send a Brigadier General with four regiments at or near Grand Cairo. Simon Cameron, Secretary of War."[2]

Cameron's telegrams initiated an event sequence Illinoisans anticipated, as many of the state's southern inhabitants had secessionist sympathies. Even an awareness of Cairo's strategic position could not have prepared its residents for the shock of waking to numerous undisciplined but enthusiastic armed men and the initial noise, confusion and mountains of haphazardly collected war supplies. Governor Yates acted immediately, and only 9 days after the Fort Sumter surrender several hundred primarily northern Illinois troops reached Cairo by train.[3] By May 10th, over 5000 soldiers had arrived at Camp Defiance, a Union encampment just within the Ohio and Mississippi levees' junction.[4]

Billeting the multitude was daunting, and prices rose on nearly everything for both the military and town residents. The Saffords' former Shawneetown neighbor Mary Cunningham Logan personally observed the situation when she arrived with her husband, now Colonel John A. Logan, and his Thirty-first Illinois regiment in summer 1861. She recounted in her autobiography:

"...The sudden concentration of thousands of men in the little city, with its half-dozen small hotels and overflowed surroundings, rendered existence…a problem…'

'Transportation was inadequate to the great number struggling to reach the point from which the great army was eventually to move. Habitations of houses or tents were not obtainable for all these civilians and soldiers congregating there. Quartermasters and commissaries were inefficient, and without any conception of the requirements of a great army and its followers. One single-track railroad with insufficient rolling-stock was to carry all the men, all the supplies, all the horses, all the ordnance and freight necessary for the immediate organization and equipment of the Army of the Mississippi.'

'The river steamers were of the most primitive character, and, though busy night and day, were unequal to the prodigious emergency…The continuous trains going and coming kept the people along the line of the road in a state of feverish excitement, and impressed them with the stupendous nature of the preparations for the conflict."[5]

The *Chicago Tribune* gave the following saccharine disinformation to northern Illinois readers:

"The troops are all in good health, and in the best of spirits. The most thorough discipline is cheerfully submitted to. Comfortable quarters are being provided and each day brings large supplies to minister to their wants and happiness. Out of so large a force, but twenty-three men are reported upon the sick list."[6]

Contradicting that rosy report, Mary Logan noted decidedly different camp conditions:

"…almost every spot of dry ground around the city was covered with the white tents of the boys in blue. The novelty of camp life soon vanished; attacks of illness, unavoidable with so many together in an inhospitable climate, and the discomforts that beset them, brought on an irresistible longing to return to home…"[7]

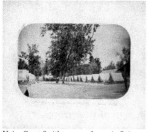

Union Camp Smith was one of many in Cairo, June 1861. Library of Congress Prints and Photographs Division, 2010648626.

For the most part the men were young and unused to fending for themselves. Most knew nothing of cooking let alone how to keep an orderly camp. Homesickness wasn't the only variety visited upon the soldiers, as the Illinois 31st regiment experienced a measles epidemic:

"Thousands of troops were housed in tents and barrack-type sheds along unimproved streets… Sanitation facilities were practically unknown, and before long the fever-ridden campsites held vast numbers of sick soldiers for whom improvised hospitals could provide only the crudest care. Beds, made of cornhusks or straw, had no sheets and were laid on the bare ground. Medicine and hospital supplies were scarce, and some of the so-called doctors were untrained. Nurses were usually convalescent soldiers, and generally unsatisfactory. Trained male nurses, the only ones authorized by army regulations, were simply unavailable. The food was the same unpalatable fare prepared by the men on active duty, and was served on unclean tin plates. Throughout the wards filth predominated, and the unbathed patients had nothing to wear but their dirty underclothing. The pungent smell of the sick, of grimy bodies, excrement and stale food, was all but over powering. Death came day after day from dysentery, pneumonia, and typhoid, largely because of unsanitary conditions, medical lethargy or incompetence."[8]

If Cairo's already unhealthy climate wasn't enough to incite the various epidemic diseases, exploitation in food, clothing and anything else needed for camp existence was enough to make anyone figuratively sick. Union uniforms were made of, "shoddy:"

"Shoddy consists of the refuse and sweepings of the shop, pounded, rolled, glued, and smoothed to the external form and gloss of cloth but no more like the genuine article than the shade is like the substance…Our soldiers on the first day's march found their clothes, overcoats, and blankets scattering to the winds or dissolving under the pelting rains."[9]

Unscrupulous vendors with fat government contracts short-changed the military, while deteriorating horse carcasses added to the town's stench. The Civil War offered ripe ground for profiteering, but no record exists of the Saffords' participation in activities deleterious to soldiers' provisions or welfare. On the contrary, Mary, Alfred and presumably Julia Safford aided the Union cause significantly. As well paid bank cashier, Alfred gave generously of his money and time as later noted by a U.S. Sanitary Commission inspector.[10] Meanwhile, Mary's thoughts turned to poor young men who battled disease for months before battling Confederates. Her initial efforts:

"She had heard of the suffering in the camp hospitals, and earnestly desired to smooth pillows, stroke fevered brows and read consoling passages from the Scriptures. This role of the ministering angel, very popular in fiction and poetry of the time, was one that many well-meaning girls aspired to play…Washington's improvised hospitals suffered from a perfect plague of angels, smelling salts in hand, drawing their skirts daintily about them, shrieking and fainting at the sight of blood. Cairo, a much smaller place, had only one angel, Mary Safford."[11]

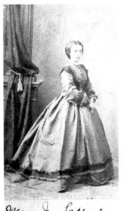

Mary Jane Safford, early 1860s. Photo John Sartain used for engraving in Linus Brockett's book on women's Civil War service.
Courtesy Cairo, IL, Public Library.

Due to Mary's charm and social standing, her efforts for sick soldiers were highly noticeable and publicized. Although physically delicate, she flew determinedly down a path that led other, "angels," to shriek and fly away. With her family tradition of boldly treating medical problems and a natural urge to serve, Mary made a fine candidate for more useful nursing but never enrolled in Dorothea Dix' Army Nursing Corps.[12] A further report:

"When the hospitals at Cairo began to fill up, it was but natural that Miss Safford should feel that duty called her there. We had read of women nurses in Soldiers' hospitals, but as yet the reality was unknown in America. At first she only asked admission to the wards to carry flowers and kind words to the sufferers, but at length she began to speak to the men about their wants, and then asked permission to supply them. The surgeon in charge had been attached to the army for many years, and belonged to what is called the old school of practice. For a long time this new nurse had so arranged her visits as to avoid meeting him, fearing that he might not approve these modern ideas concerning woman's mission, and that he would interdict her visits. One day however, as she was entering the hospital with her basket of flowers she met him face to face… he said to her slowly…'Ah, Miss Safford…I wish to say that your flowers and kind words are doing more good than my medicines. I hope you will feel free to come as often as you can.'" [13]

Illinois ministers spread the word of Cairo's soldiers' dire situation. At the Galesburg, Illinois, Brick Congregational Church in May 1861, Reverend Edward Beecher shared a letter from Dr. Benjamin Woodward who voluntarily accompanied five hundred Galesburg men to Cairo just after Ft. Sumter's fall. His story corroborated others' descriptions of Camp Defiance's horrid conditions:

"The army doctors were expressly classified as surgeons, not physicians. Their business was the care of wounded men after battle. Soldiers were not supposed to be sick. Succumbing to civilian disease in camp carried a strong suspicion of malingering to the army mind… If a stricken soldier survived his illness…he regained his own strength only by callously ignoring the needs of his sicker comrades. If he died, the government generously shipped his body home for burial, free of charge."[14]

By the time Reverend Beecher read this letter, Galesburg already had received two of her sons, "free of charge," due to illness, and congregants were indignant. Rather than wallow in anger, they collected over $500 in pledges of medicines, clean linens, hospital supplies and food. They elected 44-year old church member Mary Ann Bickerdyke to transport supplies to Cairo, oversee distribution and start what eventually became an over 4 year commitment to help, "her boys," receive adequate care.[15] With the exception that Mary Ann Bickerdyke and Mary Safford were both patriotic and cared deeply for the soldiers' welfare, the two Marys were virtual opposites. Mary Safford was refined and physically delicate. Bickerdyke was, "large, heavy, with, 'muscles of iron and nerves of steel,' a dynamic personality."[16] Author Young further described her:

"...possessed of an arsenal of ungrammatical eloquence which she used whenever an obstacle blocked her path, as when a doctor asked her by what authority she was appropriating hospital supplies. She replied, 'From the Lord God Almighty. Do you have anything that ranks higher than that?' " [17]

In June 1861, Mary Ann Bickerdyke arrived by train in Cairo as an unpaid volunteer nurse without appointment and unattached to any specific corps of relief. Mary Safford was still on a mission of smiles and flowers, but Bickerdyke recognized in her the potential for a good nurse:

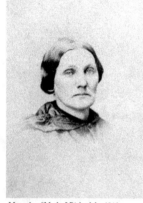

Mary Ann "Mother" Bickerdyke, 1860s. Courtesy Cairo, IL, Public Library.

"...the two women worked well together, complementing each other's efforts, and bringing a measure of cleanliness and comfort where there had been nothing but squalid misery. Miss Safford's money, or her brother's, was freely spent where it would do most good. The handsome Cairo mansion was frequently used as a convalescent rest home."[18]

Although the Saffords initially lived in the bank building, their eventual, "Cairo mansion," stood at the now vacant southeast corner of 4th and Washington Streets, at most a mile from Camp Defiance. Perhaps they also entertained the group Mary Logan described as Cairo's, "new army," of anxious friends and relatives.[19]

Yet a fourth Mary worked toward similar goals in Northern Illinois. Chicago women's relief groups functioned in an uncoordinated manner to send troops boxes of clothing, food, hospital supplies and, "comfort bags," of other sundries. Wife of Universalist minister Daniel Livermore and co-editor of Chicago's Universalist newspaper *New Covenant*, Mary Ashton Livermore presided over one of these groups and traveled to Cairo to investigate and publicize its desperate conditions. She commented on Mary Safford's work for the soldiers in classic words subsequent authors have used to characterize her as a little charmer used to having her way:

"If she was not the first woman in the country to enter upon hospital and camp relief, she was certainly the first in the West. There was no system, no organization, no knowledge what to do, and no means with which to work. As far as possible she brought order out of chaos, systematized the first rude hospitals, and with her own means, aided by a wealthy brother, furnished necessaries, when they could be obtained in no other way.'

'Surgeons and officers everywhere opposed her, but she disarmed them by the sweetness of her manner and her speech; and she did what she pleased. She was very frail, petite in figure as a girl of twelve summers, and utterly unaccustomed to hardship."[20]

Livermore seemed to describe an innocent teenager rather than a twenty-nine-year old woman who had experienced pioneer hardships, family deaths, a major flood, and somehow survived Shawneetown's school students. However, at 4' 4" tall, Mary Safford did qualify as petite. Livermore was fascinated by the cultivated socialite but also acknowledged, albeit in less flowery English, Mary Ann Bickerdyke's herculean efforts on the soldiers' behalf. Safford and Livermore became fast friends and later cooperated in women's rights promotion.

Cairo was particularly uncomfortable both for the military hordes' presence and for the beastly hot weather as noted by correspondent Albert Deane Richardson:

"June 8. The heated term is upon us... At eight, this morning, the mercury indicated eighty degrees in the shade. How high it has gone since, I dare not conjecture; but a friend insists that the sun will roast eggs to-day upon any doorstep in town... The raw troops on duty, who are sweltering in woolen shirts and cloth caps, bear it wonderfully well.'

'A number of Chicago ladies are already here, acting as nurses in the hospital...this tender care for the soldier is the one redeeming feature of modern war." [21]

Commencing in June 1861, the United States Sanitary Commission, led by a group of physicians and other prominent men, oversaw delivery of supplies for the hastily assembled troops otherwise neglected in proper personal and health care. As the organization evolved and confidence in its fulfilling a mission of shipping necessary items to the troops grew, smaller relief groups merged with it, and Mary Livermore and her friend Jane C. Hoge became leaders of its Northwestern Division that included the Chicago area.[22] Commission personnel reported to the military both camp conditions and needs for maintaining healthy troops. Livermore's prior Cairo report prompted Commission President Reverend Doctor Henry W. Bellows, John S. Newberry, MD, and associate W. H. Muzzey, to visit Cairo where they met Mary Safford at the end of June.[23] Previously, military nursing was performed by untrained male troops, and Bellows' letter to military medical personnel promoted women nurses' being allowed to continue their efforts.[24] Chicago's Sanitary Commission branch began sending supplies:

"Whatever Miss Safford and Mother Bickerdyke called for –from a surgeon to a lemon—was dispatched to them by the women of Chicago by the next train on the Illinois Central."[25]

The only hospital in Cairo at the war's start was called the Brick Hospital.[26] The Sisters of the Holy Cross led by General Sherman's wife's cousin Mother Angela Gillespie ran the approximately 100 bed facility with an eye toward cleanliness and tender patient care.[27] What, if any, role Mary Safford served at the Brick Hospital is unknown. Although various sheds, private homes and hotels sufficed poorly as Cairo's additional hospital space, it wasn't until much later and after Mary Safford departed Cairo that a true military hospital appeared.

Camp nursing work occupied most of Mary's summer, but in August her brother Joseph Brewster Safford died in his mid-40s in northern Illinois.[28] While Mary and Alfred coped in Cairo, A. P. K. was among the second wave of silver miners headed to Unionville, Humboldt County, Nevada Territory, hoping to profit from the Comstock Lode. It is unknown if any of these remaining Safford siblings attended their brother's funeral.

On September 4th, Brigadier General Ulysses Simpson Grant arrived in Cairo and established his district headquarters office and living quarters at Alfred's bank.[29] The Saffords lived in the bank initially, and later correspondence shows Grant knew them. He appreciated Cairo's strategic location and, with his West Point education and 1840s Mexican War experiences, now began his first district command including Cape Girardeau and Bird's Point, Missouri, as well as Cairo and Mound City, Illinois. Two days later, without firing a shot, his troops occupied Paducah, Kentucky, and then

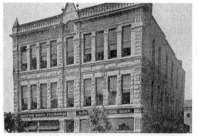

Cairo Bank building where Grant had 2nd floor headquarters near Alfred Safford's office. Cairo Custom House Museum, Cairo, IL.

controlled Fort Holt near Cairo. This prevented Confederates' overrunning an area more sympathetic to the South than to the Union. Before his troops occupied Paducah, Grant became aware of 4000 Confederates at Columbus, Kentucky, on the Mississippi River's eastern bank about 20 miles south of Cairo.[30] Rebel troops approached within 15 miles of Paducah just prior to Grant's taking it, and he was anxious to roust the remaining enemy near Columbus. As the impending war involved both land and water engagements, the Army and Navy needed to function cooperatively, and Commodore Andrew Foote assumed command of all Naval forces near Cairo.[31] It is unknown if Mary Safford knew him.

Mrs. Logan mentioned many soldiers' and officers' families' staying in Cairo's immediate vicinity. However, Grant's September 20th response from Cairo to his wife's inquiry about joining him reflected his hesitancy:

"I dont know what to say about your coming. I should like to have you here and at the same time I feel that I may have to leave any day. I am in most excelent health, work all the time scarsely ever getting a half hour to take a ride out on horseback.—Evrything looks quiet here now but it may be simply a quiet before a storm.'

'Cairo is not half so unpleasant a place as I supposed it would be. I have a nice office and live with the members of my staff immediately back of it."[32]

By late October, the chaotic mix of military camp activity, troop transport boats, ironclad gunboats' patrolling the rivers, supply barges, railroad trains, support personnel, potential spies and the threat of several thousand nearby enemy troops must have kept the Cairo residents and troops alike on edge in suspense. Their wait was short as recalled by Grant:

"About the first of November I was directed from department headquarters to make a demonstration on both sides of the Mississippi River with the view of detaining the rebels at Columbus within their lines. Before my troops could be got off, I was notified from the same quarter that there were some 3,000 of the enemy on the St. Francis River about fifty miles west, or south-west, from Cairo, and was ordered to send another force against them…My force consisted of a little over 3,000 men…We dropped down the river on the 6th to within about six miles of Columbus…'

'…after we started I saw that the officers and men were elated at the prospect of at last having the opportunity of doing what they had volunteered to do—fight the enemies of their country.'

'…I speedily resolved to push down the river, land on the Mississippi side, capture Belmont, break up the camp and return."[33]

Belmont, Missouri, is directly across the Mississippi from Columbus, Kentucky, and today is a flat farm field without evidence of the conflict now called, "The Battle of Belmont." At that time two gunboats accompanied Grant's troops and fired on Columbus while Union troops attacked the enemy camp at Belmont.[34] The gunboats' booming noise carried well over the Mississippi's waters to soldiers' worried friends, relatives and sweethearts 20 miles away.

Mrs. Logan narrated:

"All the next day, the 7th of November, 1861, the sound of cannonading told sadly and painfully that the battle of Belmont was on. The streets and levees of Cairo were thronged with anxious people trembling for the morrow, knowing only that some loved one was in the fight…Hour after hour rolled slowly away, and still no tidings save the continuous knell of the cannon's roar."[35]

General Grant's description continued:

"The officers and men engaged at Belmont were then under fire for the first time. Veterans could not have behaved better than they did up to the moment of reaching the rebel camp. At this point they became demoralized from their victory and failed to reap its full reward."[36]

Grant's word, "demoralized," is a polite euphemism for his troops' orgy of looting after a perceived easy victory's following only two hours' battle. While the Union troops brazenly celebrated, stealthy groups of Confederates crossed the Mississippi, imposed themselves between Grant's soldiers and their transport boats, and blocked the exit to Cairo. The novice soldiers' seemingly easy conquest transformed into a bloody battle. Its high cost included around 345 dead, 715 wounded, and 463 missing soldiers.[37] Both sides declared victory. Grant recounted:

"You see my army was a green one. The boys were never in a fight before…They met the rebels, ran at them and whipped them with an ease that astonished themselves. They were exultant…I had just about as little command over them as a herder has over a wild drove of Texas steers."[38]

Previously, the soldiers' main health problems were medical rather than surgical, but now battle wounds compounded prior months' illnesses. Mary Logan recounted the returning warriors and Cairo's concerned citizens:

"Finally, toward the early dawn a light like a meteor was seen to dart round the bend, another and still another came, until at last the outline of the fleet could be seen…After the prisoners were all off, the civilians who failed to see their friends in the lines were allowed to go on board the boats, to find them among the wounded, dying, or dead…'

'Tenderly covering the faces of the dead with anything we could get, and trying to soothe the suffering of the wounded, brave men and women worked unceasingly until ambulances and wagons came and took the unfortunate ones away to the hospitals which had been hastily prepared for the sick and disabled so suddenly assigned to them. Hotels and private houses had been seized, and the inefficient purveyors and quartermasters had put them in as good condition as the meager and ill-assorted supplies would permit. For days and weeks physicians, surgeons, and volunteer nurses kept their constant vigil, trying to save as many as possible from the roll of the dead."[39]

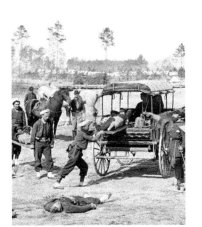

American Zouave unit soldiers demonstrate use of ambulance to remove the wounded from battlefield at unspecified location. Library of Congress Prints and Photographs Division, 2003006453, Civil War glass negative LC-B813-7381.

Mary Safford and Mary Ann Bickerdyke were among those who worked unceasingly and had prepared for the incoming wounded:

"Mrs. Bickerdyke and Mary Safford were waiting at the dock, surrounded by every wagon, buggy, handcart and wheelbarrow they could scrape up. Miss Safford had arranged with Cairo friends to take the wounded officers into their spare rooms. The enlisted men were hurried off to the inadequate camp hospitals."[40]

After having faced their first battle horrors, the wounded then confronted the equally horrific handling by surgeons untrained in treating extensive traumatic injuries. Mary Logan continued:

"Inexperienced surgeons were too hasty in making amputations, and needlessly sacrificed limbs which might have been saved."[41]

Though small in stature, Mary Safford became larger than life in reports of her

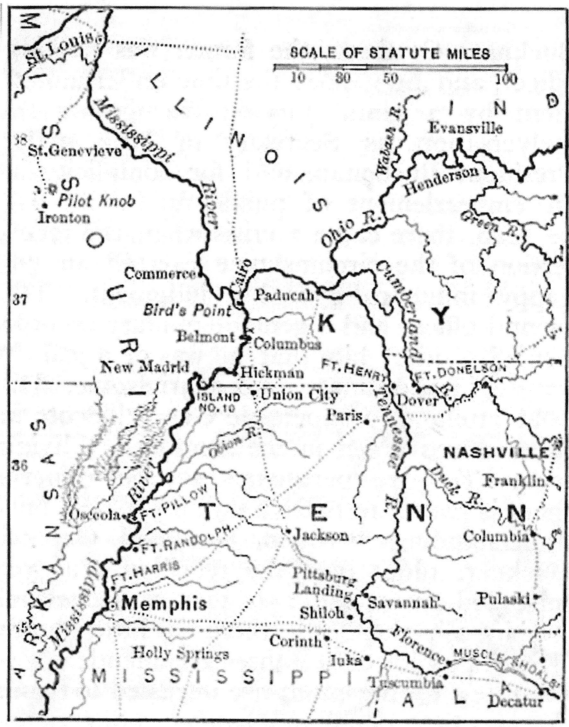

Western battles' sites, Belmont, MO, Fort Henry and Donelson and Savannah, TN. Walke, Henry, 'Operations of the Western Flotilla," Century Magazine, 29:3 Jan 1885, p 424.

intrepid activities after the Belmont battle. The perceived degree of peril she suffered was directly proportional to the number of years passed between the battle and its narrative. Six years after the battle, Linus Brockett wrote of her heroism when tying her handkerchief to a stick as a truce flag while she ministered to wounded on the Belmont battlefield.[42] Twenty-six years later, Mary Livermore embellished the same story with bullets' whizzing past poor Mary.[43] On the battle's centennial, author Fischer added a, "keen wintry wind," to Livermore's account.[44] Although Mary Safford never wrote of this event, 27th Illinois Volunteers member and diarist Private Edward W. Crippin, who fought at Belmont recorded the battlefield sights:

"All over the Battle field they scattered and in heaps the dead and the dying Friend and Foe lay in close proximity to each other. Some torn asunder by cannon balls some with frightful wounds here and there in different parts of the body. Some were killed out right with musket balls through the temples or forehead others with limbs torn completely off suffering the most torturing agonies 'twas a most horrible sight to contemplate."[45]

Certainly, Mary viewed the battle's gruesome maimed and dead in Cairo. The sight of young soldiers' bodies' deteriorating where they fell in battle would have left a strong impression on even the staunchest soul. Other reports of Mary's involvement leave a question about the Belmont battlefield story's veracity, as her prior routine's description was more that of a generous soul's fulfilling recuperating patients' requests and lifting spirits:

"...Pretty Mary Safford, unflaggingly pursuing her angelic activities, was responsible for much of the hospital's favorable publicity. Miss Safford hung the white lace curtains at the bare windows, and saw to it that there were flowers or autumn leaves in season to brighten the dreary wards. Miss Safford's Sunday afternoon prayer meetings, with sacred music and guest preachers, were well thought of." [46]

Her true Battle of Belmont experience lies somewhere between the brave little soul's searching the battlefield and the delicate lily's hanging lace curtains while practicing smile therapy. Either way she contributed to the soldiers' mental and physical health. Initially, she and her friends were classified officially as lady, "hospital visitors," good to cheer the patients, feed them broth, write letters for them, but not good enough to combat infection. However:

"Working with Bickerdyke in the hospital tents, Mary learned to set aside the inhibitions and artificialities of the traditional lady. She learned to discard superficialities…and to come to grips with the essentials of life in the dirt and blood of the wards."[47]

Around this time Julia Grant undertook the mammoth job of traveling from Galena in northern Illinois to Cairo with her four children ranging from 3 to 11 years.[48] On arrival the family moved into General Grant's headquarters' rooms in the bank building where Julia Grant probably first met the Saffords. Although her memoirs don't mention Mary Safford, Ulysses Grant's later correspondence confirms their acquaintance.[49]

Mary Safford's activities after Belmont:

"She continued her labors among the hospitals at Cairo and the neighborhood, constantly visiting from one to the other. Any day she could be seen on her errands of mercy passing along the streets with her little basket loaded with delicacies, or reading-matter… On Christmas day, 1861, there were some twenty-five regiments stationed at Cairo, and on that day she visited all the camps, and presented to every sick soldier some little useful present or token."[50]

Preparations for future engagements proceeded in Cairo:

"After the battle of Belmont, many more troops were ordered to rendezvous in Cairo, Illinois. General Grant was designated to organize an expedition up the Tennessee and Cumberland Rivers. During the months of December and January, in the worst weather ever experienced in that climate, the troops in great number were mobilized in and around inhospitable Cairo." [51]

Cairo was cold, wet, occasionally foggy and snowy in January 1862. Troops slogged in and out of town, traveled up and down the frigid rivers on various short expeditions and drilled for upcoming battles. The Saffords braced for a different event as Alfred's wife Julia's consumption completed the activity for which it was named, and she died of pulmonary tuberculosis. [52] Her obituary read in part:

"She…lacked but one week of being 32 years of age at the time of her death… she was extensively known by her works of Christian sympathy and active benevolence.'

'She was buried at Blue Island, near Chicago, on Tuesday; that being the burial place of some members of Mr. Safford's family."[53]

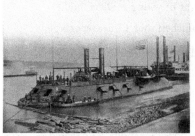

Gunboat off Cairo, IL, 1863. Library of Congress Prints and Photographs Division, 2013647496.

Around the same date, Generals Grant and McClernand with their staffs left Cairo to travel up the Ohio toward Forts Henry and Donelson. [54][55] Simultaneously, Joel A. Matteson's son Major Frederick W. Matteson arrived in Cairo with the 64th Regiment, Illinois Infantry also known as the, "Yates Sharpshooters," before moving south along the Mississippi River. [56] Concurrently, British author Anthony Trollope observed in Cairo:

"…we still found at Cairo a squadron of gun boats---if gun-boats go in squadrons— the bulk of the army had been moved…Four of these gun-boats were still lying in the Ohio, close under the terminus of the railway, with their flat, ugly noses against the muddy bank…" [57]

Likely, the Saffords traveled via Illinois Central train in accompanying Julia's body. It is hard to imagine a more wretched experience than loading a loved one's coffin upon a horse cart headed through cold, muddy streets, to a train depot on a slippery, gunboat-lined riverbank.

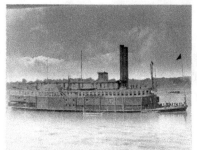

"Hospital Steamer," U.S. Hospital Boat Red Rover, 1862, for transport of wounded. Library of Congress Prints and Photographs Division, 2013647486.

Gunboats contrasted sharply with the formerly elegant riverboats now called, "hospital steamers." After the Belmont battle, Sanitary Commission Inspector Dr. Laurence Aigner leased five such steamboats at up to $600 per day and transformed them into hospital transports. [58][59] Built in 1857, "City of Memphis," was considered one of the largest and finest Mississippi riverboats and was modified to carry 750 beds as the first hospital transport on western rivers. [60][61] Now with long rows of cots in what was the salon, the ship had been:

"…of the very latest design, her paint gleamed white, her brass shown, and fancy gold leaf letters on the side proclaimed her the 'City of Memphis,' most luxurious of the Mississippi passenger boats built for fashionable travelers just before the war… thick carpets still covered the floor and fine curtains hung at the windows"[62]

The boat's prior notoriety arose from its 1860 pilot Samuel Clemens' colliding it with another vessel in New Orleans. [63] By the time Mary Safford helped transport patients on the same steamer, the man who became Mark Twain was nowhere near Cairo.

Fort Henry was on the Tennessee River's eastern bank approximately 60 miles upriver from its junction with the Ohio. Twelve miles northeast of the Tennessee's mouth is that of the Cumberland River also flowing north into the Ohio. Before twentieth century development, these two rivers were the Ohio's largest tributaries and were thoroughly navigable. Using many of the various steamships including the, "City of Memphis," as transports and seven Cairo gunboats, Grant and Foote moved 17,000 men approximately 100 miles to a position near Fort Henry to commence hostilities on February 6, 1862.[64][65][66] Grant planned a joint attack by land and water, but due to impassible muddy roads, only Foote's gunboats participated in the battle. Confederate General Lloyd Tilghman surrendered and sent his approximately 2,500 men to Fort Donelson before Grant's land troops even reached Fort Henry.

Although one of the first significant Union Civil War victories, it involved casualties. Reputedly, the gunboats took hits, and a Rebel shell ripped an ironclad's middle boiler causing significant damage with scalding steam's killing or wounding 48 men.[67] Sanitary Commission workers transported burn victims on the, "City of Memphis," to hospitals in Paducah, Kentucky and Mound City, Illinois.[68] No record exists of Mary Ann Bickerdyke and Mary Safford's involvement with the hospital steamer at this juncture, but as they were highly active in patient care and evacuation just a few days later, conceivably, they assisted after the Fort Henry action, too.

Fort Donelson was 11 miles east of Fort Henry on the Cumberland River's west bank. Grant took the fort in a complicated bloody battle during excruciatingly cold, wet conditions over eight days that ended with Confederate General Buckner's surrender on February 16th.[69] Dr. Aigner arrived on the, "City of Memphis," two days ahead of other hospital steamers and single-handedly dressed wounds day and night before assistance arrived.[70] Reputedly, Mary Safford and Mary Ann Bickerdyke were aboard the steamer for its five trips' transporting patients to the hospitals at Mound City, Cairo and St. Louis.[71] Although exact numbers are unknown, the Union had around 500 dead, 2100 wounded and Confederates between 1500 to 3500 casualties.[72] Lying in alternately frozen or thawed mud, the wounded were in abysmal condition while waiting helplessly for days without even the most basic first aid or provisions.[73] Private Crippin's diary revealed Cairo's weather then, "commenced storming, sleeting and snowing with the wind in the north," and remained very cold.[74] Mary Logan elaborated:

"The storms of the winter of 1861-2 were unprecedented, being especially wild during the month of February. Everything was covered with ice and snow; night and day a raw, cold wind blew such bitter blasts that men and animals could scarcely stand against its force. They had to move about or freeze to death. More than one of the brave men in the siege died from the exposure they experienced. Their clothing was frozen on them. Officers and men fared alike during the entire siege of Fort Donelson..."[75]

The Sanitary Commission's John S. Newberry, MD, who met Mary Safford on his June 1861 inspection of Cairo's facilities, wrote of the conditions:

"Our steamer was moored alongside of the 'City of Memphis,' on which were, at this time, two hundred and fifty or three hundred of the wounded...'

'We found the cabin floors thickly crossed with the wounded men, and others were constantly arriving from the various places where they had been deposited when taken from the field of battle. When received they were laid side by side in juxtaposition, part on the floor and part on mattresses. Our examination showed that the individual condition of the wounded men was deplorable. Some were just as they had been left by the fortune of war four days before; their wounds, as yet undressed, smeared with filth and blood, and all their wants unsupplied. Others had had their wounds dressed one, two or three days before. Others still were under the surgeon's hands, receiving such care as could be given them by men overburdened by the number of their patients, worn out by excessive and long-continued labor, without an article of clothing to give to any for a change, or an extra blanket, without bandages or dressings…with few medicines and no stimulants, and with nothing but cornmeal gruel, hard bread and bacon, to dispense as food."[76]

Lack of candles nearly caused conflagration of the, "City of Memphis," when, "helpers," possibly lit bonfires on deck for light or cooking.[77] Preparations of the supposedly, "equipped," hospital transports were sadly lacking, and Mary Ann Bickerdyke, Mary Safford, and other medical personnel had few supplies to meet great needs.

Accounts of Mary Safford's hard work on behalf of the wounded men included:

"…standing in the snow, her slight form whipped by the wind directing men who with pick and axe pried and hacked the wounded out of the mud into which they had frozen fast…'

'…She was coughing, feverish and threatened with imminent collapse…But she went on doggedly, supported by the mountainous force of Mother Bickerdyke."[78]

Bickerdyke's biographer elaborated:

"Mary Safford did good work on the five journeys she made with Mrs. Bickerdyke, to the military hospitals at Cairo, Mound City, St. Louis and Louisville. She held herself remorselessly to the task until the last man was safely stowed at Louisville. Then she went home to Cairo and a nervous breakdown."[79]

Fischer's short biography of Mary Safford explained further:

"…Mary was too sensitive to her surroundings—the revolting heaps of human arms and legs (amputation was the surgeon's rule of thumb), the stench and the moans of the sufferers. Mother Bickerdyke watched Mary's appetite fail, noticed her disturbed rest, her troubled face.'

'Hoping that a change of location would help to ease the tension, she took Mary along on her evacuation trips aboard the, 'City of Memphis.'…But the working conditions were actually the same—the undressed wounds, smeared with filth and blood…Mary became exhausted, for even the lighter work on the hospital ship was too demanding for her rapidly fading strength. She was forced to return to Cairo. When her strength returned, she resumed the less strenuous role of nurse's aid in local military hospitals…"[80]

The nurses cared for the Union's wounded and for many Confederates. Major General Halleck's correspondence to military and medical personnel after the Donelson battle confirmed the Union's policy of treating wounded, friend and foe, alike.[81] Approximately two-thirds of the 21,000 Confederates who fought at Donelson became prisoners and soon arrived at Cairo before transfer to the various prison camps throughout Illinois and neighboring states. With the attendant commotion, Mary Safford's recovery must have been difficult and was short-lived, as an even larger battle loomed.

In 1909, C.R. Woodward wrote of his Cairo experiences in a book that included Mary's photo with the label, "very strong, liberal-minded woman."[82] He recounted an incident at a social event at the town's best hotel:

"A Little Turnstile, with Safford at the Wheel.'

'One night, while attending a party at the St. Charles (now the Halliday) General Grant appeared at the door of the ballroom and said to Mr. Safford, who was dancing a quadrille near by: 'I want to send several little boats up the

Cumberland and Tennessee rivers, at daylight, and we want $10,000 or $12,000 cash.' Mr. Safford excused himself from his partner and said to me: 'Woodward, please take my place until I return.' " [83]

Presumably, Alfred provided the cash that enabled Grant to, "send several little boats," up the rivers, as the Battle of Pittsburg Landing also called the Battle of Shiloh was imminent. Despite Mary's exhaustion after the Donelson battle, she traveled to the region with Alfred as Ulysses Grant wrote to his wife March 24, 1862, from Savanna (sic), Tennessee:

"Mr. and Miss Safford are here, or rather at Pittsburg nine miles above here." [84]

Grant wrote Julia again on April 3, 1862, from Savanna:

"Mr. & Miss Safford were up here and returned a few days ago. I sent my watch by him to be expressed to you." [85]

Reasonably, Grant felt secure entrusting a valuable heirloom to the Saffords. For safety, Julia and the children moved to her in-laws' home over 500 miles away in Covington, Kentucky.[86] The Saffords possibly accompanied Sanitary Commission provisions.

Meanwhile, General Grant assembled his force that, with General Buell's Army of the Ohio, and General Pope's Army of the Mississippi, comprised the approximately 65,000 Union men who faced approximately 45,000 Confederates under Generals Albert Sidney Johnston and Beauregard.[87] Commencing Sunday, April 6th, the two-day battle saw fortune of war pass between sides with multiple land and gunboat activities' resulting in a Union victory at a cost of almost 24,000 casualties.[88] Sanitary Commissioner Dr. Newberry described the scene:

"...Depending upon the large stock of stores forwarded to Pittsburg before the fight, we had little to supply the pressing wants of the wounded at Savannah...We therefore hastened forward on Sunday morning to headquarters at Pittsburg Landing. The scene that here met our eyes was one to which no description, though it exhausted all the resources of language, could do anything like justice.'

'For the space of a mile or more, the bank of the river was lined with steamers, closely packed together, loaded with troops, stores and munitions of war...'

'To one standing on the bluff overlooking the landing, the scene below seemed one of wild and hopeless confusion... the countless throng of army wagons floundering through the mud, now interlocking, now upsetting with their loads; the wounded, borne on ambulances or on litters to the boats; the dead, lying stiff and stark on the wet ground, overrun with almost contemptuous indifference by the living; the busy squads of grave-diggers rapidly consigning the corpses to the shallow trenches—all this formed a picture, new, horrible, and never to be forgotten... "

"Previous to our arrival and in company with us, there had come to the relief of the wounded in the battle of Pittsburg, quite a fleet of hospital boats...'

'These, each marked with its yellow flag, lay moored among the steamers which lined the shore. They had come freighted with stores, surgeons and nurses, and afforded commodious and comfortable quarters to thousands who, but for them, must have endured incalculable suffering in many cases death itself."[89]

Mary Safford participated in nursing and patient transport at Shiloh while on the hospital steamer, "Hazel Dell."[90] Whether she regained her strength before traveling to Tennessee is questionable, as Bickerdyke's biographer Baker wrote of Mary's appearance after the battle:

"Miss Safford had risen from a sickbed to do it, against her doctor's advice and her brother's pleadings. She had been ill since Donelson, unable to eat, her sleep broke by remembered horrors. Nevertheless, when the call came she gathered strength to answer it.'

'Mrs. Bickerdyke did her best to spare the girl. But there was no way of sparing anyone in the rush of evacuating the wounded. Again the hospital steamers plied the rivers, distributing the victims among the permanent hospitals...'[91]

Apparently, on one such trip Mary saved the life of a captain with the Fifty-Seventh Illinois Volunteers:

" 'God bless Mary Safford!' he writes. 'She saved my life. When I was wounded at Shiloh I was carried on board the hospital boat, where she was in attendance. My wound got to bleeding, and, though I was faint from loss of blood, I did not know what was the matter. She found it out, for she slipped in a pool of blood beside my bed, and called a surgeon to me, just in time to save my life. Gracious! how that little woman worked! She was everywhere, doing everything, straightening out affairs, soothing and comforting, and sometimes praying, dressing wounds, cooking and nursing, and keeping the laggards at their work. For herself, she seemed to live on air.'

'...They brought Sam Houston's son aboard, wounded, a rebel officer, wearing the Confederate uniform, and ordered one of the privates removed from a comfortable berth he had, to make room for this young traitor. You should have seen Miss Safford! She straightened up, as if she were ten feet tall, and declared, in a grand way, that 'the humblest Union soldier should not be removed to make room for a rebel officer, not if that officer were General Lee himself!' She stood by the berth, and looked so resolute that they were glad to find another berth for Sam Houston's son. I do not wonder that all the boys called her 'the Cairo angel!' "[92]

In April 1862, representing the Northwest Sanitary Commission, Mary Livermore and Jane Hoge visited Cairo on reconnaissance for Commission supplies' proper utilization and were impressed by Mary Safford's supervision of it. On observing the wounded brought to Cairo's hospitals via the transport boats, Mrs. Hoge noted:

"Miss Safford, of Cairo, met many such fearful processions...With a calm dignity and self-poise that never blanched at any sight of horror, with a quiet energy and gentle authority that commanded willing obedience, she gave her orders to the nurses, dressers and stewards, till rapidly and imperceptibly she brought light out of darkness, and order out of confusion."[93]

Various sources suggest Mary Safford served both at Cairo's facilities and on the transports. Chicago's well-known Unitarian Reverend Robert Collyer wrote to the *Chicago Tribune* editors of her participation in transporting wounded:

"To Pittsburg Landing and Back. An Interesting Letter from Rev. Robert Collyer. The Sick and Wounded. Chicago, April 17, 1862—, Minister at large mentions that 'on our boat, the Hiawatha, Miss Safford of Cairo, whose praise is in all the hospitals, cheerfully volunteered to help us...' "[94]

A week later, the *Chicago Daily Tribune* contained a further testimonial from Dr. H. C. Gillett who also journeyed on the, "Hiawatha:"

"Under the direction of Miss Mary Safford, they prepared food for the sick and wounded, bathed their wounds and washed their powder and blood-stained faces...'

'What Miss Nightingale has been to the British Army, Miss Mary Safford has been to the American. Since the commencement of the war, she has devoted her time and energies gratuitously to this labor of love. I can assure the benevolent that contributions sent to her care will be applied with economy, and distributed where most required, and when this wicked rebellion is crushed out, the name of Miss Mary Safford will be immortalized in American history like that of Miss Florence Nightingale in that of England. Dr. H. C. Gillett" [95]

New York Tribune war correspondent Albert Deane Richardson traveled the Tennessee River following the Pittsburg battle and saw crowds of primarily women of the Cincinnati, St. Louis and Chicago Sanitary Commission branches.[96] Likely, Mary Livermore and Jane Hoge took that same boat while on their inspection tour. Possibly, Mary Safford was with them, but Richardson failed naming her or the vessel upon which he traveled. However, he reported Reverend Collyer's Sunday evening prayer meeting. Although no record of Mary Safford and Richardson's acquaintance exists, she knew his wife Abby later. He shared many meals with his friend Ulysses Grant, was privy to Grant's strategy and even received his tip to wait for the Donelson attack rather than rush to New York to report the Ft. Henry victory.[97] Later, Richardson penned Grant's biography but mentioned neither Alfred nor Mary Safford. Undoubtedly, she and Albert crossed paths given his and Alfred Safford's mutual friendship with Grant.

After May 1862, no additional references to Mary Safford's nursing career surfaced beyond vague reports of her having yet another breakdown.[98] In 1866, when Frank Moore solicited Mary's story for his book on women's Civil War involvement, she described her truncated nursing experience:

"I was obliged to you for the mention you desire to make of my efforts in our great national struggle for the establishment of freedom and unity, and yet my work was so early nipped in the bud by impaired health, and I was obliged to leave the scene of action to other hands not more willing but stronger, that it seems scarcely worth the while to mention what I began and others finished." [99]

Presumably, Mary returned to Cairo for immediate rest, but within two months her life changed dramatically. Concurrently, brother Alfred continued as Cairo's banker and assisted Grant in providing funds for his wife.[100] Meanwhile, brother A. P. K. shared his Unionville, Nevada Territory, tent with a man named Gorham Blake.[101]

4 ACROSS THE POND

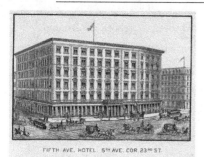

Fifth Avenue Hotel, New York City.
Taylor Map of New York, 1878.

The prior months' excruciatingly ghastly events now past, Mary Safford's life changed so drastically in summer 1862 that even she must have questioned her new reality. Likely, Alfred determined her only path to health existed far from Cairo. On July 3rd, Mary, Alfred, Isaac Bush Curran, and Joel A. Matteson's daughter Clara were in New York City's posh Fifth Avenue Hotel.[1] All but Alfred applied for passports, but he served as witness for Curran while he, in turn, witnessed for Mary and Clara who turned eighteen the prior day. For this only legal documentation of her age, Mary Safford swore under oath she was 24 years old and born December 31, 1837, though multiple records suggest otherwise. She was not ignorant and would have known her birth year but was starting a lengthy overseas trip with the wealthy, image-conscious Mattesons.[2] As a 24-year-old *companion* for their two teenage daughters Mary would appear more a peer than would a 30-year-old spinster. This, "white lie," allowed her beginning adult life anew in more ways than one, and her diminutive size allowed her passing for 24. Mary's speaking both French and German and celebrity as, "Angel of Cairo," provided added attraction for her inclusion in the Mattesons' entourage. Alfred Safford also witnessed passport applications for Joel Matteson, his thirteen-year-old daughter Belle, and Mrs. Matteson in Saratoga Springs, New York. The Mattesons planned their European trip to avoid the Civil War's dangers and thought hostilities would end soon.[3]

Four Matteson daughters and two sons lived to adulthood. Elder daughters Mary Jane and Lydia married bankers employed in Matteson's institutions, and elder son Charles was cashier in Matteson's Peoria bank.[4] The pretty younger daughters Belle and Clara participated in the family business by having their engraved images on several denominations of notes issued by Matteson's banks.[5][6] Presumably, any bank note with Matteson family members' images was redeemable at any Matteson bank and functioned locally as pre-Civil War currency.[7] Son Frederick Matteson was not involved in the family business yet, as he attended Yale before the war.[8] Against his mother's

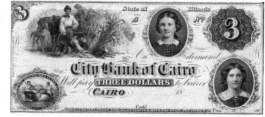

Joel A. Matteson's bank scrip: City Bank of Cairo $3 Bill with engravings of Clara and her mother Mary Matteson. Toppan, Carpenter & Co., New York & Philadelphia, likely late 1850s. Courtesy of ha.com.

wishes he quit school and joined the Union Army where Joel, at cross-purposes to his wife, secured a commission for him as Major in the Yates Sharpshooters. Mary Matteson sent Frederick a chainmail shirt for protection from Confederate bullets.

A Matteson entourage photo includes Mary Safford, although Clara Matteson Doolittle's reminiscences fail noting her but mention Joel's friend, "General Curran."[9] Silversmith Isaac (Ike) Bush Curran came to Springfield, Illinois, in 1840.[10] After his wife and newborn baby died in 1847, he mingled with Springfield's politicians including Governor French who named him Illinois' Quartermaster General.[11] From then on Ike was, "General Curran." His jewelry store

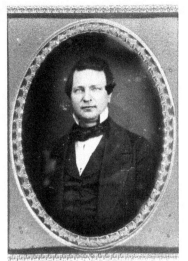

Isaac Bush Curran, Joel A. Matteson's friend and 1862-4 traveling companion. Abraham Lincoln Presidential Library & Museum.

and residence, across from the Illinois State Capitol, was a popular place for gatherings of the politically elite including Mary Lincoln who reputedly attended dances there and would have known both Curran and the Mattesons.[12] In February 1862, Ike sold his store, and in April, Abraham Lincoln nominated him as United States Consul for the Grand Duchy of Baden, to reside at Carlsruhe, Germany.[13] On this European excursion, 43-year old widower Curran escorted the Matteson ladies and Mary Safford to places they desired seeing but the Governor did not.[14]

While awaiting passports, the Matteson party could enjoy a variety of New York sights including P. T. Barnum's American Museum with its controversial, "What Is It."[15] In an August 1871 report, Mary Safford wrote, "Dear Madame von Littrou has taken me round such as Barnum did with his What-is-it," in recounting an Austrian woman's introducing her to prominent Viennese people.[16] Mary's choice of subject for this analogy is a bit odd since the What-is-it was a black man dressed as an African man-monkey described as, "lively and playful as a kitten."[17] Perhaps Mary had only heard of the What-is-it and not seen him, as she staunchly believed in racial equality.[18] If the Matteson party's departure date was beyond July 11th, they could have seen Mary and Tad Lincoln who traveled to New York to attend a mass recruiting rally in Union Square and toured the ship, "Great Eastern."[19]

Clara's narrative failed giving an embarkation date but noted the group's sorrow on learning of 23-year-old Major Frederick Matteson's August 8th death of typhoid in Corinth, Mississippi.[20] "When we had been in London four weeks a cable came announcing his death in camp... My two older sisters and brother were at my brother's bedside

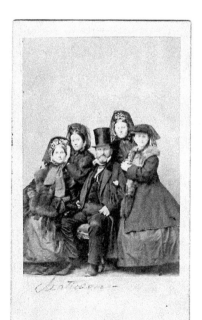

Governor Matteson's family and Mary Safford (standing at right) on grand tour. Abraham Lincoln Presidential Library & Museum (NI-4084).

before his death but it is doubtful if he recognized them...we were so sad that we did not enjoy the journey as we would have under different circumstances."[21] The event likely elicited guilt for Joel who had obtained Frederick's commission. Sadly, chainmail shirts don't prevent typhoid.

Sanitary Commission worker Mary Livermore was associate editor of the Universalist and reform publication *New Covenant* and wrote patriotic articles' encouraging women's both supporting war efforts and foregoing fashion obsessions.[22] Shortly after arriving in England, Mary Safford began sending articles to *New Covenant* under the heading, "European Correspondence." Her London column chronicled observations of the British Museum's many historically significant items including Martin Luther's Bible, Shakespeare's manuscripts, and what she said interested her most, "a letter written by Columbus soon after his discovery of America." Also impressive was a letter, "from Washington in reference to military affairs." Mary's educational and entertaining column tended to exaggerations' rivaling Barnum's when extolling museum specimens' origins:

"The drawings and engravings are arranged to show the wonderful progress in the art, commencing with the rude etchings of Holbein, Robers, Hogarth, Vandyke and Reynolds, until their sketches become, 'chefs d'ouvre,' the perfection of life and beauty.

All the known 'ologies are complete in rare and exquisite specimens from every portion of the universe. The minerals, alone, cover sixty large tables, besides filling shelves, nooks and corners.'

'With the Elgin marbles I felt a degree of familiarity, having read so much of them. And yet it seemed more a dream than reality, that I was looking upon portions of the Parthenon, the work of Phidias, executed more than 400 years B. C.'[23]

Fourteen months later, she saw the rest of the Parthenon in Athens.[24] She provided further lengthy description of the British Museum's antiquities including Egyptian artifacts:

"Their dead are here exhibited in great numbers, the linen bands with which the mummies are wrapped, as white and perfect as if it had been months instead of centuries since they were swathed...I saw a mummied hand so arranged that a gem of a ring protruded from one of the fingers. Mummied animals are numerous, comprising jackals, cats, snakes, crocodiles, the heads of rams, the sacred Ibis..."[25]

Some readers might consider Mary's coolly objective mummies' description macabre, but, apparently, she found these items more fascinating than disgusting. Possibly, her experiences with the war's sick and wounded tempered any revulsion at the sight of ancient dried human and animal remains. After experiencing the worst specimens of man's inhumanity to man, Mary may have found the, "other Egyptians,'" extreme care and respect for the dead refreshing. She also wrote of their toiletries, items to which she felt American women could relate:

"...the fashionable belles of that day were adept in the use of rouge and powder—."[26]

In conclusion, Mary reported attending the church services of Charles Haddon Spurgeon:

"...like his originality and off-hand American style of delivery. It is astonishing what an audience he draws. His church seats six thousand. I went, the first time very early and in the rain, but found the steps to the church and side-walk a dense crowd of people, waiting admittance, and hundreds stood during service who could not find seats."[27]

Described as a, "young Calvinist," Spurgeon was one of London's most popular preachers since John Wesley and gave weekly sermons in his immense Parthenon-like Metropolitan Tabernacle.[28] Even with London's marvelous diversions, Mary's sentiments remained with the war's medical needs at home, and she noted her original intent in European travel was to recuperate that she might reprise her Cairo role. From her column's postscript:

"I wish our poor sick and wounded soldiers could have a cold, bracing climate like this in which to recuperate. I do not get any hospital news from the papers. I do not think I can reconcile it with my conscience to be away long, if the war continues, and I get strong so that I can endure as I have done. My heart yearns daily to add my mite to the heavy burden of labor that has to be borne by a few. May God give strength to those who work and bring speedy peace to our dear land."[29]

Clara recounted the party's continued travels:

"... after a stay in London of several weeks...purchased an enormous landau and beautiful horses and as there were six in our party we had plenty of room, making use of the footman's seat, and the one beside the coachman and, as the latter declined to go at the last minute, my father and a friend of his, General Curran, who accompanied us, drove and we had a really more comfortable time, although we were so sad that we did not enjoy the journey as we would have under different circumstances. It was an ideal way to travel through beautiful England. We spent each night in some picturesque little town and a little longer in Canterbury. We drove on board the steamer at Dover and drove off at

Calais and proceeded on our journey to Paris in the landau."[30]

Clara's, "six in our party," included the four Mattesons and Isaac Curran, but she never names Mary Safford. Perhaps Clara considered her merely an insignificant chaperone. Possibly, Mary's only reason for travel was therapeutic. Her diagnoses ranged from exhaustion to more serious problems:

"She was herself suffering from a severe injury to her spine, the result of excessive labor and exposure in the field and hospital, and her physicians declared that nothing but complete rest and absence from her work would save her life. Accordingly her brother sent her to Paris, where she submitted to the most painful treatment for the cure of her disease."[31]

Unfortunately, Mary's *New Covenant* columns that might have reported her Parisian activities are unavailable. Perhaps she actually rested. In the city where English was not the first language, Mary spoke French as taught in Vermont and Montreal.

The group spent a month in a Parisian apartment formerly rented by, "the manufacturer of Singer sewing machines,"--likely Isaac M. Singer who fled the United States in 1862 on bigamy charges.[32][33] The Americans then moved to a rather conservative home in Passy, a fashionable area with villas and chateaus among woods and vineyards between Paris and Versailles.[34][35] From 1776 to 1785, Benjamin Franklin lived in Passy where he installed his printing press, became the toast of Parisian society, and practiced diplomacy as America's Ambassador to France.[36][37] French writer and Union sympathizer Victor Hugo drew an image of Franklin's Passy house and sent it via U. S. Consul at Paris Bigelow to the 1865 New York Sanitary Fair's sale to raise funds for Union troops' provisions and hospitals.[38] Although concurring with Hugo's views, Mary did not meet him, as he lived in exile on Guernsey while at odds with France's Emperor of the Second Empire Napoleon III also known as Louis-Napoleon Bonaparte.[39] 1862 was a banner year for Hugo, as his masterpiece *Les Miserables* first appeared in print with English translation soon afterwards. It was available in Paris, and probably Mary and the Mattesons knew of it and the public's negative feelings toward the emperor.[40] Napoleon III and Hugo's shared antipathy is not surprising, as the former sympathized with the Confederate cause and would have helped the South had it been safe for France to do so.[41] Both French and British interests supported the Confederates, and, in early 1863, British shipyards actively constructed rebel ironclad boats and recently launched the Confederate battleship, "Alabama."[42] The visiting Americans needed to keep a low profile to not further aggravate ill feelings toward the Union.

Second Empire Paris was currently undergoing elaborate renovations. Courtesy of the emperor's plan, tourists enjoyed wide Parisian avenues with grand views of monuments and impressive buildings while the Parisians received tremendous government debt and forced relocation of poorer inhabitants.[43] The Matteson touring party kept touch with other Americans and with U. S. friends and family through services of John Munroe and Company with its offices in New York, Boston, London, and Paris.[44] The banking firm provided circular letters of credit, a forerunner of the modern day ATM.[45] By registering their Parisian addresses, tourists could utilize Munroe's mail forwarding service.

Beyond Clara's and Mary's short initial reports, the party's excursion record is silent until Flora Payne's Paris arrival in early February 1863.[46] Born in Cleveland, Ohio, Flora celebrated her 21st birthday with seasickness on her Atlantic crossing but was ready to tackle the, "Grand Tour," in a grand way with the Mattesons.[47] She attended Cleveland Seminary for Young Ladies and then New York's Spingler Institute for Young Ladies.[48][49] Headmaster Abbott

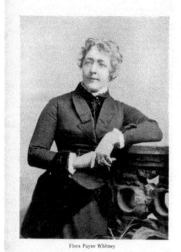

Flora Payne (later Whitney), Mary Safford's travel compa
January 1863–November 1864. Hirsch,
Mark D., William C. Whitney: Modern Warwick,
Archon Books, 1948, p. 50.

remembered her as a, "High-spirited girl played havoc with Spingler's discipline."[50] Her brother Oliver served in Yates Sharpshooters with recently deceased Yale schoolmate and friend Frederick Matteson but after Frederick's death transferred to an Ohio outfit.[51] Flora lacked Oliver's formal Yale education but received an analogous one through private tutoring at Harvard's experimental women's seminary taught by Professor Louis Agassiz in Cambridge.[52][53][54] There she occasionally raised the devil by leaving school without permission and embarking on scandalous adventures. Her father was wealthy lawyer and later Ohio U.S. Senator Henry B. Payne, a fellow law student and cousin of Joel Matteson's hero Stephen A. Douglas.[55][56] Flora's oldest brother Nathan also served the Union Army.[57] Henry Payne's former law partner Henry V. Willson accompanied Flora from New York to England.[58] Knowing Curran assisted the Mattesons on this tour, Flora assumed Ike would meet her in Paris but was surprised at her reception:

"…As I entered 'Gov. Mattison (sic)' I said, 'Miss Payne', –Clara threw her arms round me and Belle followed with a hug. This seemed to suggest something too to the Gov. and he kissed me. You can imagine my relief and delight to find myself so cordially welcomed, all fears vanished, I felt among friends– Mr. Curran and Mary had gone to the Louvre, in case I should be overlooked at the station."[59]

Flora soon met Mary Safford and wrote of her:

"My room mate is Mary Safford and I am entirely delighted with her, a girl of strong conscientious intelligence, enthusiastic, impressable (sic) nature, an earnest inquiring mind. She suits exactly the best part of me and I know that my daily contact with her will be of good to me."[60]

Likely, Flora knew of Mary's Civil War nursing experiences and may have thought Mary was near her own age. Nothing in Flora's letters suggests Mary ever intimated her true age or hid it. Flora described the Mattesons and their Parisian life:

"Clara is very pretty, gay and social, Belle original and affectionate. Mrs. Mattison (sic) very lovely and not in the least haughty or difficult to approach. The Gov. cordial and very kind but somewhat different from what you have described him…We live very simply…The Gov forwarned me that I must not expect much on the table as they live plain and had but two meals a day, but the plainest cooked in the nice French fashion gives you a hungry relish for everything."[61]

Soon after Flora's arrival, she and Mary Safford attended a Protestant French church then visited the Hotel Dieu, a venerable old hospital extending along the Seine with wards for each gender on opposite riverbanks.[62] Why the women chose touring hospital wards is curious, but perhaps Mary was familiar with the institution for having received treatment there for her reputed spinal injury. Perhaps she wanted to compare the ancient institution's facilities with those of Illinois. The women then toured the Cathedral of Notre Dame:

"We ventured in carelessly wandered through its magnificent domes, gazed up at its ancient windows, crossed ourselves and went out and walked home along the Seine."[63]

Using Paris' easily navigated omnibus system the women headed to, "the College where we go to lectures," near the

Sorbonne.[64] Women weren't allowed in Sorbonne classes, but the nearby College de France admitted women since opening in 1530.[65] Flora's initial typical activities with Mary:

"Monday morning breakfast at 8 o'c, walked down to attend lectures at 12, and 1 o'clock, walked home by the Seine to dinner at 4… In the evening went to a reception at Dr. McClintock's, quiet and pleasant…Tuesday morning Mary and I went to school in the morning, two doors from here. Walked to the College, wandered into several old churches, took a most delicious dinner at the café on the Rue de Montesqueu near Palais Royale…Mary and I walked home through the gas lights on the Seine. Wonderful how one can walk here. You seem to lose all consciousness in the wonder of sightseeing and you don't think of fatigue till you reach home. Had a quiet evening with our French teacher. She comes in when we have no other engagement. This has happened but once since I have been here. Wednesday went to school, then walked to the Arch d'Etoile to make the ascension as the day was clear and promised a fine view. This is the handsomest and proudest looking monument in Paris."[66]

"Dr. McClintock," above was John McClintock, DD, LLD, American Chapel in Paris' pastor whose New York *Methodist* newspaper columns kept Americans apprised of Europeans' fluctuating opinions on the Civil War.[67] As might be expected, the Americans of this particular social stratum kept close contact in Paris. Among the Matteson party's Parisian hosts were then current Ambassador to France William L. Dayton and U.S. Consul John Bigelow both strong Union advocates and Lincoln appointees.[68] [69] While the Matteson women may have associated with them on a more casual basis, Joel Matteson and Curran's interactions with these diplomats would have been far more serious. Napoleon III outlawed political rallies and other gatherings for dissemination of ideas that might oppose his rule, so dinner parties, especially with wine and dancing, were prime places for a camouflaged exchange of ideas and political news.[70] Flora, Mary, and Mrs. Matteson had direct personal interests in war news and ample opportunity to acquire it.

In a letter to her father, Flora waxed eloquent about the Arch de Triumph and lamented America's only grand monuments' being rivers and mountains. However, she closed with the thought that America had a monument that Paris lacked, and that monument was—Liberty. Possibly, one of the College de France professors inspired that comment, or perhaps she and Mary inspired a professor, especially one named Laboulaye.[71] Despite French governmental support for the Confederates, many Parisians admired America, its founders and their principles. Among admirers was College de France's popular teacher Edouard Laboulaye.[72] John Bigelow's respect for him likely led Flora, Clara, and Mary to attend Laboulaye's lectures, a safe haven for Americans with abolitionist ideals.[73]

Flora wrote to her father:

"We talk as much French as possible and find time to attend two Lectures a week- especially on Monday those of Mr. Sabolaye (sic). His name should be known in America – there is something about him that recalls very agreeably my impression of Prof. Agassiz the same charm of face, sympathetic eyes, and a deep quiet enthusiasm of manner that wins interest in his subject – The History of the United States – and which he handles in such a way that shows him a deep and liberal thinker – it is very gratifying to meet one who thoroughly knows and appreciates our history. His Lecture room is crowded, which shows some interest in America in these foreign parts. We three girls have been in love with him from the first – we desired some vent for our feelings, so last Monday on our way to the Lecture we bought a beautiful bouquet of choice flowers to present to him placed a card in it with the inscription 'To Monsieur Saboulaye. An expression of thanks from three young American friends.' We arrived early and gave it to the Porter desiring him to place it on the desk in the Lecture Room – to our great surprise he demurred and finally said he did not dare to – he had never heard of such a thing being done before and he could not do it without permission from the Government, for it might get into the Papers and cause trouble. We did not desire to get the good man or the College into trouble, so we finally consented to his compromise of leaving it in the little ante room and Mr. S. should decide what to do with it... feeling almost traitorous we took our places, when the great good man appeared we imagined pleasure at something lurked in the speaking muscles of his mouth, but we were quite unprepared for what followed. He took his seat amid the plaudits of his audience, and in his simple quaint dignified way said – I cannot give it to you in English as it was in French – 'In coming into my cabinet today I found for me a very charming basquet of flowers with a card from

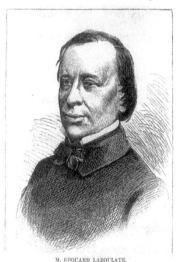

M. EDOUARD LABOULAYE.

College de France American History lecturer Edouard Laboulaye. Harper's Weekly, 15 Dec 1866, p. 789. Library of Congress Prints and Photographs Division, 90708091.

three young American friends. The young girls wished it placed on my chair, but as the French are not used to the custom they might think there was something mauvaise about it. I understand it – it is a very vrai American custom, to me it is very touching, showing that they felt my interest in their unhappy country.' The Audience greatly applauded, we three sat blushing, when some one called out 'You had better tell us how to do in France,' 'America teach France' etc – now came cries of 'the door' 'the door' 'put him out Gendarmes Gendarmes', a scene of terrible confusion would have ensued but Mr. S. quelled it by a few quiet words, that it was an honor all to himself, & now we must return to America.' We think we will not attempt it a second time lest there should be out and out rebellion- a smaller thing than a flower has caused a revolution when people are so ready to take umbrage at an insult to national honor."[74]

Just as Victor Hugo supported the United States Sanitary Commission by donating historically significant items to the New York Sanitary Fair, Laboulaye raised Commission funds by gathering autographed manuscripts for auction in 1863.[75] Later, along with sculptor Frederic Bartholdi, Laboulaye was best known for conceiving and promoting a gift for America, a statue called, "La Liberte Eclairant le Monde," or, "Liberty Enlightening the World."[76] The finished Statue of Liberty graced New York harbor as of 1886.

Flora and Mary did as much Parisian sightseeing as possible before late March 1863 when Governor Matteson announced the party would leave for Spain soon.[77]

"Mary and I have been waiting for a pleasant day to take a trip into the country, but the chilling weather has forced us to confine our time to Churches & Museums – two days, that is from one till 4, we have spent in the Louvre trying to harmonize it....We have not yet visited all the schools of Paintings, we only go when in artistic humeurs.'

'Last Tuesday we visited the Imperial Stables..."[78]

One Sunday they had what Flora called a, "delicious time," by contrasting two funerals. One wealthy decedent had a sumptuous 5000-franc funeral at the Madeleine church and interment at Paris' Pere la Chaise Flora described as:

"...a most dreary hotel like cemetery, all the vaults like little houses, whole streets of them, in them hang yellow wreaths around some rude image of the Virgin, or the Savior on the Cross."[79]

On the same afternoon at Pere le Chaise's paupers' side the women viewed a 10-franc funeral with a bare wooden cross, a rough board coffin placed in a ditch, and true mourners who loved the deceased. Flora's narrative of another adventure may have shocked her family, but they were likely jaded to her exploits:

"This last Sunday we spent in a way that shocks myself to remember–went out about 20 miles to the Village of D'auvray, beyond St. Cloud, to the first race of the season – a Steeple Chase…There was a gay crowd present, gaudy equipages got up for the occasion, many women without hoops, plenty of Champagne in their carriages to entice the young men…We stayed till three races were over, saw several ditched and thrown, arms broke, blood spouting from mouth and nose, one killed I believe – altogether a barbarous spectacle, one thing only can be more savage or exciting, a Bull Fight in Spain."[80]

Although minor when contrasted with Civil War carnage, the sight of, "blood spouting from the nose and mouth," and, "one killed," may have stirred Mary's memory, as these horse races occurred around the Shiloh battle's first anniversary. While Flora could barely imagine sights more, "savage or exciting," Mary certainly could.

The women planned an outing to Normandy and Brittany in mid-March 1863, but cold, bleak weather prevented it.[81] Instead, they traveled southwest of Paris with Isaac Curran and Benjamin Bates, Flora's newly acquired special friend who assisted through her transatlantic seasickness and later journeyed to Italy to consider building railroads. Thus, the group consisted of 21-year old socialite Flora, 43-year old widower jeweler/politician Curran, 31-year old Mary who posed as 25, and the enterprising Mr. Bates of undetermined age. The unlikely quartet left Paris March 24th, as Flora described:

"Tuesday morning we started, sturdy looking voyageurs, as I shall describe – Myself, cloth dress, shaved off from the graceful American sweep so as barely to touch, also the sleeves have been managed down into tight ones, little black sack, bought in New York proved invaluable, round black hat, over my shoulder slung a little leather bag, that we had manufactured for such purposes with great care, containing night dress (flannel) toothbrush, comb, one clean collar & handkerchief, shawl slung across other shoulder. Mary ditto, only she is a little thing & looked very queer & cunning. Mr. Curran had on a rowdy brown old American hat - red scarf on neck, cane, bag over shoulder, looking as he always is comfortable and good natured. Mr. Bates is so fine & large looking that he did not need the aid of any baggage to attract attention, so put his tooth pick in his pocket - for the sake of the looks however, I allowed him to carry my sack & even sometimes my shawl."[82]

Flora's calling Mary's look, "queer & cunning," likely meant unique and cute. Throughout her letters, Flora meticulously described their own fashions and that of the natives of whatever country they visited. Mary's involvement in the 1870s dress reform movement possibly began with knowledge of practical dressing she acquired while traveling. The young women packed light and the men lighter, but even today's most ascetic tourist would bring more than a toothpick for an overnight jaunt.

The group rode atop a horse-drawn rail car to Versailles and traveled through the laundry district of Paris and saw:

"…great vineyards of sheets and shirts…it is carried out and along the Seine, and it is one of the 'sights' on certain days to see the washerwomen lining the banks & beating the clothes on its rough stones."[83]

They stopped at Versailles' Hotel de France and, "arranged for quarters for the night, Mary & I taking a room with one bed, the gentlemen one with two."[84] That afternoon while touring the Palace of Versailles they decided its finest paintings were by Horace Vernet, court painter of Louis Phillippe.[85] Flora's description of Vernet and Napoleon III's relationship:

"...he was employed by the present Emperor before his death, but they had a falling out, imperial wished to be made the leading figure in some Picture, Painter said, 'Sire I paint for posterity not for you' – whereupon he was dismissed. Mary who is a little orleanist tells this with great gusto."[86]

The above suggests Mary supported the idea of more liberal rule than monarchy offered.[87] Meanwhile, Isaac Curran's diary entry was far more terse and included on March 24th:

"I ought probably admit that part of the pleasure I find now on this visit is derived from the joy Miss Flora expresses so beautifully in her every word and step!"[88]

At this point Curran was impressed with Flora while Flora was taken with Benjamin Bates. Unfortunately, Mary's thoughts to complete this potential ménage a quatre are unavailable. However, the tone in Flora's letter (albeit to her mother) suggested they maintained strict decorum. Flora recounted their evening meal included, "good wine," and that for amusement they read to one another until 9PM bedtime.[89] The next morning they, "had a jolly cosy breakfast," in the gentlemen's room before walking to St. Cyr to board a train to Rambouillet where they toured what Flora called one of France's oldest chateaux. They then stopped overnight at the Maison d'Or and had chicken dinner, considered an extravagance. At Fontainbleau the next day, they took a room at the Hotel de France and toured the, "cosy and homelike," 1900 room Fontainbleau Chateau before returning:

"...we started to walk to Paris. All was in our favor, sun & pleasant shades. ...the idea suddenly took us to make the rest of the way by water. We sent out for a man to row us, he came, a one eyed gray haired old fellow, who said he would take us to Corbeil 23 miles for 25 fr...You may imagine the fun we had in the moonlight, our old guide was a case down on the emperor, down on all royalty, nothing but the pure republic – tried the Marsaillaise for us, his arm would leave his oars & fly up in violent gestures. You can imagine the fun we had – had some brandy cherries along, that helped to keep us merry, when it grew cold we had shawls & two gallant gentlemen to hold them around us."[90]

Unfortunately, Mary Safford's impressions of the adventure are nonexistent, and Isaac Curran's diary has no entry for that evening. In fact, his entries cease until after the Matteson entourage left Paris. A true gentleman uses discretion in his journal entries.

5 PROCEEDING ON THE GRAND TOUR

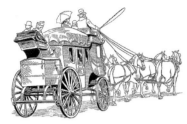

Before leaving Paris for Spain, Mary and Flora imagined themselves penniless and desperately leaping to their deaths in the Seine only to be fished out and removed to:

"…that dreadful Morgue – it is a very respectable low stone house, near one of the bridges, we passed it always on our way to Lectures…one day we girls being by ourselves went in – it is one large room lighted strongly at one end. We looked through an iron grating, there were raised tables beyond, elevating the head. The clothes of those found hung all around. Three bodies were there, a stream of water constantly dripping on their upturned faces. I cannot think of them as human creatures, they were too ghastly

Diligence type of stagecoach.

and discolored, with such a livid light on their faces. We looked about a minute, then fled…"[1]

Morbid curiosity brought Flora into the Morgue, but Mary knew death's image first hand. Flora never wrote of Mary's recounting Civil War experiences, and likely she never did, choosing instead to enjoy the European tour. From this point and in her later correspondence, Flora called her, "Midge," but this nickname never appeared in Mary's correspondence or elsewhere. Flora reported their preparations before embarking on an independent 400-mile journey from Paris to Bordeaux:

"…Midge & I cut down to the shortest. We left our trunks at Monroes (sic)…we wont see our trunks till we get to Geneva, where we put on stouter clothes for mountain wear. This is what we have done – I dont say the rest have, they are more stylish, and have innumerable quantities of silk dresses that they like to air."[2]

Neither woman was poor, but both were practical and pared their baggage to travel frugally:

"We left Paris about 11½, took second class cars…We did not venture to talk much, holding ourselves very discreetly, as it is not usual for young ladies to travel alone much…We amused ourselves between a little Spanish Grammar and the outside country…"

"…one modest gray haired old gentleman just returning from his first trip to Paris, was very much amazed at our travelling alone – he had never heard of such a thing, thought it must require a great deal of courage…our independence amuses the French very much, a few nights before leaving Paris we were dining out where there were several old ladies & married ones younger – they made us describe over & over again how the young ladies did in America – that they were allowed to go out alone, and have as many beaux and as much fun as they please but I told them after we were married it was as strange for us to go out with another gentleman as it was here for them to be seen with their husband, that we devoted ourselves to our families, 'Ah' said they 'you don't hurry to get married do you?' "[3]

After 5 days, Flora and Mary felt completely comfortable traveling independently:

"We are highly delighted at the success of our trip & having proved that we can travel alone. We have met with almost uniform kindness, have been imposed upon nowhere … do not be at all uneasy at our independence, we are very discreet & well behaved & nothing serious as yet has happened – have to go to bed early as we do not dare to be seen after dark."[4]

Upon rejoining the Matteson party in Bordeaux, Mary and Flora ceased carefree travel and moved from economical lodgings to the Mattesons' expensive hotel.[5] The city's reputation as France's, "Hell," of criminal activity gave reason for Flora and Mary's remaining inside well before dark and probably worried Flora's mother despite the young women's purported, "discrete & well behaved," demeanor.

Mid-afternoon April 17th, the entourage piled into a large French stagecoach called a, "diligence with coupe," and headed toward Madrid:

"...went along quietly through the rich grain lands of France, the blue lines of the Pyranees (sic) before us, as if beckoning with their enchanted peaks – the whole passage across was charming, on one side the unending mountain ridges with soft clouds rolling down their summits..."[6]

"...conductors changed and mules put on –night fell, a cold mountain rain drizzled down & we were in for fun, which we had watching our strange team of 10 or 12 mules dashing along, a strong head light cast a weird glow on their shaven backs, resting on the cowled out-rider who guided us over most darkly yawning precipices, every ten miles fresh relays were attached & new drivers...smoking we dashed into high walled towns, through the dark narrow streets up to the station, a whistle, an appearance of a scowling face, a banditti whispering & on we would gallop."[7]

The tempestuous ride continued until early morning, keeping Mary awake and making Ike vow that if he survived he would never again be caught in a diligence at night. The haste was necessary for their catching a train to Vallidolid where, despite the rush, they had to wait:

"...we had a funny time with the crowd of curious peasantry around – poking fun at the beasts (they may have called us), not a soul to speak English or French & the Gov shouting aloud his orders, for he even still holds to the opinion that to hear is to understand ..."[8]

Two days later, they arrived at the Madrid home of U. S. Minister Plenipotentiary Augustus Koerner, Matteson's Lieutenant Governor in the 1850s.[9][10] Flora reported their finding here a new guide:

"We leave Madrid tomorrow evening, expecting to be in Cordova on Sunday, for an extra travelling companion we have nephew of Washington Irving, a Van Wirt (sic), a nice fellow who is anxious that we go straight on with him to Granada, where perhaps for the sake of his Uncle they might give us rooms in the Alhambra – he is attached to the Legation."[11]

"... a most invaluable compagnon de voyage – he is a nice harmless young man...he kept with us to Cadiz, where he left us to go to Gib. by boat.."[12]

Later, Koerner remembered Irving Van Wart's joining the Matteson party and dressing in, "...a full Andalusian costume."[13]

At Madrid the party drank delicious mountain water, potable without wine that otherwise served as a weak disinfectant for foul drinking water. However, Ike may have run afoul of Madrid's water or food as noted in his diary entry the day the group left:

"An awful thing to be always remembered of the night ride from Madrid was my having a sudden attack of colera morbus—my sufferings were intense, intestinely—and no accommodations, took the outside of cars..."[14]

Fortunately, the others did not suffer Curran's malady, but all were glad to leave Madrid's dry dust. Although Van Wart proved useful for his Spanish fluency, Joel Matteson's pigheaded insistence on the Europeans' needing to speak English was both annoying and amusing as he tried purchasing bullfight tickets.[15] Apparently, the, "Ugly American," was alive and actively establishing his stereotype in the 19th century. Wisely, both Mary and Flora began studying Spanish on the train to Bordeaux and found the Spanish people equally willing to converse in French as in Spanish.[16] As it was, the bullfight was postponed, and the young women never saw one. The tour continued through hilly, picturesque La Mancha, and at Cordova local sightseeing included a donkey/mule ride to the mountains above the city:

"...robed for a donkey ride to the mountains, sans crinoline....Nine donkeys awaited us, blinking patiently in the sun, a sort of a crossed chair was placed upon them, cushioned with pillows & adorned with a saddle cloth from the brilliant calico coverlids of our beds. We sat sideways perfectly helpless, with only a stick to guide our mules, & hit them across the ears when they would crush us against a wall..."[17]

Moving then to Seville, Mary and Flora thoroughly explored historical sites and searched for paintings by Spanish baroque painter Bartolome Esteban Murillo. In addition to their walks at what everyone else considered siesta time, the girls took evening strolls through Seville's fashionable districts but soon learned that, unlike southern France, Spain was not a place for women's independent touring. However, the two already planned unfettered travel in Switzerland:

"We are on our way to Switzerland to settle somewhere. I want to make many tramps there on foot, & Mary & I had intended to join a gentleman, a friend of hers but unfortunately single...it is very galling to have to lose time, that is everything to me, but nothing to those I am with..."[18]

Their goal of sightseeing efficiently and economically conflicted with that of the affluent Mattesons who preferred a more leisurely tour. Also, the women felt confined by the era's conventions, as an unrelated single male failed meeting the prevailing times' definition of, "proper traveling companion," even for liberal-minded young women. The, "gentleman," Flora mentioned was Illinois geology Professor Joseph H. McChesney.[19]

The party visited Cadiz in southern Spain and boarded the steamer, "Sevilla," on May 8th for an excursion. Escort Curran noted Flora, Clara and Belle's sleeping while:

"Mary dancing hornpipe on Captain's Deck----Hoops, they having been discharged and stowed on first deck... Mary is asleep on a coil of rope on the poop deck..."[20]

Unfortunately, the diary's pages are faded and partially illegible, but Mary's dancing and removing her encumbering skirt hoops was significant enough to warrant notation in Curran's otherwise tersely worded record. The party disembarked near Spain's southern tip and on May 9th toured Gibraltar where Curran recorded their seeing:

"Many Moors with turbans on their head—some white and some more red and their faces are all colours – some black as night, some brown..."[21]

Only Isaac Curran's diary recorded this portion of the trip when at least part of the group visited Tangier, Morocco, on Africa's north coast, as he noted:

"...carried on back of Moor from boat to shore up through the street! Such a town, the Lord save us..."[22]

The following day they toured the Moorish market, saw numerous camels, donkeys, vegetables, goats, cattle, and:

"Now a man on black horse rides through the crowd hollering Allah! something..."[23]

Curran, Mary and Flora rode mules from Tangier to Light House Cape then proceeded to Cape Spartel's Cave of Hercules to see men cutting millstones above two huge rock-lined caves that opened to the ocean.[24] Traversing 20 miles of, "beautiful sand beach," they returned to Tangier via a road through the plains and:

"On this Coast is sand in hills, sand plains and sandstone mountains. The coast is often the scene of shipwrecks –

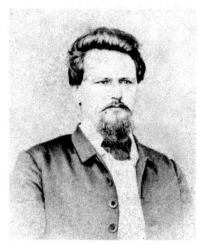

Jesse McMath, U.S. Consul Tangier, Morocco, 1863. From the collection of Dr. Philip Abensur, Paris, France.

Monsoons - Stopt to dine under an olive tree, by a mineral spring! Good lunch with Consul McM and his interpreter…"[25]

These men were U.S. Consul General Jesse H. McMath and U. S. Consulate General Interpreter Moses Pariente.[26] McMath's later accomplishments included helping broker the cooperative agreement between the Sultan of Morocco and numerous other nations for establishing the Cape Spartel lighthouse for international maritime safety.[27] [28] On May 12th, Curran recorded walking to Mt. Washington with Mary and Flora at 4:30AM presumably because the northern African coast's warm weather necessitated the early start.[29] Mt. Washington was not a mountain but Consul McMath's house located on the, "Old Mountain," a lovely residential neighborhood just west of Tangier and overlooking the Straits of Gibraltar.[30] After almost reaching the house, the trio encountered a rainstorm and they:

"…took refuge in the house of Sir John Hay Her Majesty's Consul in Tangier. Sent in our Cards and were invited in – and refreshed with English Tea…and stopped at the house of the Interpreter who has one of the most delightful places in the vicinity just enough sea beach to match his land and garden."[31]

Sir John Drummond-Hay was the British Consul at Tangier, and although the Americans may not have met him, just seeing his remarkable home as he described it would have been a treat:

"On entering the house a great stuffed hyena, grinning round the angle of the staircase, greeted each new comer—frequently to the dismay of a native, who took it to be a living beast.'

'A balcony, or rather verandah, from which could be seen the bay and the opposite coast of Spain, ran the whole length of the house on the upper floor in front of the drawing-room windows, and overhung the little garden…Here was kept the tame leopard in 1858, and later several mouflons and gazelles; here, too, young wild boar and porcupines had their day."[32]

Danish author Hans Christian Anderson visited Hay's home five months earlier and wrote:

"The stairs and corridors were adorned with skins of wild animals, collections of Moorish pottery, spears, sabers, and other weapons, together with rich saddles and horse-trappings, presents which Sir John had received on his visits to the emperor of Morocco.'

'In this house there was every English convenience, even to a fireplace …"[33]

After leaving Sir John's home, the American trio stopped at the garden of interpreter Moses Pariente, a wealthy Tangier merchant and founder of the Moses Pariente Bank, the town's oldest.[34] [35] [36] He had many homes some of which he rented out.[37] Curran's diary noted Pariente's residence's view but not his political ones.

The next day Curran rose at 4AM to travel by donkey to old Tangier with Mary.[38] After difficulty with ornery donkeys' kicking, balking, and the, "heathen Haman's," exchanging them for equally bad ones, the two rode to the old town. In addition to being a morning person, Mary was adventurous and rode beyond his sight. She was not above solo exploration in a foreign land where a woman alone was nearly unknown. The Moroccans likely found her more a curiosity than an object of prey given her confident demeanor and potentially absurd appearing western clothing unsuited to the climate. Following their morning's exploration, Mary and Ike returned to the hotel and by 10AM boated to Gibraltar, less than 20 miles away. Flora's letters resumed with a description of the reunited party's exhausting and dehydrating climb of the British fortifications at the 1500-foot Rock of Gibraltar.[39] Perhaps in her forwarded mail at Gibraltar, Mary learned the news of her brother Alfred's marriage to 26-year old Anna Candee on April 7th.[40]

The Americans then traveled to seaport Malaga where Irving Van Wart rejoined them and fulfilled his promise to accompany Mary, Flora and Clara on horseback to inland Granada, a distance by current roads of about 88 miles.[41] Curran noted the event:

"15th May Malaga Mary Flora and Clara, left this morning on Horseback for Granada – Mary not looking well, I fear will have a hard ride today."[42]

He and Matteson rested in Malaga while Mrs. Matteson and Belle rode by diligence to Granada. Meanwhile, Irving Van Wart and three gentlemen friends intended riding horses from Tangier to Tetuan, Morocco, but errant luggage sent them scrambling to Malaga and bypassing their Moroccan adventure. Flora described the young men's dilemma:

"…by some mistake of their courier their baggage had not come, & being young men, very fond of their shirt collars, they went straight on to Malaga after it –we joined them there by boat & then took our famous ride to Granada."[43]

Flora recounted the, "famous ride," with Irving Van Wart and three other young men in a letter to her mother:

"We were ready for anything, and six A. M. was arranged for the departure. At that time we young ladies were all up, dressed sans crinoline…rolls of loose white muslin around our hats, as preventive of sun strokes. We found the steeds at the door but the gentlemen had not yet appeared – first came Irving, the lord of the day, for he rode his own horse, having concluded the purchase of what he fondly thought a fine black creature, saddle new & clean, blankets strapped on before & aft, himself spurred and expecting to ride a sensation thro the town. Mr. Fearing came next, looking as always rosy & good humored, then Mr. Bowden, a nice young fellow, lately come over here to travel & lastly arrived Mr. Hazeltine, a gentlemen! that had been worrying all this time over his cravat – they were all college chums at Harvard, where I knew Mr. Fearing…Mr. H. is now an Oxford student, with a few English airs put on and a languishing attempt to part his hair down the middle, otherwise original & well behaved….I cannot boast much of our steeds, not the Andalucian (sic) ponies I had pictured with flowing tails & proud high step, they were rather used up, with high shoulder blades & thin chests and most unchristian trots – but sure footed for mountain traveling – imagine us away, two guides with sumpter horses on before."[44]

In summary, this grand adventure's participants were Mary Safford, Flora Payne, Clara Matteson, three American upper crust, unmarried, recent Harvard graduates plus Washington Irving's flamboyant grand-nephew, two guides with two pack animals and an assembly of not terribly attractive borrowed horses. The prohibition of young women's traveling with unrelated single males seemed to have flown out the window. Flora continued:

"The morning was bright, our way lay along the coast and our spirits rose in our saddles. The hissing surf attracted the gentlemen, and they left us for a bath, when they overtook us, their moist look bespoke their enjoyment & much to our satisfied delight the part had been washed out of Mr. H's hair & Mr. Irving's collar was not quite immaculate. About 10 o'c reached Velez Malaga…and ordered breakfast…which consisted of fried eggs & chocolate …with some pickled beefsteak & salmon, discovered in the saddlebags, made quite an agreeable meal."[45]

After breakfast the group rested until 3PM, headed for their overnight destination of Alhama de Granada, Spain, but greatly underestimated the time necessary for their horses' navigating the narrow mountain road:

"Our path now lay directly across the mountains, no travelled road but a mere muleteer path. Our horses picked their way carefully up the rocks and thro streams that came rushing down the Mt. side, the same one crossing our way a dozen times...Olive orchards and sweet little towns freshened the valleys...we went in file, our way one jagged ascent & descent like the steps of a crumbling stair case, now along precipices steep and dangerous, now in dark ravines, no habitation of life, save here & there a lonely Atalaya or watch tower...here and there the ominous cross startled us in the ghostly starlight, fatal monument of wayside murder or robbery and now the gentlemen talked in low whispers, casting fearful glances into the shadows, revolvers were cocked, plans laid for disposing of the ladies in case of banditti and restrictions laid on our talking – this was too much for us, careless of and amused with our danger, and ever & anon you would hear a giggle and a silvery peal of laughter, leaving its echoes behind, our cavaliers would draw up close, begging us for Gods sake to keep quiet so we would till the ridiculousness of our silent file would again provoke rebellion."[46]

Finally, near midnight the wary and weary travelers reached their destination:

"Found a cosy little posada, stumbled over sleeping mules & men up the stairs into our room, found it neat & clean, with a great earthen basin for a wash tub, and on the little beds sheets & pillow cases all ruffled & embroidered. What a sweet rest we enjoyed tho I confess we would have relished more of a sheet and less of a frill – 15 hours had we been in the saddle & we were somewhat sore the next morning."[47]

If Mary was ill before the ride, she must have been miserable after it. The next day, as most paused to eat oranges near a cool stream, Flora and Mr. Hazeltine rode ahead and arrived at Granada:

"Off my horse I could with difficulty totter to my room, gasped out 'bring me strawberries & lemonade,' when they came, a whole platter full & a whole pitcher full, finished both and took a hasty bath & went to bed. Mary arrived at 5, & Clara at 6. Bell and Mrs. Mattison (sic) came in the evening diligence, leaving the Gov & General to rest at Malaga."[48]

After their harrowing riding adventure, Mary and Flora's stay in Granada was delightful to a point:

"Our Hotel was right under the shade of the Alhambra...We inhabited the same spot where stood the house of 'Pedro Gil,' the stout little water carrier, immortalized by Irving & Mary and I were quite sure ours was the very room (and truly so, as far as its poverty was concerned) where his vain wife showed herself at the window decked out in the jewels of the Moslem treasure."[49][50]

In Granada the four young men treated them:

"There the young men...treated us young ladies to a most famous dinner – it was a most elegant little affair, they somehow managed to have their dinner in a Spanish olive oil district, cooked a l'anglaise, the sweet mingling of the harp & bandoletti gently fed our appetite, precious wines flowed in abundance, and in the evening, to the tune of the fandango thrummed by the 'King of the Gipsies' we danced merry American dances, and went singing home, the nearest approach to a spree that we had in Spain. Irving here left us for Madrid..."[51]

After returning from the evening's fun, the women should have slept well. However, the Alhambra's famous fountains interrupted restful sleep:

"...this fountain was right under our windows and however charming, not at all conducive to slumber – my imagination aided by the clear songs of the nightingales, might have wandered back into the ages of the Moors & heard in this the music from the silver lyre of the beautiful enchantress, but I had enough practical in the shape of innumerable fleas to keep me in the 19th century, and the next day so complained that the fountain ever after ceased at nightfall…familiarity reveals the nakedness of romance."[52]

Besides discomfort from the horseback ride, the young women suffered flea infestation probably exacerbated by corsets and crinolines. Despite this, they explored Granada and the Alhambra then returned by diligence to Malaga for further touring.[53] The return trip was likely far faster and more comfortable but not nearly as much fun.

The reunited Matteson group then took the Spanish steamship, "Guadaira," for a 1000-mile, nine-day excursion along the Spanish coast to Marseille, France.[54] Onboard, the four young women including Belle had what Flora described as the best cabin, good food and a Captain whose gallantry included introducing a few new customs:

"…he would insist at the table when we had eaten all we would, on passing us bits of dainties that we were obliged to accept, would treat us to sherry every day, that made us shudder to drink, finally he invented the idea that we must smoke – so he presented us with a bunch of cigarettes and we became quite adept in untwisting them and in puffing the smoke thro our noses."[55]

Even thirteen years later, Mary wrote of this same Spanish culinary custom:

"In Spain, at public tables, we were not unfrequently proffered a tit-bit poised upon the fork of our native neighbor seated opposite us. It was something that pertained especially to the Spanish cuisine, and he desired to call our attention to its excellence, and this was his familiar method of doing it."[56]

The steamer's several cities' stops allowed the party's touring and opportunity to catch more of the ubiquitous fleas. To remedy this:

"…some of us happen to be cold water devotees, and it is pitiful the way they suffer on those particular occasions – ex., Mary from the inner room, 'Clara'….exclamations, latter puts her head out of the door 'Mary has caught & killed 10'. I have snapped three and three more have escaped…"[57]

The flea scourge continued, but the young women maintained good humor in circumstances beyond their control.

The Americans arrived in Barcelona for the June 4th Corpus Christi celebration with its late night grand procession of elegantly robed priests, banners, music, sweet incense, crosses and three-foot long torch-like candles.[58] Although up late viewing the festival, Ike and Mary walked early the next morning before departing Barcelona. Curran's eloquent diary entry at day's end:

"This evening at the hour of sunset we witnessed one of the most gorgeous I ever beheld—and as the sun went down we saw the monuments on the dividing line where Spain and France high on the mountain tops—they stand and look like columns of gold. Mary, Flora and self saw and expressed our delight and promised to remember and speak of this one sunset way off in our distant homes when we meet in after graves! Will we ever meet in dear old America? Again that is the question. God grant we may. Tomorrow, with good luck our sail will be ended in the old ship Guadalia (sic)."[59]

The Mattesons remained in Marseille as Mary, Flora and Ike visited the Nimes vicinity for its famous Roman ruins including an old amphitheater Curran compared to Springfield's State Bank building and an aqueduct he thought looked like New York's High Bridge.[60] He noted their good health upon leaving June 12, 1863, for Avignon to tour additional Roman ruins and an unnamed museum that was likely Musee Calvet.[61] The museum housed works of French artists David, Bigand and others whose paintings are displayed there today but in 1863 were considered modern art.[62]

The American group reunited a few days later for a Rhone River cruise north to Lyon, France, famous for silk and fashion houses. Flora wrote extensively on the town's silk production, prices, dressmaking, fashions, traveling costumes and stated further:

"The one style in trimming is the entre deux, black lace insertion over color, with a ruche of the silk on either side. Mary has it on her dress, simple, straight round; lace 14 francs per yard."[63]

The women comparison-shopped, studied the various silks and trimmings, and had stylish new travel clothes made. Knowledge Mary acquired at Lyon silk and dressmaking establishments probably helped years later when she designed practical women's undergarments for dress reform promotion.[64]

On June 23rd the Americans left Lyon by train to Geneva, Switzerland, where Ike's diary pages ended although he continued traveling with the party.[65] Metropolitan Geneva disappointed Flora and Mary who had expected:

"…a place of chalets, of endless Alpine ranges, of picturesque mountaineers, the little boys all called Guillaume, apples and arrows growing on every tree, goiters as large as barrels.."[66]

The party first settled at the luxurious and expensive Hotel Metropole with front rooms' facing Lake Geneva, but soon Mary and Flora moved to the equivalent of today's bed and breakfast known as a pension. Flora elaborated:

"Midge and I have no longer a front room, and thus have lost the Lake, an untold regret. In place we have a beer garden from which the most horrid discords of music haunt our slumbers. Our landlady is a mild tempered woman, but who, of course, has to make her living out of her Boarders…Dinner at 2; soup, strong as the bones of yesterday's beef will make it, one kind of eatable meat, potatoes a l'ordinaire, cauli-flower or turnips, rice pudding or whipped cream and wormy cherries."[67]

Flora was learning the new (to her) art of economizing. Also, she admired and wanted to emulate Mary's less conventional travel mode:

"Mary & I are in a fever lest we shant see anything of Switzerland this summer… We cannot rely upon the Family for their plans are unsettled, but they cant take the journey as we want to – the girls are not strong enough for it & it would kill the Gov – it must be made on foot, with a good Alpen stock & it is not very often a chance would occur for this, but we have one, a friend of Mary's, Mr. McChester, not a young man & of considerable geological reputation, has offered to take the trip with Mary (& I am to go too) – she is independent & is going any way, sometime early in August …the Gov is awefully (sic) careful lest we should do anything to make any talk,…"[68]

Despite his unwitting participation in the Ugly American competition, Matteson felt propriety imperative. Apparently, Mary Safford kept contact with her geologist friend McChesney who in 1862 became U. S. Consul at Newcastle-On-Tyne, England, and was about 3 years her senior.[69] To 21-year old Flora, 35-year old McChesney was, "not a young man," but perhaps she thought his "considerable geological reputation," in Illinois was a good sales point for his being an appropriate chaperone. Mary's willingness to travel with an unrelated, single male only a few years her elder showed her disdain for impractical propriety. Flora's entreaties to her parents to allow this unconventional escort likely met with disapproval since the proposed Swiss walking tour with McChesney never materialized. Instead, a familiar trio toured Geneva's environs more sedately:

"Last Sunday, Mr. C, Mary and myself started on an excursion trip, the round of the Lake to Vevay… we fell in with two young Poles and became much interested in what they told us of their unhappy country. Both of them had been in the late struggles and were obliged to leave on account of their health failing. Had just been to Geneva where they had bought 40,000 arms. Not much, they said, but an assistance. They said Poland had but 50,000 men in the field…."[70]

The trio's meeting men who had just purchased enough weapons to arm 80% of the Polish Army livened an otherwise dull boat trip. A few days later, Flora complained of a stye and described Mary's Cairo angelic style care:

"…it would have been dreary enough but for my little sister of charity Mary, who read to me Kingslake's Crimea…"[71]

Mary Safford reprised her hospital visitor role for her appreciative roommate-patient by reading to her from a book Flora noted was, "forbidden in France under severe penalties," due to its political message. She recovered in time to join the group and two additional Americans, a Mrs. Stone and her 27-year old, "Byronically lame," but very interesting and humorous son for a July 4th excursion:

"We piled into our omnibus and had a warmly merry ride across the country…leaving the gentlemen to order the dinner rushed at once into the delights of the place – a swift mountain brook rolled right by…the wild beauty of these streams…as bright & cold & pure as the air of their native haunts…Joyous as itself, we bounded along after it, ever & anon washing our hands and faces & freezing our laughing lips…worked our way back to find the two young gentlemen wading…We hid their shoes & stockings, tossed their towels up in the trees & got into a regular frolic…"[72]

Two years earlier, Mary delivered 300 bouquets to Cairo's sick soldiers.[73] Where mud, misery, and nearly unbearably hot, humid weather typified Cairo, Switzerland's cool mountain streams, fine food and careless existence were the norm. Flora further recounted:

"…delicate little trout we had, exquisitely browned…& many popping bottles of mountain iced champagne…how we eat & laughed & drank, & how all that was dear to us was remembered in our toasts…After dinner came the lounging and the smoking and the joking & then the ride back, with all of us young ones up on the top of the groaning buss, how we sang!"[74]

Mary and Flora visited a venerable old preacher named, "Dr. Milan," who in youth had an active congregation but now led a simple life. Though retired, he still held Sunday services and conversed with Mary:

"…he turned to Mary & said 'Are you going to Heaven', Mary 'I hope so.' 'You hope so – now see there' said he his bright eye flashing 'the wickedness of that answer, look at her, her face shows that she is an intelligent person & yet she tells me that she hopes she is going to heaven, why says he, are you an American.' oh yes answered Mary. 'There, why did you not say you hoped you were an American, ah my dear child, are you more sure of your country than you are of heaven.' – why I know that I am going to heaven. I have known it for fifty years. We said that we would not dare to say that, but said he 'the Bible says, believe on Christ and you are saved – it is my right, I know it.' "[75]

In the next few weeks, Flora and Mary probably felt angelic while on high Alpine treks. On July 16th, the entire group except the Governor who rested in Geneva, traveled to Chamonix, France, by diligence.[76] Although deciding against climbing almost 16,000 foot Mt. Blanc, Mary and Flora did significant hiking:

"Our first excursion was to the 'Glacier de Bossons' that pours down into the valley till melting into a stream. I & Midge went a foot with our Canes, the rest on mules…The valley below grew smaller & smaller but the needle point above us seemed yet in the air – the last turn made & we made a slight descent to reach the Glacier …"[77]

The girls walked 10 miles and on another day 30 more on what Flora described as:

"…up a pine covered crag opposite Mt. Blanc. At 6000 ft we came to snow- kept on scrambling up good paths 2500 more – then, clinging to the rocks with our hands, climbed up a bare chimney-like wall…Way up on the highest needle of a crag we lay down at full length, dangling our feet over a precipice wall of 8500 feet. Just half way up in the distance to Mt. Blanc, we had the finest view…"[78]

For their next adventure, Flora, Mary, Clara, and the young Mr. Stone, hired mules and two guides for a four-day trek from Chamonix then headed around the southern side of Mt. Blanc to St. Bernard. They traveled above rolling grain fields, through high meadows of summer wild flowers, by waterfalls and pine forests before their night's rest at a primitive inn 6000' above Chamonix. The next day they rode above tree line in an alpine world of clear, crisp, cold air too rarified for vegetation. Flora recounted:

"…nothing now but patches of snow & barren poles to mark out our rout (sic), but still 'excelsior' till we came to two isolated giant peaks, the 'Col de Bonhomme' & the 'Col de Bonne Femme', sterile lovers in vain seeking to embrace each other - over the first we were to pass at its base lay a huge pile of stones, a cairne (sic) & our guides gave us each a stone to add to the pile…"[79]

Despite a wild descent, sure-footed mules delivered their riders safely to the French and Italian border at the Col de la Seigne, and they proceeded to Courmayeur for overnight rest before heading down the valley of Aoste:

"…one of the most luxuriant valleys of Italy, closed right in between ridges of mountains, 5000 ft each side, the glacier at one end, sending its fertilizing streams through the midst…We ate apples & peaches, but in this flush of nature what becomes of man – oh how appallingly deformed & horrid – what burdened beasts to inhabit such Paradise. We saw a few of them along the wayside, one frightened my mule so that he threw me off…"[80]

The travelers were seeing Aoste's famously deformed residents. In this isolated mountain valley, a dietary iodine deficiency and additional hereditary factors led to many inhabitants' enlarged thyroids, hypothyroidism, dwarfism and mental deficiencies.[81] The condition evoked the visitors' simultaneous pity and morbid curiosity:

"… they are all cretins, which is ten times more revolting – they are stunted & dwarfed, & their meaningless faces most disgustingly idiotic – the dull vacancy of soul & body…& it was such a silent hideousness. There was no sound anywhere – it was as walking thro' a city of the dead…"[82]

The shocking sight of these poor people contrasted markedly with their surrounding idyllic mountain scenery, and vowing never returning to Aoste, the party resumed traveling. On July 24th the four travelers plus guides rode mules through skin-soaking cold rain to the St. Bernard monastery where Curran and several monks greeted them. As no wood was available to heat bath water, the already soaked young ladies took cold baths before joining him, the Mattesons, and a new traveler in the monastery's parlor:

"I sat next to a Mr. Peyton from Virginia, a C.S.A. man sent abroad as a representative, the Gov had picked him up at Geneva and had made a boon companion out of him. It is a sad thing to relate that the Gov & Mr. Curran are both of them slight sympathizers with Secesh…sometimes we have quite bitter quarrels."[83]

Given Mary's sympathies and Flora's brothers' current Union Army service while the war raged at home, the image of Matteson and Curran's fellowship with this traitor likely offended both girls and possibly Mrs. Matteson. However, the reality of visiting the historic and holy monastery overshadowed political discussion. While touring the site, Mary and Flora found an aged St. Bernard dog and learned of young monks' laboring in this forbidding climate and altitude for only 10 years before returning to a quiet life in Martigny. Not all of the monks' rescue attempts were successful:

"Afterwards we went to the Morgue – one side lie a mass of whitened bones, arms & legs & sculls (sic) ghastly grinning – the building is small, with a grate at each end so that a strong current of air blows through, thus drying up the bodies without decaying them – there are about 8 bodies within preserved in the position in which they were found, shreds of white garments still cling to them through which the dried bones show most revoltingly…"[84]

The Matteson group sans Mary and Flora took carriages to Martigny where the entire party was to reassemble for a 5 P.M. train ride to Villanueve. Whether avoiding Matteson for the moment or from their sheer independent natures, the young ladies walked different routes. A comedy of errors ensued, with fearful Flora's sitting by the roadside and singing psalms, while the guides, Clara and Mr. Stone searched for her and Mary. Meanwhile, assuming Flora was still behind her, Mary took another path and ended up with a bloody nose courtesy of a kicking mule. Regrettably, in all the confusion the young women forgot their money was in baggage the Mattesons took to Villanueve. With just enough in their purses to pay the guides, the women borrowed money from their understanding landlord and caught the next day's train.[85]

The reunited party continued through Berne, Switzerland, and missed by one day seeing Henry Ward Beecher.[86] By August 2nd they visited Interlaken where Mary likely had her first exposure to a destination health spa for consumptives. A week later, after hearing alpine horns in Lauterbrunnen and seeing Grindelwald's impressive snow avalanche chutes, the party traveled by train and diligence to Lucerne, Rigi, Zug and Zurich.[87] This seemingly alphabetical order of villages' tour ceased near Ragatz where the group visited an even more significant health resort at Pfeffers hot springs:

"We passed thro long, low corridors, like those of an insane asylum, meeting invalids of the lower classes …Formerly, patients were let down by ropes and staid for a whole week under the hot water….we all went in to take a bath—a delicious marble-lined tank with the warm water pouring in all the time…staid in for an hour and when we came out, felt so glorified that standing on the verge of the chasm, Midge said, 'Come, Flim, let us go over. We shall never be so clearly prepared for heaven again.' Fortunately however, we decided on going to breakfast…"[88]

Mary's comment to Flora about, "going over," likely referenced the concept of, "cleanliness is next to godliness," or, "we better die now since we'll never be this clean again!" Choosing breakfast over suicide, their godliness did not stretch far enough to prevent others in the party from criticizing their missing church. At least their fleas had the day off.

After a little over a month in Switzerland, they moved to Baden Baden, Germany, at tourist season's height. Known for its healing baths, upper class visitors, and gambling houses reminiscent of those at Saratoga Springs, New York, Baden Baden was:

"…a place so hot with wickedness that the very springs boil with loathing and hiss as they touch the impure air. Yet is it most charming in its situation and singularly healthy in its climate…"[89]

Mary, Flora and Clara practiced, "royals watching," on the English next door neighbors, but, to the girls' dismay, the young heir to a title and fortune turned out to be merely a small red-haired boy. They followed the King of Russia for a short distance as he shopped in town one afternoon, but he only gave them a, "kingly stare," while they, "returned with our Republican one."[90] The young women came upon the historical, "Maison de Conversation," an elegant gambling establishment that Flora described:

"Gentlemen are obliged to throw away their cigars and take off their hats…and after all, this enforced politeness is but a mask to conceal vileness. Thus doubtless when Satan gives tea parties, which he must sometimes do for the old tea drinking ladies of his court, his ministers concealing their tails in their glowing liveries, stand each side of the dread entrance & usher in the company with the most grace of the modern court….In the center of this room is the 'Rouge et Noir' table, covered with green baize divided off in drawn lines…pools for the cards are between and heaps on heaps of shining lucre…" [91]

Despite drinking liquor and occasionally smoking, Mary, Flora and Clara felt gambling unacceptable. In this den of iniquity they also saw:

"…plenty of those sad women who have sold themselves for gold & have come here for excitement…They are everywhere flitting about in their exquisite dresses & their jaunty sans souci airs…Outwardly they all seem gay as the sunshine, that is joyful alike to all, the pure & the impure. You pity them yet you would not touch them, dowered with a fatal beauty, taught to cherish it & make it tempting by all the allurements of manner & dress, for a few short years they have flattery & carriages & jewels & good dinners & then they die. Few live to be over thirty, except some that are spared to show however fair the beginning, how horrid the end of vice."[92]

The American girls seemed more to pity than condemn the women who in this pre-antibiotic era often met an early demise from venereal diseases. If the, "sad women," did not die young, skin lesions, heart defects, and neurological deficits from such infections as syphilis left them in a degenerated state. Years later, Mary Safford was involved with prison reform work and referred to these girls as, "Magdalens."[93] Her later compassion for fallen women may have sprung from her exposure to them at places like Baden Baden. Whereas many reformers lacked opportunities to encounter even high-class prostitutes, Mary witnessed them here.

The party advanced to Heidelberg and Frankfurt to watch a ceremony with the Emperor, Kings of Bavaria, Saxony, Wertemburg and all the Grand Dukes in full regalia.[94] In early September, the travelers boated the Rhine River from Bierach to Cologne and passed Carlsruhe where Curran was to have assumed his consulate, but he continued traveling.[95] At Cologne, he, Mary and Flora briefly parted from the Mattesons:

"…Midge & I & "Ike" seceded at Cologne. Tis not often we have the courage to do this, for the Gov has one marked peculiarity, he don't wish anyone to see what he does not…He is never happy long in one place, that torture of an uneasy conscience, & you know men's evil deeds live always. He has enemies here, who have spared no pains to sow far & wide the slanders against his name – it has yet not affected our relations with others but I fear for it in Rome."[96]

Both Flora and Mary knew of the controversy surrounding Governor Matteson and other Illinoisans. The infamous 1859 scandal involved Matteson's purported defrauding the state for over $200,000 of Illinois-Michigan Canal scrip.[97] A Sangamon County, Illinois, Circuit Judge rendered a verdict's requiring Matteson's fully reimbursing the state, but the case's final settlement did not occur until April 1864 and involved sale of much of Matteson's property to repay the state. Thus, while traveling in Europe, likely, Matteson was in ill humor as he not only grieved his son's death but potential loss of family property and fortune. Perhaps even old friend Ike felt relief at short respites from him.

The reassembled group proceeded to Prague and then to Vienna's Hotel Archduke Charles located about two miles from the city's Allgemeines Krankenhaus or General Hospital where Mary did post-graduate medical study six years later.[98][99] After touring a few days, they boarded the steamer, "Hildegard," for a four-day Danube River cruise through southeastern Europe. Leaving in fog at 4:30AM and traveling around 150 miles, the boat anchored the first night in Pest across the river from Hungarian capital Buda. The cities had numerous cigar factories, and Hungary had, "the entire monopoly of the Tobacco trade."[100] The American women and girls spent the night in a boarding school dormitory with women from a variety of countries including:

"…two Bulgarian sisters, cross legged on their berths smoking tiny cigarettes,…Armenians and French & Germans, some fair, some dark, and they all gabble in the oddest languages – and I fall to sleep dreaming the times of Babel are come again.'

'This is the first time we have been among people really new to us, taking neither manners nor dress from the English nor French, but have an entire way of their own."[101]

Truly, the Americans experienced vast cultural differences among their boat's first class passengers' including an Eastern Orthodox priest, a wealthy English-speaking Russian family from Odessa, a Moldavian princess, the Parisian criminal lawyer Monsieur Isaac Moise Adolphe Cremieux with a client, and Turkish Admiral Mustapha Pasha, President of the Arsenal Council who, "owns several Palaces and oh, ever so many wives."[102]

Cremieux was French minister of justice, very active in the French provisional revolutionary government of 1848 and known for his work fighting anti-Semitism in North Africa and Europe.[103] Called the, "French Abraham Lincoln," the man's 1848 Cremieux Decree declared an end to slavery, mostly of sub-Saharan Africans, in all French colonies."[104] The document was comparable to Lincoln's Emancipation Proclamation but predated it by 15 years. Flora's letter to her parents further recounted the famous 68-year old lawyer:

"…Monsieur Cremieux, one of the most distinguished men in France, the renowned Parisian advocate, the great criminal Lawyer…Many the dark to him personal pages he unfolds to us. He has suffered too for his liberal opinions, was thrown into prison in 1850…"[105]

Mary, Flora and Monsieur Cremieux's potential conversations on slavery's abolition, anti-Semitism, political imprisonment, and the French Revolution must have been fascinating, while Cremieux may have relished an attentive and intelligent young female audience.

Scenery improved as the boat left Austria, crossing Bulgaria through high, rock-walled gorges, and, by the fourth day, white minarets appeared just before the party disembarked at Cherenovada. After a short steamer excursion across the Black Sea with a rousing round of seasickness and subsequent arrival at Pera, "swarthy Turks in white trouser bags and turbans," rowed the party ashore.[106] Such was their entre to what Flora called Stamboul or Constantinople (now Istanbul) where the group stayed in dingy, inconveniently arranged rooms of Pera's Hotel D'Angleterre on Istanbul's European side. As Mary Safford and cohorts crossed the Bosphorus' narrow waterway, the Asian segment of their Grand Tour commenced.

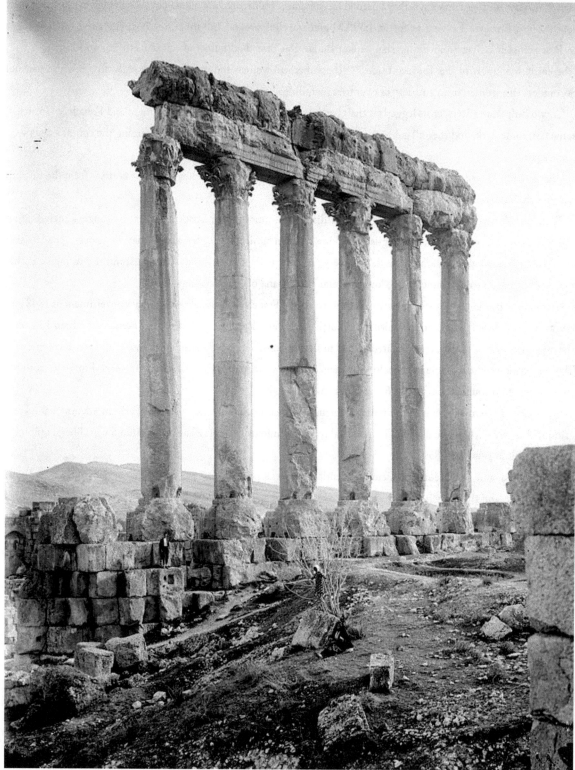

Baalbek. Man at base of far left column demonstrates the ruins' massive size. Matson Photo Collection. Library of Congress Prints and Photo Division, LC-DIG-09490.

6 MIDDLE-EASTERN JOURNEY

In Autumn 1863, the Americans toured Istanbul with help of a, "dragoman," a guide/interpreter supposedly knowledgeable of the city and facilitator of travel through its crowded, confusing streets. Flora elaborated:

"We have a guide, else you could not possibly find your way through these tangled threads of streets. These dragomans are called one of the three curses of Constantinople, for they are as plentiful as fleas & thro' nature & education will cheat you, speak all languages & profess to be able to take you anywhere in the city, tho ours got lost several times."[1]

Istanbul's Christian and Muslim inhabitants exhibited a palpable mutual antipathy:

"We pass thro' the main street of Pera – this is built on the opposite side of the valley formed by the Golden Horn & is the quarter of the Franks, where they form an aristocracy by themselves, for no Christian is allowed to live in the city of the Faithful, & truly he would not..."[2]

The group viewed people of numerous ethnicities, clothing styles, behavior, languages and economic conditions. Here they saw the typical Turkish woman's costume of form-fitting clothing, white veil drawn across the face, bare ankles and, "yellow slippers without heels."[3] Touring the huge domed mosque formerly known as St. Sophia church, they were amply impressed with its mixed Christian and Muslim décor with little done to hide evidence of the former. Quickly, they learned to haggle with bazaar merchants who routinely treated customers to Turkish coffee, tobacco, and dishonest dealing. One evening American Consul Charles W. Goddard called and complained that due to the Turks' laziness and dishonesty his was, "the most disagreeable consulate in the world."[4] He provided tickets to Istanbul's first horse race courtesy of the Sultan who, for the first time, provided entertainment for his countrymen. In 1876, Mary Safford wrote of this:

"...now Arab blood was pitted against English jockey and the French steed.'

'The race course...had every appearance of a spent crater...The ascending, and in places quite precipitous, natural walls, that nearly enclosed it, formed an admirable amphitheater upon which the immense audience was placed, tier upon tier, to the very summit.'

'There was the green, white, and yellow turban of the Turk, indicative of the number of times he had made a pilgrimage to the sacred shrine of his prophet; the Persian, in his flowing, rich robes; the Greek, with his outstanding white skirt, his gold-laced, slashed jacket, and his tasseled fez; the merchant from Thibet, dressed in his richest stuffs,- -in fine, it was as if the whole world had arranged for a dress-parade, where all of the costliest and quaintest garments were exhibited.'

'A Swiss chalet had been built upon the most favorable site from which to view the race for the occupancy of the Sultan. It was beautiful in its graceful proportions and exquisite finish in different woods.'

'We observed on either side of the door two stalwart men standing, holding by the horns two rams, and wondered what part they were to take in the performance. Soon an open carriage, drawn by four magnificent horses, was seen to approach. In it was Abd-ul-Aziz, dressed in a plain civilian suit with the usually worn fez. As soon as he touched foot to the ground, the rams were slaughtered, and their blood was sprinkled upon the places where he trod. This blood sacrifice was made in honor of his divine origin, as successor in regal line from Mahomet.'

'Ranged in a semi-circle in front of the chalet of His Serene Highness, were a dozen or more of carriages, shaped something like hollow pumpkins, gilded, and fragile enough to have conveyed so many fairy queens, instead of the wives of the Seraglio. Each carriage was drawn by six jet black stallions, handsome enough to have been Landseer's best models. At the head of each horse walked a eunuch.'

'The women of our party were privileged to walk near, and along the line of carriages, and to gaze in upon these Circassian beauties, purchased for a price, the slaves of a supreme ruler. Their faces were covered with so thin a material that we could see their rich olive complexion, with its peach-blossom tint, which we could not vouch for as the gift of Nature. Their dark, lustrous eyes, gleaming through the opening of the covering to the upper and lower portions of the face, could be compared to nothing else but the liquid, expressionless eyes of the gazelle.'

'These caged prisoners seemed as curiously to gaze at us as we at them. We had seen some of them in their own home; so that our curiosity was tinged with an inexpressible sadness at the fearfully inert lives they were condemned to live. One of the illustrious number addressed us in French, and asked if we were English, and we interchanged a number of casual interrogatories. We afterward learned that this wife was an especial favorite of His Highness, and that he had granted her request to learn French and music. And then followed the terrible sequel of what a little learning did for her. She eloped with her French music master, and escaped to Paris. No doubt that proved an effectual quietus to all other favorite wives affected with strong-minded tendencies."[5]

As disenchanted Consul Goddard refused attending, for all practical purposes the Matteson party and Mary Safford were America's only representatives at this auspicious event and had elevated seats in the area reserved for ambassadors. Constantinople's Greek Patriarch, numerous other important personages and royal harem women passed before them. Aside from the blood sacrifice, the horse races were no different than elsewhere. Sultan Abd-ul-Aziz's regime's innate brutality haunted him years later when he died violently.[6]

Mary, Flora and the Matteson girls were privileged to visit the Sultan's harem, and Mary wrote of this in an 1869 women's suffrage journal:

"Our native cicerone conducted us to the palace, and left us at the entrance of a spacious court, in the charge of an attendant upon the household who spoke French. By him we were shown into an ante-room, where we waited until he had announced us. We then followed him into a small room, with alcoves upon three sides. In these alcoves, reclining upon couches, were the inmates of the Harem. They were variously occupied, one in adding an extra touch of henna to her finger nails; another in cutting the designs from bits of flowered silk; a third was at her favorite occupation— preparing candy. A brazier stood upon a tripod before her couch, and she was lazily shaping the sweet compound with more the air of a time-killer than that of one designing to accomplish aught.'

'Their gross, uncouth figures were covered with illy-shaped robes of thin material; the braids of their black hair were disheveled; the barbarity of barbarism was typified in the massive appendages that dangled from their ears; bracelets were upon both wrists and ankles; rings in profusion were upon their fingers; their bare feet were carelessly slipped into sandals;--making a tout ensemble indicative, in the highest degree, of vulgar, low-bred luxuriousness. Upon being presented to them, they expressed much cordiality, and beckoned us to sit beside them on their couches. The red hair of one of our party gained for her the greater share of attentions. They were curious to know if any application would convert their own jet black locks into so beautiful a color. From the surprise and admiration they manifested, it seemed they had never looked upon the like before. Our complexion, features, and dress were marvelous to them, and we thought to add to their surprise by telling them we were from America, but the name had evidently no significance for them. They made no inquiries respecting our county, our home, or our customs---only our apparel excited their inquisitiveness. The effect of this aimless life was visible upon all the inmates of the Harem. Not a countenance was lighted with intelligence. Large, lustrous eyes; long, silken lashes; arched eyebrows, pearly teeth, alabaster complexion—these fairest daughters of Circassia were to me, compared with thinking women, as wax fruit to nature's own sun-ripened." [7]

After visiting the Howling Dervishes, religious men who performed exhausting ritualistic rocking and vocalizations and then seeing equally active Dancing or Whirling Dervishes, the Americans were not convinced to convert to such a fatiguing religion. [8]

On a rainy October 27th, the group left Istanbul by boat for a surprisingly smooth voyage through the Sea of Marmara, the Dardanelles and the Aegean Sea, as weather cleared. Passing several famed Greek isles, their craft anchored at the Piraeus harbor where English, French, Italian, and German warships gathered peacefully to honor the newly arrived 17-year old Danish Prince William Christian, soon the new King George I of Greece. The Matteson party appeared coincidently for the events surrounding the new monarch's appearance at Athens:

"We were just in time for the celebrations...We took carriages to the town, some six miles from the entrance, driving through the Piraeus, that is a busy place with modern houses and a population of 5000...evergreens & wreaths adorned & festooned the streets & served as frameworks to photographs of the fair young King...There was everywhere an attempt at a happy greeting...Found a nice hotel; secured rooms at $2 ½ a day, a little dearer because of the festivities..." [9]

They toured Athens, climbed the Acropolis, and, unlike earlier tourists, consciously chose neither to deface the Parthenon nor to remove souvenir marble bits:

"...one guard has followed us about most uneasily – he thinks we are very hard to get rid of, cannot understand carrying away ideas as specimens instead of stones. As we rise to go, shouts draw us to the walls, a rolling tone of cheers from the people gathered around the Assembly house, whence the young king is coming from taking his oath. There is the jingle of voices & music, a noise of happy rejoicing...'

'After dinner the whole town was afire with illuminations...Every house was blazing with a brilliant beauty that was magical – everywhere was the name & the picture of the young king in circles of light & evergreens..." [10]

On Sunday, November 1st, Mary and Flora, with Bibles in hand, headed for Mars Hill to stand in the Apostle Paul's pulpit and re-enact preaching his sermon:

"...no wonder it was such a solemn sermon, for it was a mighty solemn place...the deaconesses of our party gave us much approbation for our early rising – how could we help it, so near to Mars Hill & Paul that one might almost be persuaded to become Christians!" [11]

Whether Flora and Mary reenacted for historical or religious purposes is debatable, but later the entire party attended elderly missionary Dr. King's Sunday services in Athens where he had poor success in making converts from the Greek Orthodox faith. [12] The next morning he introduced the Americans to Professor Koeppen, the new King George I's private tutor in Greek. Previously, the older gentleman taught History and Modern Languages at Pennsylvania's Franklin & Marshall College and wrote the comprehensive *The World in the Middle Ages*. [13] Despite his lofty position, the dapper professor eagerly gossiped about the new King:

"...he is a high gay spirited boy, fond of the chase, of swimming & all many amusements...If he succeeds at his royalty he is to marry the Princess Helena – Queen Vic. with her usual discretion & love of match making allowed them to fall in love with each other at his sister's wedding, but it is to be kept in the bud till the Kingdom is safe."[14]

After three days in Athens, the party left by steamer for Smyrna, took a train to an active archeological dig for the Temple of Diana at Ephesus, Turkey, and then took another steamer to Beirut, Beyrout or Beyrouth as Flora spelled it or Beyroot as Mary Safford did.[15] Despite spelling discrepancies, all agreed the city was in Syria, not Lebanon as now. Traveling in autumn's, "season of rains," the rough steamer passage led to group seasickness and Flora's comments on the journey:

"Midge is the first one to fail & she really has a suffering time of it, tho' she sings out as cheerily as a martyr at the stake."

"...the harbor is so miserable that even little boats could not land & we were seized in the arms of one eyed savages who waded with us to shore..."[16]

After meeting the American Consul, numerous Christian missionaries, and visiting a few city sites, part of the group that included Mary secured the services of Michael Henne, reputedly Syria's best dragoman, and planned meeting him in Damascus.[17] A rift occurred in the otherwise cordial group:

"...Beyrout. There we had a difference...the Gov, who never likes to do things after the way of other people, took one of his most obstinate fits & declared that he would not hire a dragoman till he got to Damascus. In vain Consul and all assured him that one was not to be had there... so Mr. Stone, his Mother, Mary & I engaged aides to make our arrangements independent of the Gov."[18]

Mary, Flora, and the Stones traveled by diligence to Damascus on the 65 mile French, "broad, graded macadamized... Napoleonic road."[19] Leaving Beirut at 4AM, Mary noted:

"There are seen a few scattering villages of the Druses and Maronites as peacefully dotted side by side, as if there were no wrangling hatred, one for the other, a pent up fire of envy and jealousy, that is liable to burst forth at any moment, to the destruction of lives and property. The Maronites are the so-called Christians, with whom the French took sides, and the Druses, heathens, with whom England sympathized. Judging from their deeds, I think one as deserving the name as the other."[20]

Religious differences permeated the region then as now. Despite such wrangling, the locals treated the visitors well, and, after eleven changes of horses, the party finally arrived at a silent Damascus long after dark. Mary described their hotel:

"We enter from the street, a small open court, a fountain in the center—the walls painted with broad stripes of red, white and blue, through a door, into a second and much larger court, walls painted like the first, pavement black and white marble, a large fish pond in the center, fed by running faucets, with fountains at either end, and large orange trees, laden with golden fruit, and sweet-smelling flowers. One side a deep, alcoved recess, the raised floor spread with mats and divans, inviting for an afternoon siesta. Opposite is the parlor—on either side of the door the same deep niches that we see in the court, the floor raised two steps, is covered with Persian carpets. The very high ceiling is finished in Mosaic, the walls painted gaily, a favorite pattern, festoons of flowers and vines arranged on the wall to represent windows—of which there are but two, looking into the court. Divans surround the walls, and Boston rockers recall to mind 'Old Lang-Syne.' Marble tables in the center, with astral lamps, which serve for illuminators at night and you have the inventory of furnishing.'

'In the marble paved passage between the two side niches, is a running fountain. In the wall opposite, the door is a deep niche, wherein stands a mirror, and on either side, in lesser ones, are placed narghiles, silver and amber mouth-pieces, delicate little coffee cups, and silver holders, ready for use when friends happen in. Our dining-room is off from the same court, and none the less Oriental in its arranging as well as the bountifully spread table, arrayed adown its center with luscious fruits of the land, grapes, oranges and pomegranates. Stone steps lead up to a balcony, around which are our bed-rooms, neat and comfortable, and within sound of falling waters to lull us to sleep. Our Grecian host dresses true to his nationality, as does his pretty Greek wife. We take coffee or tea and bread at eight o'clock, breakfast at eleven o'clock, and dinner at seven."[21]

In subsequent days, the group toured Damascus including the horse market where they first saw Bedouins, as Mary narrated:

"…gay colored, striped or black silk or cotton handkerchief of the Bedouin put over the head, a folded half-square, and tied about with a rope, a cord, or skein of bright-colored yarn. These are the first specimens that we have seen of the real Bedouin, the wild men of the desert, whose dark faces and black, flashing eyes, make us content to keep our distance. Sole inheritors of all the rags of past generations, which they proudly wrap about them as heir looms, they could not present a greater medley of pieces and colors. Not a few are girded about the loins with skins their heads bound around with ropes. Their usual dress, however, is a loose shirt, reaching midway below the knees fastened around the waist, and a loose over-garment of coarse wool, striped black and white, wadded under the arm, or dragging along the ground. Their feet, if covered, scuff along in low boots, the sole jetting out like an eaves spout, and turning up at the toe like a scow boat.'

'Now rides by on a gaily caparisoned horse, a sheik of his tribe, known as such by the weapons of defense that he and his train carry—a spear fifteen feet long, poised in air, battle-axes, old inlaid fusils, their belts stuffed out with silver-mounted daggers and pistols. Our astonished gaze at them was equaled by their surprise at seeing us; bids grew less animated while we tarried; they neither laughed nor talked, but gave an occasional deep, gutteral grunt, and a significant glance at each other, as much as to say: 'there is no use, we have no words in our vocabulary that will do them justice.' When they passed, and our crinoline yielded to the pressure, it was evident that they were more than ever at a loss to give us a place in the human scale, and looked around upon their own tattooed, brown women, their forms but half concealed with evident satisfaction that they were not as we. Woman's curiosity so far predominated over the shy indifference of one, that she seized me to institute an investigation of my person and clothes; she felt of my hands and face as if I were wax, and she would be responsible if I cracked under her touch, possibly she felt a sympathy for me in my frailty, not less than I for her in her degradation and filth; her hair matted, a graduated band of coins pendant upon her forehead, cheeks tattooed, nose set with jewels put in with screw, arms half covered with the one loose, tattered garment, loaded with heavy silver bracelets."[22]

After this cross-cultural physical examination, the Americans resumed touring and were borne with the mass of humans, donkeys and camels through narrow, noisy, and occasionally dark, filthy, Damascus streets and bazaars. A fascinated Mary recounted:

"But within these dingy alleys and somber niches, ranged along on either side, more like impromptu stalls than anything else, are found the riches of the whole East—the silks of India and shawls of Cachmere, the carpets of Persia, with spices and perfumes from Araby. Every branch of labor is open to your inspection, for if not carried on out of doors, you have but to cross the threshold of the ever open door to see swarthy, turbaned figures squatting over their work even at blacksmithing as they sit around the forge, one works a skin bellows as you would blow a bagpipe, and the other wields the anvil, but when it comes to shoeing a horse, the trying moment comes that brings them to the feet."[23]

The tour included visits to carpenters, weavers, saddle and shoe factories, a boys' school where the teacher demanded baksheesh, a bribe for the privilege of watching their lesson, and silver workers that Mary described further:

"Now we dodge through a low doorway, and there is such a clicking of hammers and blinding of smoke that we can easily imagine ourselves in the grand workshop of Vulcan. It is the silversmith bazaar; a large area covered over with a vaulted roof supported here and there by an ancient column. Each workman, and perhaps there are fifty, sits on his own mud heap forge, crooked over a miniature furnace of glowing coals, on which is bubbling a few melted globules of precious ore. He leaves his work and reaches out to a little box securely locked, opens up to you his ready stock; there are all sorts of ornaments enriched by settings of precious stones, but that which is most lovely in your eyes is the filagree silver work. Coffee-cup holders and bracelets, delicate as if the finely spun thread had been woven. They thrust antiquities at you and have a merry time trying to convince you that they are genuine. You know at once that you are not in the presence of staid Mussulmen whose faces rarely light up with an attempted joke. All these artists and workmen are Christians."[24]

Ironically, with the Civil War's raging at home, the Americans attempted to tour the, "slave market for Caucasian beauties," but sales had closed for the day.[25] Often, both Flora's and Mary's descriptions included Biblical references, and Damascus offered opportunities for their continuing this practice. Mary did so upon seeing overloaded camels in the open-air market:

"Since I have seen the goods that are piled upon these poor creatures I begin to believe that it was no trifling affair— the royal bakshish of forty camels burden that the crafty Hazael offered the far-seeing Elisha. I do not imagine that the manners and habits of the people have changed much since that time. Every surrounding gives to the Bible a new and living interest."

"…though we zig-zag still, that we are in the street called, 'Straight.' We walk up with credulity in our faces, if not in our hearts, and peep through a grated window into the house of Judas, where was lodged one Saul of Tarsus, whom the Lord sought there through his servant Ananias, whose limb is shown within covered with the dust of ages and hung with myriad scraps of rags—Mussulman offering of respect for the worthy dead. We visit the house of Ananias—deep beneath the surface of the ground—now a Catholic chapel. The place is shown us where Paul was let down the wall from a projecting window, and where the great light, as from Heaven, shown about him. I can conceive it to have been a blinding one if the rays were more concentrated than those of a Syrian sun now. It is said that these holy places are subject to change every few years, so that we do not feel it incumbent to bow our heads with deep feelings of reverence." [26]

Obviously, Damascene tourism catered to those of varying religious beliefs, shopping styles and means of transport:

"For a turn about the city we have horses. I had an Arab colt upon which, doubtless woman never sat—with a man's saddle and halter to guide him. I have heard and read much of the poetry of motion and the sensation of being borne on the wings of the wind in riding these Arab steeds, but I must confess that my experience did not accord well with either. I only gave myself into the hands of Providence and clung closely to the saddle, letting the wild Arab go as he would." [27]

Mary did not recount Bedouins' witnessing the girls' struggle to maintain dignity when astride men's saddles, crinolines tucked goodness knows where, while riding unruly Arabian horses haphazardly through Damascene streets. Perhaps the sight amused even the stern desert dwellers. Fortunately, no one was injured. Other entertainment included an old Arab called Antika who:

"…comes in and, as from the magic depths of a Pandora-like box, pulls from his girdle and the ample folds of his loose over-garment, shawls, scarfs, caps, great varieties of jeweled ornaments, pistols, and Damascus blades with silver mountings worth the real metal. He dresses us up and parades us about in his gay merchandise, till we almost fancy ourselves heroines of the 'One Hundred Nights.'" [28]

On further touring, the Americans contrasted Damascus with the nearby arid, chalky desert and marveled how irrigation promoted life and growth. Mary's narrative continued:

"We passed through the Christian quarter—a heap of rubbish and ruins since it was demolished during the massacre, when the streets ran with the blood of four thousand slaughtered Christians—and entered at the gate of God, through which the Pilgrim caravan of seven to eight hundred makes its annual exit to Mecca; a pilgrimage requiring from four to six months, and many there be who go out that never reenter." [29]

Here Mary referenced the July 1860 Damascus massacre and did not exaggerate the extent of Christian deaths and property destruction.[30] She noted their cicerone or tour guide, "old Ibriham," was Jewish:

"Led, through the walls by the same ever-open little door, to a dark entrance cumbered with filth, where, in times of past persecutions, the family assembled that its members might be considered too wretchedly poor to be worth a sacking; again through another passage, and burst upon our view surroundings that make the age of the Califs no longer to be doubted. We are in an open court; there is the gurgling of fountains, the singing of birds, the air laden with the fragrance of the orange blossom, jassamine and white rose. The pavement is tessellated, the walls are brilliantly painted, and small saloons surround the court. You pass beyond into another; the same gorgeous display of fountains and high vaulted ceilings set with small bits of mirrors, pearl, shell and ebony. Divans about the room are laid with white Cachmere with cushions of rich Damascene silk. This was the Jewish Sunday. The mistress of the house and her daughters come toppling in on kubkobs—wooden soles on two upright bits of wood six or eight inches high, ornamented with pearl, with a worked band over the foot—which they step off from at the door, dropping down considerably in the world. They were real voluptuous Jewish beauties with full lips, large eyes, whose long silken fringes and brows were touched with kohl; their long dark hair, braided in myriad little plaits, hung down the back, the ends dangling with gold and silver coins; their heads were glittering with pearls and jewels; their jeweled fingers deeply stained with henna, and their only covering a loose sort of chemise left open in front to the waist leaving the whole form exposed.'

'Within these showy palaces they spend their days in self-adornment. I pity them and all their kind who have nothing better to live for." [31]

Damascus' inhabitants provided a rich, diverse array of costume and societal details for Mary's keen observations and reporting. Her knowledge of other cultures' couture would prove useful in her dress reform campaign years later. She wrote of men's attire as well:

"The Mussulman Sunday—the grand market day—is one of unusual interest. This is the day set apart for the women to wail over the graves; some pretend to say that they converse with their departed friends though an opening that you see in the top of each Dutch-oven looking tomb. As if intent upon giving his best robe an airing at least once a week, the Persian struts along in blue and gold, his high, black sugar-loaf, a yard in length upon the back of his head, at an inclination backward of forty-five degrees. You see plenty of spruce descendents of Ham decked out with all their characteristic fondness for finery; the Turk with his longest rich, robe; while the Jew, not to be outdone, comes out in his fur-lined and trimmed mantle. When we stop in the market and see the traffic that is carried on, we realize what a great trading center it is…On an average from three to four thousand camels arrive and depart daily." [32]

Mary visited a Damascene bookstore:

"Passing a book bazaar one day I happened to think that a specimen of Arab printing would be a curiosity, and stepping up to a niche where books were lying about promiscuously, reached forth to take up one, when I was warded off by the proprietor as if I would call down fire to consume his whole stock. Not knowing why I had called forth such indignation; I appealed to the guide, when he told me that Christian money could buy anything but books lest perchance they contain the name of Allah or his prophets, and cannot be profaned by Christian hands. I said to him, poor bigot, and left him to moulder and grow dusty with his sacred books." [33]

Mary, Flora, the Stones and newly acquired companion Le Baron Ferdinand d'Houtpoul headed from Damascus toward ancient city Baalbek's ruins, but Matteson, having previously refused hiring a dragoman in Beirut, now inserted his family onto the others' adventure. [34] Mary described guide Michael Henne's November 22nd arrival:

"Sunday evening our dragoman arrived, whom we had engaged to meet us here with equipments for tent life and who had insinuated himself into our good graces when we first arrived at Beyroot (sic)…at a cost of five dollars per day each, everything furnished. Monday morning we were up in good time for a general move; we blockaded the streets with our grand trains, as you can well imagine, when I tell you that we had in all twenty eight mules and horses, and with ourselves, dragoman guard and men, twenty-eight. I should think that the like had never been seen here before, by the crowd that gathered around us. We have never tried our horses and know not our fate—we have a long day before us, the road is good for some miles, and it is suggested that we make the most of it. The dragoman leads off; we let loose the rein; one is thrown; horses are changed, saddles are girted anew, and again we make a cavalry dash, and off rolls poor Mrs. S—a second time, the unfortunate one, as before—now badly bruised; but she mounts again, and now we move on, somewhat tempered in our speed. When you once understand these Arab horses they are easy to manage, and pleasant to ride. They are not used to bit nor whip, but are urged, checked and guided by a rod poised in the hand. They walk well, are good pacers, and run with the least encouragement, but woe to your equilibrium when they stop as they do instantaneously, by slip of the hind feet and brace with the front." [35]

With that less than propitious start, they began the two-day trek north to Baalbek. Mary summed her obvious delight in her travels:

"Traveling is very much like amassing wealth—the more one has the more one wants." [36]

Unfortunately, this was the last of her surviving newspaper accounts of Middle-Eastern travels, but Flora's letters recorded the group's progress. Five dollars per day per person in 1863 bought great food and accommodations but less comfortable transport:

"...it was delicious to find how magical Michael's saddle bags were – cold chicken, eggs, bread, confitones, figs & coffee. We eat with an appetite despite sores and aches, half an hour was allotted to a cigarette & a nap, & up again we mounted our fearful steeds that not having lunched as we had, were less inclined to be merciful to our tender flesh – and we had a hard jog over hard stones for about four hours, when we struck down into the plain of Zebdany. The smoking blue light revealed the village but something white in the trees this side called forth a shriek, 'the Tents, the Tents' – pistols were fired & soon we were in the midst of quite an encampment – the American Colors waved over one...Our tents were something gorgeous, flaunting red peacocks...with here & there bunches of brilliant roses... here was 5th Avenue style – lights down the center, napkins, wine, soup, three courses of meat, pudding desert (sic) and coffee, all cooked deliciously, more than we could eat...some crept off after dinner, the rest indulged in a game of Euchre, till 9 o'c when we all left to wrap the drapery of our couch around us & lie down to pleasant dreams, on the soft springy mattresses." [37]

Proceeding in drizzling rain, over stony mountains, the group, according to Flora, felt like, "nine insane spirits seeking a holiday in Hades," but their second night's stop offered much less elegant accommodations:

"a bleak little convent...a room that had to commend it a roof, & windows that were windowless opening on all sides to the view...but it was comfortless & we wished we were in the Louvre or even in Cleveland rather than sitting shivering here by the ruins of Baalbek..."[38]

Baalbek proved intriguing:

"...had intended to give two hours the next morning to the ruins & hasten on, but some of us got so entangled in their splendor...that we gave the word to stay, & stay we did, tucking up our skirts and doing the ruins thoroughly. There was once here a prosperous city, in the palmist days of the Phoenicians, one of their holy cities, for they built here a Temple to their God – the Sun- and called it the Heliopolis of Syria."

"...stones...so Cyclopean are they in their immense size – three that once gave the name to the Temple of the 'Three Stoned' that measured respectively, 62, 63 & 64 ft. To believe, we paced them, their thickness 13 feet...In the quarry near by lies a stone almost quarried, measuring 68 feet, that never took its destined place – perhaps even the Cyclops bent under such labors.'

'...all underneath this were vaulted passages..."[39]

The Baalbek tour was thoroughly enjoyable once the Mattesons and Curran, disgruntled by rain and lacking appreciation for the ruins, returned to Beirut. Mary and Flora celebrated Thanksgiving by eating, "a hot camp dinner," and illuminated their tent, "with a bowl of blue burning punch."[40] They toasted to, "health and glory of our brave armies, & to our Union now and forever..."[41] Though physically far from the Civil War, their thoughts did not stray far from it especially with direct family involvement. Flora's brother Oliver lately received a bullet wound in battle.[42] Also, the Mattesons' sons-in-law along with Mary Lincoln's brother-in-law Ninian Edwards and her niece Julia's husband recently signed a contract to provide Union Army supplies in Illinois.[43] Though safe from the American war's conflict, the travelers experienced potential desert dangers from lone, armed Arabs on horseback. Mindful for their own safety,

Mary's group headed toward Beirut:

"...we were delighted yet tired with our tent life in Syria...having experienced rather a hard wet time it was unanimously voted that the state of the country was too dangerous for a trip across the interior, and as we did not care to be sacrificed in some miserable maronite massacre, we decided to take the boat to Joppa, & cross to Jerusalem on the usual pilgrimage donkeys."[44]

Storing most of their baggage at a convent, the reunited American group rode on horseback and donkeys from Beirut to the Plains of Sharon and stopped for the night at the Convent of Rama.[45] They found comfortable lodgings, clean beds and a hearty breakfast before remounting and donning India rubber overcoats for the rest of the ride to Jerusalem. A party of young English Officers accompanied them part way to where serial watchtowers marked the road. With relatively good weather in this usually rainy season, the Americans elected momentarily postponing Jerusalem sightseeing and diverted to Jordan, the Dead Sea and Jericho with the guidance of dragoman Michael. He charged everyone an extra three dollars/day in bribes for safe passage through hostile country.[46]

At daybreak, Mary and Flora preceded the others on foot, exited through Jerusalem's massive stone Jaffa Gate, and accompanied by a Frenchman familiar with the region, descended the steep hill leading from town and past various Biblical and historic sites. They headed toward Bethlehem, only 5 miles away. Eventually, the others on horseback and donkeys caught up, and group discussion ensued on whether they were on a religious pilgrimage. They concluded their mission was secular as:

"...pilgrims of history, and with the Bible for our Book, search out places, that age alone should consecrate..."[47]

Through Bethlehem's narrow, dirty streets the tourists attracted:

"...groups of natives...bothering that we should buy the ornaments of wood & pearl made by the workman here... They followed close at our heels to the convent, or rather Convents, for around this contested spot, the three – Greek, Latin & Armenian – cluster close, each the jealous guardian of the 'Cave of the Nativity' that is the oldest special locality fixed upon by the Christian church."[48]

Bethlehem's natives were persistent salespeople, as Flora added, "we went out of Bethlehem strung with beads and pearly devices of virgin scenes and nativities sufficient to have opened a bazaar."[49] At Bethlehem's Grand Basilica, also called the Church of the Nativity:

"With tapers in hand we followed down a flight of steps & came to the Chapel, a low vault hung with tapestries,– we descend into it by a step – it is a hole in the rock – push back the gorgeous tapestries & it shows itself rough and unhewn – a marble trough now marks the spot where the manger lay – over it burn silver lamps that through silver gratings dimly lights up a picture behind that represents the scene..."[50]

Only the men were admitted into the Convent of Mon Saba, while Mary and the other women stayed in tents pitched by the dragoman and ate a, "meal of many courses with a change of plate for each." They slept poorly that night, "because of the terrible jingling of bells the donkeys kept up, and the ravages of sundry starved regiments of fleas out on a foray from the neighboring Convent."[51] The men slept equally badly, as Mr. Curran came to the women's tents around 1:30AM thinking it was departure time and rousted everyone for breakfast. The amazed dragoman and his disgruntled men hastily prepared breakfast, packed everything and then realized it was too early to dare travel Judea's hill country. As beds were already packed:

"Not being a place to lay our heads we literally took to the stones for a pillow. M & I crawled into a cave up over the Convent – it was as stern and frightful a desolation as we ever witnessed, the death deep ravine, the grim hangings of the Convent walls, dim lights glimmering in the dome, the faint weird voice of midnight vespers, & shining down fitfully, the red crescent of the old moon and the full morning star – now and then breaking the timid silence would rise the wild cry of an Arab shepherd or the monotonous chant of some passing pilgrim – frightened and cold, we fairly went to sleep, till roused at 5½ to mount our horses."[52]

Waking on the wrong side of the rock, the now disagreeable travelers rode through rocky canyons, past black caves and old tombs until arriving at the Jordan River Valley. After two hours, they reached a Bedouin encampment where the dragoman acquired additional guards for the party's safe passage through dangerous territory. Flora recounted their new protectors:

"...The bare legged tawny skinned tattered creatures came out with their dogs to hoot and howl at us. In the center of all this filthy misery, on a little rise of ground, stood pawing a white Arabian horse, waiting for the sheik, for he joined us here with his escort, as we were nearing the boundaries of the hostile tribes – we made quite a parade, the Sheik on his beautiful horse, in the dress of his people – a striped calico shirt bound with a girdle, a tattered over cloak, his bare legs stuck in boots turning at the toes that he plunged to the heel in his stirrups, a bright handkerchief bound round his head with a rope of Camels hair, and his locks matted over the bronzed face shading the curiosity of the quick eye. He was handsome as they all are, with an untamed regularity of face that submits to no description. His only weapon was a long lance, measuring 15 ft. made of cane, light and tipped either end with a point of iron - this he carried across his shoulder or grasped in the middle, making it quiver as a magnet needle...Now he would ride by our side mimicking our shrill notes or chanting low monotones of his own. Now he would dart off, play around us with his threatening spear, and in a moment with a low cry, sink into some ravine or pace the edge of some precipice...Now way off we would see him, motionless – horse and rider – against the sky, spying the land if any dwelt there who ought not. He was a sheik over a tribe of 500 men, 300 white, 200 black, once slaves. We had three with us, called soldiers and as tawny members of a legion as you could imagine – their ragged cloaks had no sleeves & showed their bare muscular arms to the shoulder; their legs and feet were to match, and they carried in any way that was the easiest a rusty flintlock..."[53]

Accompanied by these guardians, the Americans reached the Dead Sea that, although beautiful, was not tasty:

"...dipping but the tips of our fingers we touched them to our tongue – no fountain in Hades, no waters of Marah could be more tormentedly horrid, not saltish alone but brackish and bitter, and so nauseous that though we scrubbed our mouths with sand and sputtered and spitted, it was hours before we could forget the taste."[54]

Unsatisfied at merely tasting the Dead Sea, the party swam in it:

"And now we were determined to test again its reputation in its buoyancy, so we all went swimming – that is, not to belie that word we undressed and went out into the sea...we all of us just bobbed up and down like corks, it was just like being on a huge life preserver, we could not sink and our swimmers could not swim...the most fatal thing that could happen to you was to have your head occasionally duck under the brackish water – it would enter your eyes, agonizing them with pain...When once on shore we experienced all the discomforts of a Dead Sea spree – our skin stuck all over and itched most ruefully, as though we had been slowly roasting before a hot fire..."[55]

At least the saltwater bath forced the flea contingent to abandon its human hosts. The entourage continued riding over desolate and inhospitable desert, past swamps and eventually to the Jordan's willow and tamarisk-lined banks. Appreciating the significance of River Jordan baptism, the group chose recreating Biblical events to sooth their skin after the Dead Sea swim but had a somewhat less than religious experience:

"…it was a most laughable sight our baptism in the Jordan – the waters are very very cold flowing from snow tipped Hermon, and the current rapid and dangerous – we baptized our toes for a long while, wondering if that would not do, but finally though heartily opposed to the doctrine of immersion, we did get in all over and sat down in the water…We all dipped too & played around in the water, dashing it at each other, laughing and freezing in the same breath…"[56]

Not all was fun and games that afternoon for:

"…while we were at our watery devotions one of the guard had drawn a knife on the dragoman & threatened to kill him, which had it been done we had run the chance of lying as a memorial, with the stones of the 12 Tribes of Israel, at the bottom of the Jordan. A few accidents have happened, chiefly to Americans, who reckless & boastful that they are wiser than custom, ride through the plain without an escort – one was murdered & two, while bathing, had their horses and clothes stolen & travelled to Jericho in a worse plight than a certain man who fell among thieves." [57]

Fortunately, these wary Americans had hired guards, albeit of questionable reliability. The tourists rode from Jericho through the miserable village Riha where a mob of filthy children pelted them with rocks. Despite this and recurrent flea infestation, the party camped there that evening before venturing through Judea's hill country:

"…frightful in their desolateness… are the favorite hiding places of the wild tribes, and we kept close together – occasionally from behind some projecting rock, the gleam of a matchlock would catch our eye and fever us for a moment, but it turned out to be nothing…but had we been without our trusty Sheik, we might to this day lie drying on the burning hill tops…" [58]

With that dramatic flourish, Flora concluded her reassuring letter to Mother, and the party concluded its perilous desert venture with safe return to Jerusalem where their tour guide was the American Consul's Jewish brother Mr. Moeser, a well-educated and good lecturer.[59] By now it was early December 1863, and the group toured sites associated with Christian, Jewish and Moslem traditions. Passing through the Damascus Gate on the city's north side, they entered a narrow opening where, by candlelight, they ventured under the Haraam, the site of the Temple. Emerging from underground they found:

"…footpaths across corn fields & olive groves to the Tomb of the Kings, where M. de Saulcy at the head of a band of Frenchmen are excavating. They were just opening a staircase leading to the arch of the entrance, & were taking casts for the Louvre of the work of the listel (sic) – wreaths of fruits and flowers. We entered underground an antichambre, from which branched off smaller ones, set with niches, some having 3, some 5 and 8, & they opened an infinite series one behind the other. Before we left the city they discovered a beautiful sarcophagus, containing the perfect outline of a female form – on touching the air it vanished into dust. They are confident she belonged to the Family of the Kings. Leaving the enthusiastic Frenchmen at their work, we walked on for miles & miles through Cave tombs…"[60]

Famous French archeologist Louis Felicien Joseph Caignart de Saulcy researched and provided Holy Land antiquities for the Louvre from several sites including Baalbek and Jerusalem.[61] His peers questioned his interpretations of findings as when he claimed discovering Sodom's exact site. A prolific writer, his 1866 volume *Les Derniers Jours de Jerusalem (The Last Days of Jerusalem)* appeared just a few years after Mary and the others saw his excavations.

After liberal baksheesh changed hands, the party visited the Mosque of Omar at the site of Solomon's Temple and then visited the Holy Sepulchre.[62] Again, locals assailed them with tourist trinkets, as the tourists mingled with numerous pilgrims' passing through hallowed sites. For being in such a holy locale, not all was at peace in the American group's relations:

"We kept the peace till we got back from the Jordan – at Jerusalem – where we had an awful fuss, & verily had there been a steamer convenient Mary and I would have shipped for home... M & I went to the Sepulchre & up on Mt. Olives to pray & decided that though we were not in the wrong we would go on our knees & make up, so after an aweful (sic) high talk it was settled & we have just all of us been sweet enough to make a pie of since...Gov. as he himself says is the easiest man in the world to keep in a good humour if you will only pet him. Now you might be willing to do this at all times to a man you thoroughly respected – even then at times it might try your nerves..."[63]

The Jerusalem visit potentially ended harmoniously, but the party split for the overland trip to Joppa. Flora, Mary and Mr. Stone went ahead:

"Mary & I & Mr. Stone made it in one – it was a pretty hard ride, for we had men's saddles & had to manage it as best we could to go easy. ...and we got a fright –At the loneliest pass two Arabs came up on their horses, wild ugly looking men – they insisted on riding near us & attempting a conversation, till finally they stopped on ahead of us. I was sure this was a critical moment & stuffed my watch & ring out of sight. Now Mr. Stone had to jump off to set his girth to rights, they came back to see what was the matter and asked me what time it was."[64]

With the danger behind them, the reunited group endured Joppa's bad weather and bleak accommodations for over a week while awaiting a steamship to Alexandria, Egypt:

"This is the most forsaken place I ever was in, & the winds & the waves & the monks have made it as sad as it is gloomy – the Convent is perched high up on a crag with as much of the town as there is around it, but we have not been down once – so you can imagine what prisoners we have been peering out of our grated windows...my room – a stone floor, as dusty as it is cold, ceiling rough white washed boards, two iron frame bedsteads fastened by clamps into the wall, one two-foot window, barred – gives a view over the roughest line of sea sweep that can be, one three-legged stool for the washbowl..." [65]

Monastic life was unappealing to these less than ascetic travelers who, after a month's spiritual feast and physical fast, anticipated a more genteel experience. Finally, on December 20th they arrived in Alexandria, Egypt, that had, as Flora said, "signs of civilization that made us feel like savages."[66] Only two weeks earlier, the women sat astride men's saddles on Arabian horses' running through the Syrian desert but now rode an omnibus on pavement to the Hotel d'Europe.[67] Their Holy Lands' experience provided new perspective on mid-19th century women's fashion follies as Flora recounted after watching, "fashionable," European tourists in Alexandria:

" '...Oh see that lady she has hoops on', - 'How she looks', and we laugh to kill ourselves over her hoops. They impressed us with the same ludicrous cumbrous sense of unfitness as they might have done Cleopatra who would surely have failed of Caesars hard heart in such a structure, and 'see her bonnet, how it tips on the back of her head', and 'how she walks', and we watch these few civilized natives with much more interest as curiosity seekers...the bare dark-limbed Israelite with their grace and beauty exposed, looked not half as ridiculous as this waddling ship of a woman."[68]

Both Mary and Flora had grown acutely aware of impractical dress modes, and after spending weeks in regions where the natives' couture fit the climate, both women rebelled against senseless, western women's fashions. Although laughing at, "civilized fashion," they readily accepted civilization's diet and described their Alexandrian breakfast as, "...the first good meal we had had for two weeks..."[69]

By train from Alexandria, they passed inundated farmland and numerous poor villages, "...even more wretched than Jericho, merely a scraggling collection of mud hovels with domed roofs..."[70] Muddy, flooded village ruins, blue clothed natives and laden camel trains destined for the town of Suez appeared before the pyramids signaled arrival at Cairo, about as far removed culturally as in distance from Cairo, Illinois. They reached Shepheards Hotel:

"...the crash hotel, Englishy, but stylish off from the main street in a grove of Acacia trees, fronted by a broad piazzo (sic) with a stand below for carriages and donkeys."[71]

Shepheards was the place to see, to be seen, and was well decorated for Christmas. That day Mary and Flora arose early, and as she said:

"In the morning Mary and I trotted around in our night dresses looking like ghosts caught by daylight on a spree and inaugurated celebrations by knocking them all awake with a 'Merry Christmas'. Mr. Curran presented us with half a glass of punch to keep us merry."[72]

After spending Christmas on a blazing-hot desert donkey ride to the, "Petrified Forest," the group returned to Shepheards for, "a blazing plum pudding for dinner...that made all the English cheery and sent us to bed with an indigestion."[73] The next day some of the Americans climbed all, "480' 9", of Cheops' pyramid according to Flora who recounted the climb down:

"...all we have to do is to jump jump jump and keep our heads from reeling. It takes us about 15 minutes and we are shaking hands with our friends below who have been congratulating themselves on their disdain of the climb..." [74]

The young women went on a hands and knees' exploration of the pyramid's interior and were disappointed at its insignificant contents. Had they worn them, hoop skirts and stiff crinolines would have hindered that endeavor although Mary's short stature likely helped her. Cairo's many splendors included a less than enchanting night at the opera.

Just as the Americans experienced historic events such as the Sultan's first horse race in Istanbul, here, too, they came close to witnessing a notable event. Flora's narrative:

"One more excursion you must hear about, and that is to Suez. Took the cars at 8 A. M., 2nd class of course and had a nice ride ...caught sight of the Red Sea – not at all bloody colored as we expected...Met quantities of French and English gathered here the day before to inaugurate the opening of a new canal just finished by the French – merely a sweet water one running inland some 18 miles till connecting with a large branch from the Nile, the water was let in for the first time yesterday and muddy as it was, it seemed a treat to the poor people who were scooping it up in baskets and cups as though every drop was precious. The Grand Canal that they made such a fuss about is merely engineered will follow the course of this for some miles, thus supplying the workmen with water. Nothing is done yet beyond a mere commencement, and if you could see the way they work with hands and baskets, instead of shovels and wheelbarrows, you would think it some generations yet before ships shall sail from the Mediterranean into the Red Sea. Some gentlemen old me that it was all a talk anyway, merely political and will never be finished."[75]

Suez Grand Canal between the Red Sea and the Mediterranean opened five years later. With the prior day's excitement, dignitaries and tourists crowded the Suez area. The next morning the Americans headed for the Israelites' Red Sea crossing site, then hiked through hot desert to Moses Wells. While seeking refreshments the thirsty group found a place seemingly fresh from an English comedy:

"Had a very hot walk across the desert sinking ankle in the warm sands to the welcome oasis of the Wells…A hotel here had been advertised at Suez – we found a neat room and a stupid landlord. 'Have you bread?' 'No', 'butter', 'no', 'what have you then', 'nothing' – well, emphatically you don't know how to keep a hotel 'absolutely nothing', 'nothing but brandy and sugar'. Oh bring that – we are hungry and heated with our desert wandering and all partake heartily… passage across the desert was not a very straight one, and we youngsters with shrieks of fun follow their trail imitating it in all its inns (sic) and outs."[76]

The brandy's effects likely lasted well into the evening when they returned by boat to Suez and failed in attempting singing "Hail Columbia." The next morning they celebrated 1864 New Year's Day in Cairo with, "a fat turkey," before leaving Egypt and the Middle East.[77]

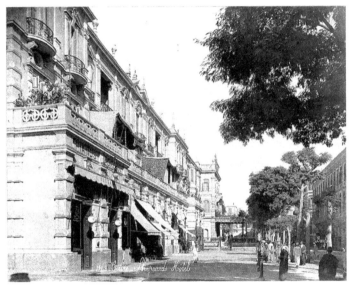

Shepheard's Hotel, Cairo, Egypt, c. 1870s.
Library of Congress Prints and Photographs Division,
2004668082.

7 BACK TO EUROPE

In early 1864, the Americans cruised the Mediterranean to British ruled Malta. Rough water kept all but Isaac Curran below decks with seasickness, and, if it weren't for his throwing a flaming tablecloth out a porthole, this book would end here.[1] Landing at Valletta, Malta, they noted their accommodations' impressive cleanliness contrasted with that in all recently toured countries. Proceeding to Catania, Messina, and Palermo, they saw catacombs Flora noted as:

"...the most curious place this side Hades, like the vaults to a large hardware store, lined each side with long boxes, some large, some small, & above them stuck in stocks, were forms of the dried dead dressed up as though living – a grinning scull (sic) above two skeleton feet...And on shelves above are groups of children, standing – dancing – sitting in rocking chairs or gathered around some prim boned matron."[2]

As Mary Safford saw far more macabre sights after three Civil War battles, mere catacombs' contents likely did not bother her.

Toward Naples, Italy, unusually choppy seas led to renewed seasickness before safe arrival at the Hotel d 'Amerique with its good food and Mt. Vesuvius views. During their rainy 2-week stay the Americans moved to what was deemed Naples' premier boarding house but found meals especially meager. They saw Naples' Campo Santo Vecchio cemetery's 365 pits--one for each day of the year. Daily, uncaring officials clumsily heaved paupers' dressed or nude corpses into that day's designated pit. At night, attendants threw lime over the lot, sealed the tomb, and, after 365 days, removed comingled dust and dried bones. Even 35 years later, Mary found Naples' practice shocking and adamantly promoted cremation for the dead.[3]

After viewing this horror, the party took a four-hour tour of nearby Pompeii and Herculaneum on a rainy, cold February day before advancing to Rome. They planned remaining until just after Holy Week, but after initial sightseeing, half of the group including Mary was sick, and the rest were exhausted:

"...a great trouble this last week has been the sickness of Mary, now lying on the sofa by my side, where she has been for eight days, so I have been a good deal with her. It is an entire prostration of her nervous system combined with an attack of Roman fever that is quite prevalent. It is a sore trial to be sick in Rome and she feels very blue." [4]

Possibly, American Embassy physician Dr. James B. Gould treated Mary. The old adage said, "When in Rome, do as the Romans do," and possibly, she acquired then common Roman Fever, a form of malaria.[5] Before its cause was identified as the parasite Plasmodium, Roman physicians believed the disease arose from swamps. These bred mosquitoes that spread the protozoan, but in 1864 no one knew it or that some Plasmodium species can hide in the body only to cause disease relapses decades later.[6] As Mary's tendency to be overactive led to resultant ills, her Roman Fever episode was possibly a turning point in her future health although she was blissfully unaware of it. "Nervous prostration," in itself was a symptom of Roman Fever, as malaria occasionally produces neuropsychiatric effects.[7] Flora reported Mary, "has been so imprudent and hurt her eyes and health so much that I should wonder if her brother makes her come home this fall."[8] However, Mary recovered and traveled several more years.

Roman Easter was subdued by Pope Pius IX's illness, but the next week Flora and Mary viewed him at St. Peter's.

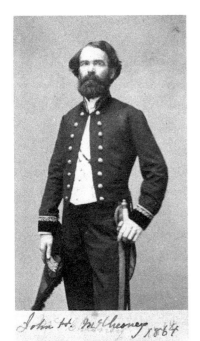

Joseph Henry McChesney, 1864. G. Penabert & Co., Paris, Increase Allen Lapham Collection, Wisconsin Historical Society Image 45226

After Holy Week the Mattesons left for Florence and Switzerland where Mrs. Matteson remained several months while the girls attended school.[9] Ike Curran left concurrently, but Flora and Mary remained in Rome for renewed sightseeing.[10] Strained relations with Joel Matteson had deteriorated further, and his own problems necessitated his return to Illinois. Among these were his sons-in-laws' scandalous mishandling and loss of the Union commissary contract with pending litigation and his son Charley's ruin from whiskey speculation.[11] [12]

Although Flora was uncharacteristically hesitant on their solo travels' propriety, Mary was undaunted and encouraged at Mrs. Matteson's advice to continue, especially in view of local assistance:

"Mrs. Gould is the wife of the American Physician, a perfect lady and the leader of the American world here. Her patronage is the best we could have in Rome. Mary had an introduction to her and as soon as she became convalescent she took her right into her house and from the first has insisted that we should stay...she knows so many people, she thinks she will have no trouble to find us friends to travel with, & if we should happen not to, we would take a respectable courier, which is the way the English women travel, & then we could have no trouble."[13]

Emily Bliss Gould founded several schools for destitute Italian children, and the Goulds' social position provided many valuable connections helpful for Flora and Mary's travels.[14][15] The woman introduced them to her guests as, " being under her care," and showed general kindness.

In March 1864, Mary Safford's Illinois geologist friend, now U.S. Consul Joseph McChesney, visited Rome. He and Mary toured Rome briefly:

"A friend of Mary's Dr. McChesney, is here just now. He is Consul at New Castle England, 40 years old perhaps, & is well known in the scientific world, having written a book on fossils & named some 40 species. He is a charming, intelligent man & he promises Mary & I that if we come to England this summer he will take a geological tour with us through the island..." [16]

Flora failed mentioning if McChesney visited Rome on business or specifically to see Mary, but the couple's being out alone together, his staying to supper and his taking Mary on social outings suggest the latter.

Mary and Flora continued their Roman holiday with a three-day trip to the Sabine Hills and a day at the Sistine Chapel before leaving in mid-May to head north toward Florence to escape Rome's heat, malarial danger and ubiquitous fleas. Possibly, Mrs. Gould supplied their new companions including New Yorker Mrs. Hayward, her daughter and four young men. For the trip to Florence the group contracted with a tour company that charged $16/person for 5 days' food, lodging and transport. Not everyone behaved well, as in response to an innkeeper's substituting raw beans for the

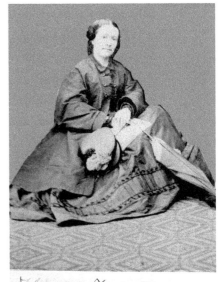

Mary Jane Safford, May 1864, Florence, Italy. Courtesy Cairo, IL, Public Library.

tour company's promised fruit, some of the travelers shot the beans at each other and at a poor greyhound.

Beyond Rome, they left Papal-controlled lands, entered what was then a unified Italy, and, in showing their passports, cheered, "Viva Victor Emmanuello – Viva Garabaldi," men considered Italy's liberators. The coach followed a route past spectacular waterfalls, but, on the way to Perugia, translation problems resulted in Mary and Flora's hiking 5 miles as the other tourists rode. At Etruria the group saw a recently discovered Etruscan Necropolis where inside an elaborate tomb's funerary urn the party found nothing but, "nice ashes inside, no nasty dead mens bones!"[17]

The tourists rented apartments by Florence's Arno River, and further economizing through communal dining allowed wine with all meals and numerous tender Florentine beefsteaks. After touring the Ponte Vecchio's stone mosaic shops, the group headed to the Campanile, the high bell tower where the party, "went up 414 steps, the steepest climb after the Pyramids & it brought us out way above the Bells…"[18] 19th Century Florence was an artists' and writers' colony. With an introduction probably from Mrs. Gould, the party called at retired actress turned writer Mrs. Anna Cora Mowatt Ritchie's villa in the Bellosguardo hill neighborhood once inhabited by Nathaniel Hawthorne and James Fenimore Cooper. Mrs. Ritchie requested they return for tea later when she could introduce them to the, "handsomest young man in Florence." Sadly, nothing further of him appeared in Flora's letters.

Although Mary and Flora preferred Rome, they enjoyed Florence's numerous historical sites and free admission at the Uffizi Galleries. There they saw the Venus de Medici said to have been a model for all sculptor Hiram Powers' nude female statues.[19] Born in Vermont, the famous Powers lived and worked in Florence since 1837.[20] Here he found fame for his celebrated yet controversial 1844 marble statue, "The Greek Slave," a 5'5" nude woman held to a post with sculpted marble chain and said to represent a Christian Grecian maiden, held captive by Turks in an 1820s Constantinople slave market.[21] Abolitionist Powers' statue copies toured English and U.S. cities, and American abolitionists quickly advertised the statue as a metaphor for slavery.[22] Both Flora and Mary would have known, if not seen, this statue at one of its exhibitions or may have read Elizabeth Barrett Browning's sonnet inspired by it.[23] Powers' workshop attracted fashionable American tourists, and Mary and Flora were no exception:

"…a visit to Powers Studio – it lies at the back of his garden through the fragrance of its roses. He opened the door for us & might be one of his workmen…he seemed to take a fancy to us …& we had a quick visit… Around the walls are models of works that have gone before, limbs & legs & arms, tiny hands & plaster casts – how could one help it but be an artist in such an air sprinkled with the dust of Carrara's precious mines!"[24]

Powers enjoyed visiting with Mary and Flora and shared Lincoln's classic joke:

"He had just heard his last joke, how he would like the liquor that Grant got drunk on for all his generals, & though not the latest to us we had to laugh a good half hour over it."[25]

The girls were amply impressed with the studio's statuary where both, "Eve Repentant," and, "Genius of Calafornia (sic)," were available for sale. A simple bust cost $1000 then, but Powers discounted for payment in U.S. dollars. As they departed:

"He followed us to the outer door, plucking us a flower for memory & showing the direction to his son, a photographist who, he said 'was wicked enough to sell his Father.' "[26]

As seen in the following photograph, Mary Safford visited the nearby photography and sculpture studio of the, "wicked," Longworth Powers.[27]

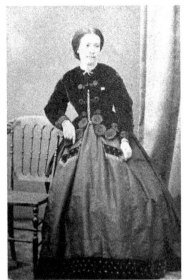

Mary Jane Safford. On reverse is, "Dr. Mary J. Safford, Dec. 31, 1864? Freres Powers Photographie Americaine 103 Via dei Serraglia Florence." Courtesy Cairo, IL, Public Library.

Across the street was sculptor Larkin Goldsmith Mead's studio.[28] With Hiram Powers' encouragement he traveled from Vermont to Florence in 1862.[29] Flora reported their seeing Mead's partially finished sculpture of a soldier's holding a small girl on his knee. This likely was the start of a well-known marble work called, "The Battle Story," or, "Returned Soldier."

Companion Mrs. Hayward received news requiring immediate departure, but the young women continued touring the Arno River valley.[30] Traveling alone with four young men was of questionable propriety, but the women were undeterred. The hot Italian summer was upon them, and they made the best of it while traveling via third class rail. Today's northern Italy was Austrian in 1864, and Italian rail lines stopped at the Po River from where the group proceeded northeast to Venice. Austrians ruled there, too, and Venetians despised them. Much of southern Italy was united under Garibaldi and Emmanuel in 1860, but Venice remained Austrian until the 1866 Treaty of Prague when Venetians welcomed their liberator Victor Emmanuel. However, 1864's oppressed Venetians were cautious as Mary and Flora learned when questioning their tour guide about Emmanuel:

"He put his finger on his lips, and looking distrustfully around as tho' a spy lay hid in each stone of the Doges' Palace, hushed us up—that it was treason to pronounce that name in Venice."[31]

The relatively peaceful European experience 21st century tourists take for granted was not usual for 1860s travelers, as kingdoms maneuvered for governing positions. Though Mary Safford was inured to war from her experiences just two years earlier, she undoubtedly shunned revisiting them, and the young women restricted their remaining Venetian visit to sightseeing without politics. After several days, they boarded a train to Verona to see Shakespeare's Juliet's fictional tomb. There an entrepreneur offered her, "burial site," as a tourist attraction that led to the following exchange:

"...so, holily we tread through the Cabbage Garden, not a very solemn entrance, said we, but never mind, sweet peas and potatoes in all but the name, are just as good as roses and lilies. Now—came a strong smell, healthful, to be sure, but not very poetical, as though we were coming to a barnyard. Never mind, who knows but that she may have been fond of horses! Come into a stable, out and out. 'There,' said the shirt-sleeved, dirty boy, 'there is the tomb of Juliet.' 'Where, you wretched boy?' 'There.' 'What! That old trough that has watered the stable horses these 20 years?' Oh, ye Gods! We laughed at the sell, and beat a retreat. So much for Juliet. Romeo they have entirely neglected."[32]

After the young men accompanying Mary and Flora departed at Lake Como, the women truly traveled alone. They went to the Tyrol, now a western Austrian region and, in trying to reach Innsbruck, Austria, through lack of guidebook and language skills, traveled to an entirely different place as noted by Flora:

"...they put us in a private carriage—and where do you think, to our amazement, we found we were going? Over the Stelvio the highest Pass in Europe. Had as much idea of going to the moon as there when we started. Oh, it was grand! Austrian carriage roads all the way. Wonderful thing at the top, went through banks of snow 20 feet high, and down the other side."[33]

Stelvio Pass is indeed Europe's highest mountain pass, and the twenty-kilometer, switch-backed Imperial Stelvio

Road designed in the 1820s is still considered a civil engineering masterpiece. Fortunately, a friendly Dutchman assisted the women who stayed near Davos, Switzerland, rather than Innsbruck that evening.

Their independent journey included a Rhine River cruise and visits to Munich, Cologne, Brussels, Waterloo, and Antwerp.[34] In a July 1864, "Letter from Miss Mary J. Safford," to Livermore's *New Covenant*, Mary wrote of enjoying travel independent of the entourage:

"We never traveled more happily than now, as we have no one to dictate. We see all of interest, and meet with nothing unpleasant from being alone. People sometimes express surprise, but when we tell them we are American women, they seem to think it all right, and say the American ladies are very brave. I am rejoiced that we have the credit of having some sense, and are able to act as if we are responsible human beings, and not put together to act like noodles in show cases."[35]

In response to the magazine's editor's query about her personal health, Mary wrote:

"I suppose, from your queries on the subject that the ever interesting theme, viz: health, remains open for discussion, but I shall say little about it, as I shall declare that I am well when I come home. My eyes give me much uneasiness. I am very careful of them. I go to bed as soon as it is dark, write very little, read never, except when I am obliged to glance at guide books, and if rest is what they need, think I ought to feel the effect soon."[36]

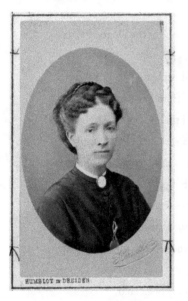

Mary Safford, Dresden, Germany, 1860s. Note china pin at neck and spectacles. Abraham Lincoln Presidential Library & Museum, Wallace-Dickey Collection-NI-3775.

Flora, too, complained of eye problems caused by Egypt's, "horrid air," but hers resolved.[37] Mary could have suffered aftereffects of Roman Fever or from desert wind and sunburn. Photographs taken before and initially on the Grand Tour show her without glasses, but later photos show a pair of oval, wire-rimmed spectacles tucked into her dress.

Aware her letter might appear in *New Covenant*, Mary wrote of English coverage of American war news:

"We cannot believe anything first reported, coming through the corrupt English. I wish the bottom of the little mean island would drop out, and the whole people be sent to render an account before a just tribunal."[38]

Her recent Waterloo experience may explain her current dislike for the imperious English:

"The great interest in Brussels was the battle-field of Waterloo, twelve miles distant. An old sergeant who was in the battle, shows it off, and I could fully understand and appreciate the horrors of the scene from past experience. There is a museum upon the spot gathered by an English Colonel, who lived here and died not long since… There are guns, swords, pistols, some that belonged to distinguished officers, balls, shot, shells, coins, some doubled and some pierced by balls, buttons, riddled hats. One I noticed with matted hair still clinging to it. Pieces of uniforms, trappings of horses, a silver spur of Napoleon, marked N, which he doubtless put to good use when he turned Paris-ward, and a copper camp kettle of his with his initial N…Wellington's headquarters is one of the shrines where the English pay special devotion. And Napoleon's the resort of the French. In reading over an account of the battle which was written by this same officer, who gathered together the museum, a concise, true account it seems as if our present crisis is something akin to the turning point of that eventful battle, which changed the whole phase of Europe. I never realized, before, how unjustly the English arrogate to themselves all the credit of that victory. All Europe combined with them to crush out Napoleon, and the Prussians gained the victory. Yet it is all we with John Bull."[39]

The women then visited The Hague and Amsterdam before sailing from Rotterdam to England. On their July 17th arrival, U.S. Consul at Newcastle-On-Tyne Joseph McChesney took them directly to the, "Temperance Hotel," run by a, "ponderous English landlady."[40] Rewarded with this consular post for campaigning for Lincoln in 1860, the geologist now kept his promise made in Rome to guide Mary and Flora through England.[41] [42] He provided the women an intriguing expedition far afield from usual Grand Tour sights:

"Monday morning we started for Monk Wearmouth to visit the most extensive Coal pits in the world & we went down the deepest...– put on miners' dresses, rolled up our sleeves, took lanterns, got into a tub, ducked our heads & descended 1800 feet – 3 minutes. I thought I was dead, pinched Mary & was astonished to find myself alive – when I dumped on the bottom."[43]

They visited Britain's largest iron works, toured the annual Agricultural Show with animal and machinery displays, and followed this with a, "hasty visit to the Chemical Works." McChesney certainly knew how to show a girl a good time, and, given his guests' geological and scientific interests, he probably did.

The women began a rail trip to Northern England and Scotland with visits to friends, croquet and nightly toddies, then toured a series of Scottish cities before rejoining McChesney for a boat trip to Inverness. Walking miles through Scotland, they studied important rock formations then hiked to Oban, the last mile barefoot despite the rain and cold. That night they could not rest since, "...some of Mr. Mac's Geological friends had arrived & we had to entertain them till late at night."[44] Oban ran rife with geologists that summer, as much of Flora's writing described visiting with them, feeding them, and, "geologizing." This locale on Scotland's northwest coast gave opportunity to visit the small islands of Iona and Staffa:

"...we got in from an expedition to Staffa & Iona, to see the 1st Cross of Christianity erected in England by the Culdees & where many Scottish kings, the last Macbeth, were buried, & some Irish and Norwegian. Where formerly 700 pupils were received yearly, now a bleak deserted Abbey & the mouldering Crosses to tell its story, & then Staffa, with a tramp over the broken basaltic Columns into Fingulo (sic) Cave...on the landing Mr. Mac met us & had the tea & the fire hissing hot..."[45]

He may have offered hot tea and a warm fire, but soon Flora was alone writing as, "Midge & Mr. McChesney have stepped out to a neighbors, to examine some specimens they have dredged to day."[46] Later, Flora joined them for a glass of hot Scotch whiskey, as she noted:

"...now we are back & at the Toddy – no true Scotsman goes to bed without his Toddy & we do as they do..."[47]

Years later, Mary Safford vilified all alcoholic beverages and other potentially addictive substances in her ardent temperance lectures and articles.[48] Her European trip provided first hand research material for the physiological effects of a variety of wines, beers, hard liquors and cigarettes.

Through constant drizzling rain, Mary, Flora, and McChesney traveled to Scotland's Isle of Skye, spent several days' hiking, much of it through shallow water, and returned to Oban for continued, "dredging & geologizing."[49] [50] It abounded with fossils, and even today fossil poachers lurk in the same region.[51] The extent of Mary and Flora's, "geologizing," is unknown, but McChesney was a serious collector who published many new fossil discoveries, and his position allowed his travel for more.[52] Reputedly, his avid geological work's superseding his consular duties led to Secretary of State Seward's complaints about him.[53] McChesney's extensive fossil collection eventually resided at the Chicago Academy of Science but sadly disappeared in the 1871 Chicago Fire.[54]

No matter whether she collected rocks or not, Mary's interest was evident from her willingness to endure miserable conditions for the opportunities offered by this knowledgeable man. As Flora put it:

"…we consider Mr. McChesney such a valuable companion that we don't like to lose a moment of his time.'

'Mary & I are travelling with one portmanteau between us, containing exactly one change of clothes – quite sufficient & we flatter ourselves we look very stylish. When we go on our short trips all our luggage consists of a toothbrush & one comb between us & Mr. Mac has his Geology, bag & hammers. We are very happy & indeed I may say, it is the only time abroad that we have combined true pleasure with profit & we mean to enjoy it."[55]

On August 15th, the trio left Oban by steamship to Ireland to tour the Giants Causeway, the tongue of huge, vertical, hexagonal basaltic columns' stretching into the ocean.[56] Traveling by rail to Belfast to visit linen factories, they encountered riots between Catholic and Protestant factions in response to a Dublin ceremony honoring an Irish Catholic political leader.[57] All was calm in Catholic Dublin, but predominantly Protestant Belfast experienced much violence as Flora noted:

"Monday was the commencement of the bad riots between the pound men and the Orangemen over poor O'Connells corner stone at Dublin. The mill girls deserted their work and grouped in the streets with knives, the men gathered in lowering knots, the soldiers were paraded out… As we returned from the Consuls where we had dined, at ten P. M., they had just set fire to a hay or peat stack by the nunnery, and there was fearful excitement. I saw several men carried away with bloody heads. Firing was kept up all night. In the morning we left and then succeeded a perfect reign of terror which you must have read about, until starvation drove the mill girls back."[58]

Fortunately, Mary, Flora, and McChesney were unscathed although possibly shaken by the violence. They continued to Londonderry then took a steamer on Lake Erne and met Mr. Conolly, a friendly local Irish Member of Parliament and, according to a guidebook read by Mary, "the largest landed proprietor in Ireland." On learning they were Americans, he gave a, "cheer for the South, but so good humored you don't mind."[59] This was likely Thomas Conolly, one of Ireland's largest estate owners, parliamentary member representing Donegal and eventual diarist on his 1864 adventures while visiting the American South.[60] He hosted the three Americans at his estate that night, took them on a late night moonlit walk and flirted with Flora. Later, after stopping to kiss the Blarney Stone, their Irish tour ended with a day in impoverished Dublin that Flora called, "…that mighty town whose beggars are clad in the cast off clothes of the beggars of London…"[61]

Returning to England by steamship, the trio hiked the Cumberland Lakes District and arrived at Wordsworth's Cottage at Grasmere. After their Stanhope lead mines tour, McChesney returned to Newcastle while Mary and Flora visited Manchester's ex-Mayor whom they met in, "Beyrout," the prior winter and who provided letters of introduction for the women's cotton mill tour.[62][63] They proceeded to Wales to find slate samples and hear Welsh spoken. September 20th the women arrived in London and lodged at a small boarding house, toured the city then stopped at Somerset House to visit a Geological Survey member and see rock collections.[64] Mr. McChesney shipped the women's huge steamer trunk from Newcastle to London, and they booked it to Dover for return to Paris. The British Isles provided the most expensive part of the women's entire Grand Tour to date, and, in only several weeks, they spent $300.00.[65]

Not completely satisfied they had seen everything of geological interest, the women headed toward southwestern England's Devon and Cornwall areas for a weeklong jaunt to tin and lead mines.[66] Their visit initially hinged on Mr. McChesney's leading them through the mines. Flora described this as, "a trip into Devon & Cornwall to see the tin mines that Mary has set her heart on."[67] Whether Mary had her heart set on visiting mines or spending the last moments with Joseph McChesney is unknown, but the women traveled alone. Shortly before she returned to America, Flora summed their British Isles' excursion:

"We landed at Whitehaven Aug 25th & sailed from Dover Oct 11th, most 7 weeks just in old merry England & all that time have been hard at work; have been I think in every County & have seen it, what I think few men and fewer women ever see, in all its geological, mineral & manufacturing marvels. In England, in her igneous & sedimentary beds are found all the periods & deposits that exist elsewhere scattered over the world..."[68]

On October 11th, with their collected rocks in tow, the women crossed the English Channel from Dover to Calais without sinking the ferry. Neither Flora's subsequent letters nor Mary's writings further refer to Professor McChesney, but 9 months after his leading their grand geological tour he married 23-year old Elizabeth Studdiford in Brooklyn, New York.[69] He retained his consular position until 1869 and returned to the University of Chicago.[70][71]

Back in Paris, Mary and Flora checked into a hotel before allying themselves with newspaper correspondent Mrs. Slicker who helped them find accommodations. Flora described them:

"We have a parlor, a pretty large room – two windows, velvet covered chairs & table, mirror, sofa, pictures & fireplace – with a bed lodge adjoining & plenty of closet & packing room, for which we pay 130 francs a month. For breakfast we have Café au lait and bread, at a Café for 1 frc. & get a good dinner at an 'estainenet,' soup, two plates of meat, one vegetable, an entrement, a dessert and a half bottle of wine, for 2 francs."[72]

One of their first activities was to provide a current address and retrieve their mail at Munroe's. Flora wrote:

"...Mary, who has now to her credit $2000 at Monroe's. Her health is not strong & she does not feel yet content to return home. She is going to Berlin the day after I leave to stay there the Winter & in the Spring to Russia, Norway & Sweden, then I think in the Fall she must come home as there will be nothing left for her to see though she talks of going home by way of China & visiting a Brother in California."[73]

Mary knew she fit in neither of her brothers' worlds now, but Alfred's support enabled her continued travel. Her susceptibility to seasickness alone may have caused her deferred return to the U.S. With their impending separation, the women shopped for Flora's extravagant diamond ring, listened to band concerts at the Tuileries, and attended the theater.[74] They parted November 15th, 1864, when Flora took an express train to Le Havre to catch the steamship, "Washington," for the 12-14 day voyage to New York.[75] On parting, Mary Safford's sense of humor prevailed as noted by the end of Flora's last travel letter:

"Mary says in case I am cast away, the submarine cable better be laid in my track & run the chance of recovering my ring – she is sure all the fishes will lose their eyes if it stays below."[76]

Piscine eyesight was safe and sound as Flora returned safely to her close adoring family. Five years later, at age 27, she married William C. Whitney who became President Cleveland's Secretary of the Navy.[77] She advanced to social prominence as a Washington and New York City hostess, mother of four and promoter of the arts. In 1893, at 51 with a personal worth over three million dollars, she died of heart disease and was buried in New York's Woodlawn Cemetery.[78] Although it is hard to imagine Mary and Flora's not communicating after almost two years' traveling together, no correspondence survives. Aside from a mutual pronounced appreciation of history, art, and nature, their lives' paths diverged greatly.

In Berlin, Mary saw Dr. Graefe, whom she and Flora met briefly in Paris when he examined them among other patients at the Hotel-de-Bade.[79] Born in 1828, a professor at Berlin's Friedrich Wilhelms University, Graefe became known as the, "Father of Ophthalmology," and, though not inventing the ophthalmoscope, was among the first using it clinically.[80][81] His famous clinic was a magnet for eye doctors in training, and he was especially known for his work with lenses to assist weak sight. Mary may have obtained her spectacles from him. She mentioned him in one of her 1874 dress reform lectures and called him, "the most eminent oculist of modern times."[82]

Little is known of Mary's Berlin stay, but her essay entitled, "An Evening at a German Professor's," recounted her adventures during winter 1864-5.[83] She reported formal presentation at the Prussian capital's royal court with minute details' suggesting her personal participation. Contrasted with this was her delight at the evening spent at a German professor's home, meeting his wife, an eclectic group of friends, and their erudite conversations. Perhaps Professor Graefe or Parisian friends provided Mary's letter of introduction to the professor's home. The essay's professor was, "rich in contentment," rather than worldly goods and thoroughly impressed her:

"…the brightest luminary in the professorial galaxy. He is not only master of his own abstruse kingdom, but his broad, clear mind comprehends other realms of thought, and his ear catches the voice of humanity. He listens, he waits, and hopes for the enfranchisement of all mankind from the thralldom of tyranny, or ignorance and of superstition. The students all feel that they have in him more than a preceptor, a friend, an advisor…"[84]

Mary's description of the professor's guests gave tantalizing initials and suggested the celebrities' occupations including those of several royal visitors. Among them was African explorer B--, a student of nomadic Arabs L-- and Mrs. R--a famous female German writer friend of Goethe's. Although potentially intimidating, the throng of prominent people treated her well and probably found her war and travel stories fascinating.

The essay's highly detailed report of the professor's wife included her simple hairstyle and her unfashionable but serviceable clothing. Mary balanced this somewhat unflattering description with a list of the woman's numerous good qualities including having anonymously taken part in the thoughts behind her famous husband's writings. In later dress reform speeches and essays, Mary reiterated the story, as in her 1874 version:

"I retain as a delightful memory an evening spent at the house of a German Professor in Berlin. There were rare minds gathered together from many lands, men and women whom one had known and prized from afar… the Frau Professorin…was arrayed in a pearl-colored silk, which as I afterward learned, had been her wedding gown, made fourteen years before. Her hair, all her own, was gathered into a meager knot behind.'

'I could but make an estimate then of the probable time she had saved from those fourteen years by wearing her gown as it was first made. I felt sure, taking into consideration the matching of material, the selection of trimmings, the confabs with dressmakers, that would have been necessary to keep the dress modernized in accordance with the changing demands of the mode, that months of precious time had thus been spared…Who could tell but that those days, weeks, and possibly months, were what gave her the time, in part, to learn to converse fluently with her guests, as she did, in as many different languages as they represented."[85]

From all evidence, Mary spent her initial overseas time in observing and not in performing altruistic acts as she had as, "Cairo's Angel." Her exposure to 19th century Berlin's socially conscious intellectuals possibly reawakened her humanitarian instincts, and her later essay specifically mentioned the professor's wife's efforts in that direction:

"Weekly she gathers into her home a class of poor girls, whom she instructs in the ways of usefulness…"[86]

The Germans also amazed Mary with their non-competitive and clever conversation, irrespective of gender, "where mind met mind, and was elevated by the contact." She noted the egalitarian sense of the evening with, "…no withdrawal of the ladies to give the gentlemen an opportunity for indulgence in a solo debauch." All was the antithesis of her prior traveling companions' world.

No record exists of Mary's Berlin departure date, but sources suggest her next destinations were Norway, Sweden and Russia.[87] [88] She traveled alone, and whether her purposes were merely to meet local people or due to a recent epiphany of social awareness, she supposedly began a program of helping poor Norwegian women:

"…Miss Mary J. Safford, a young lady of Cairo, Illinois…visited Norway, and there devised ways and means for the emigration of peasant girls to the United States, where they might join their relatives who had already migrated thither. Miss Safford is one of those who will create modes of usefulness, if she does not find them already at command."[89]

Mary highlighted some of her Scandinavian experiences:

"At a country wedding that we had the pleasure of attending in Norway, many of the entremets were passed among the guests, each eating in turn, from the same dish, with the same spoon, as much or as little as he desired. The native beer of the country was drank from one glass, passed from guest to guest. At a very enjoyable entertainment given us by a professor and his family, the delightful old University town, Upsala, a like custom of partaking from the same dish with others was observed."[90]

In the 1880s, two different Norwegian writers on separate visits to America mentioned Mary. Feminist Aasta Hasteen wrote in 1880 of seeing, "the glorious Dr. Mary Safford."[91] 1903 Nobel Prize winning author and lyricist for the Norwegian National Anthem, Bjornstjerne Bjornson wrote of hearing Mary Safford lecture in 1880 and noted her travel to Norway.[92]

On Mary's steamer voyage from Stockholm to St. Petersburg, Russia, she met General and Madame Z--- on return from German health springs to his Siberian duty station.[93] They guided Mary through Moscow's educational and charitable institutions, far exceeding a usual tourist's itinerary. She wrote somewhat disdainfully about the University of Moscow's excluding women but praised the school's 200,000-volume library and its impressive anatomical, microscopical and geological collections. Her escorts showed her the, "Institution of Learning for Girls," where courses considered appropriate for young ladies included embroidery and proper court etiquette. The couple assured a skeptical Mary that the girls' education fitted Russian societal expectations as, "we consider women only as flowers scattered along the highways and byways of life, to cheer the thorny paths of men."[94]

Mary's response, as a 33-year old independent, unmarried woman:

" 'To be plucked by them,' we suggested—'worn for a day and then cast aside, if only their bloom attracts. But what of the spinsters, those who are left in the market, on the hands of anxious friends, or who are alone in the world?' "[95]

In response, her hosts next escorted her to a depressing institution for elderly spinsters.

Mary's itinerary after Moscow is unknown, but she resided in Florence, Italy, in late 1865 and spring 1866, as her signatures appear in the register of the Gabinetto Scientifico-Letterario di Vieusseux, a subscription literary and scientific library and meeting place for Italian and foreign intellectuals.[96] She paid for one month's library access each time. On December 30, 1865, she wrote an apology to U.S. Minister to Italy George P. Marsh who was inundated with her mail sent through his consulate.[97] Marsh also frequented the Gabinetto Vieusseux, and Mary may have met him there or through his friend, sculptor Hiram Powers.[98]

Reputedly, Mary assisted in organizing hospital work during the Italian war with Austria.[99] Likely, this was the Austro-Prussian War of 1866 when Prussia assisted Italy in freeing Venice from Austrian rule. Mrs. Livermore reported Mary's being in Florence assisting, "Madame Mario," in nursing Italian troops during this period.[100] Madame Mario was battlefield nurse and newspaper correspondent Jessie Meriton White Mario, British wife of Garibaldi's friend, Italian freedom fighter Alberto Mario.[101] She was the first woman to apply to the University of London's medical college but was unsuccessful in gaining admission.[102] Possibly, she inspired Mary's seeking medical education several months later in America.

Further evidence of Mary Safford's Florentine presence is in Cairo, Illinois' Public Library. Written on the exterior of a tri-folded white paper in flowery 19th century handwritten script is, "To Miss Mary Safford from Mr. Hart."

Inside is:

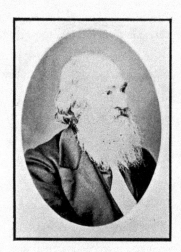

To Mary

You praise my song, "Two little trees,"
To Sister's love; nor writ to please;
Without a sprite; or Fairy;
The thought; the feeling;--landscape thine,
The memory alone is mine
That would an evergreen entwine
Around her name, Dear Mary:

My only sister.---Mary too,
Like thee, the woman, truest true;--
In doing good ne'er---weary;
Who to her kind, and Country gave
Her woman's worth,--the moral brave;
Did all she could to sooth, and save;
And looked like thee, Dear Mary.

J. T. Hart, Florence, Italy
June 9 – 1866 [103]

Joel Tanner Hart, Kentucky poet and sculptor.
Berry, Carrie William, Joel Tanner Hart, 1914 (?), Kentucky
Digital Library.

Perhaps Mr. Marsh or Hiram Powers introduced Mary to his friend, Kentucky sculptor Joel Tanner Hart, or perhaps she met him at Gabinetto Vieusseux.[104] Supposedly, he liked writing poetry more than sculpting although he did both, and, "Two Little Trees," was a poem he wrote for his niece Dian Weaver.[105] The Kentucky Historical Society now owns a portrait Hart painted of his sister Mary Morgan Hart Weaver—"Mary, too," from the poem.[106] The above previously unpublished poem suggests Hart's admiration for Mary Safford's good deeds, but the cryptic real meaning is likely summed in his line, "The memory alone is mine."

Having lived in the far western U.S. since 1850, A. P. K. Safford left in December 1865 and arrived in New York City February 1, 1866.[107][108] There, he applied for a passport on May 6th and presumably soon crossed the Atlantic.[109] He met Mary in Florence, and she hardly recognized him after over 16 years separation.[110] Probably, the siblings traveled together, for Mary knew Italy and spoke Italian.[111] A series of unsigned letters to A.P.K.'s home newspaper *Humboldt Register* dated during A. P. K.'s European trip's period told of being in Florence July 6, 1866, and described the sculpture studios of Mary's acquaintances.[112] The anonymous author was far more knowledgeable of Italian politics than the usual tourist. As the same paper previously published Mary's travelogues, likely these letters were written by one of the Safford siblings. How long A. P. K. accompanied Mary, who was in Paris during late August, is unknown as is her European departure date.[113]

8 MEDICAL EDUCATION AND EARLY WOMEN'S RIGHTS WORK

In correspondence to Caroline Marsh, wife of the U. S. Minister to Italy, Mary described the return voyage and revealed an ongoing though unidentified chronic illness:

"I have been suffering much more since I returned than I did in Europe. We had a most uncomfortable passage. I was quite ill all of the time, and went through a very trying ordeal at the Custom House in Boston which together with the fatiguing trip west and excitement incident upon getting home may be the cause of my continued suffering. I have not given myself up to complete rest as I doubtless ought to do..." [1]

Mary initially visited her Cairo family for a month but soon headed to Washington, DC, with A. P. K. European experiences broadened Mary's political concerns, as she related this visit:

"...and with an interest that I doubtless should not have felt before going abroad, since by comparison now I see everything from a much broader and more appreciative point of view. I found myself a daily visitant at the Capitol where I never wearied in listening to debates upon pending questions of vital importance to our future healthful, national development. I found more of dignified decorum prevailing the Senatorial body than I had anticipated but the legislature is sorrowfully typical of the contending elements that represent a great and growing people. I observed nothing with more satisfaction than the progressive condition of the colored people everywhere. They voted in Georgetown while I was in Washington, with a quiet demeanor, and yet, as their vote proved with an understanding of right principle, that astonished everyone. Chivalrous prejudices against them are giving place to the enjoyment of rights belonging to the human family regardless of race. Their eagerness to acquire an education can only be compared to that of a hungry man who craves food to satisfy the keen demands of appetite. I found in the schools of Washington, in the same classes, old men and women over sixty years of age, calling to aid glasses and bowed down with decrepitude, and little children of three years, learning together the alphabet. There is no bounds to their expressions of gratitude for this millennium dawn that clearly foretells a brighter day than the race has ever known. The chief gaieties of Washington were passed when I arrived so that I only had a few side leeps (sic) onto the stage of fashionable life: but saw quite enough to reconvince me of how unsatisfactory it is. I attended one reception at the Presidents and deserve the congratulation of all my friends that I made my escape unmaimed for life. Unless you have been unfortunately caught in a 4th of July mob you could form no idea of the confusion confounded upon this occasion. The crowd was most thoroughly democratic, in manner of speech, in action, and in dress: it was a scene to remember, but never with a wish to witness it a second time. It was sad and humiliating to pay ones respects to such a man as represents us at the helm of State." [2]

Mary was obviously not a fan of President Andrew Johnson. Her letter continued with a knowledgeable discussion on the U.S. State Department's involvement in volatile European politics:

"I suppose like Vesuvius, all these gaseous elements in the political crater may smolder, fume and smoke a long time yet before there is a general eruption." [3]

As she wrote from New York City:

'My brain teams with schemes for future usefulness. I hardly dare launch my boat till I am stronger and better able to endure fatigue…I turn from the pleasure living, and Mammon serving devotees of 5th Avenue to other avenues of usefulness in this thronging world of a city, and my soul thirsts to drink deep from the only fountain that satisfies that of usefulness.'[4]

Likely, before she went abroad, Mary considered her options for a fulfilling life limited. She could live in Cairo, teach school and pray a kind gentleman would willingly marry a 35-year-old spinster. Her desire for usefulness was evident in her short-lived but sincere efforts to help Union soldiers, but her small size and frail health precluded her becoming a nurse. Also, after years of Alfred's supporting her, she needed financial independence. Fortunately, contact with European intellectuals awakened her to women's professional possibilities.

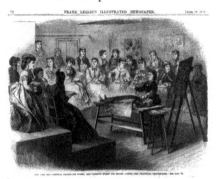

New York Medical College for Women, anatomical lecture room c.1870. Frank Leslie's Illustrated Newspaper, 16 Apr 1870, p. 72.

Conveniently, Mary Livermore's friend Elizabeth Cady Stanton was a trustee of the nascent New York Medical College for Women.[5][6] Stanton was an ally of homeopath Dr. Sophia Clemence Lozier and helped her obtain the school's charter from the New York legislature.[7] Reciprocally, Dr. Lozier was a generous donor to the suffrage movement.[8] In November 1863, president and professor of women's diseases Lozier opened her college as an all women's institution to circumvent male medical students' harassing women as routinely occurred in coeducational schools.[9][10] Although not initially labeled a homeopathic institution, many on Lozier's faculty were homeopathic physicians, and the curriculum included homeopathic principles.[11][12]

In 1868, Dr. Elizabeth Blackwell, the first woman graduate of an American allopathic medical school, founded Woman's Medical College of the New York Infirmary, an all women's allopathic institution.[13] Allopaths were called, "regulars," and had a traditional medical education previously available to men only. In contrast, homeopaths followed the tenets of Samuel Hahnemann with his doctrine, "similia similibus curantur," or, "like cures like." Considered a radical treatment approach by the allopaths, homeopathy preached treating specific diseases with infinitesimally small amounts of substances that when given in a greater concentration would produce the symptoms of that specific disease. Whether homeopathic minute doses of occasionally poisonous substances actually treated disease or whether the homeopaths' refusal to use toxic substances allopaths routinely prescribed led to patients' recoveries was debatable.

The two women's schools varied significantly in medical philosophy, but each had more stringent training requirements than the era's male medical schools.[14] Competition arising from Drs. Lozier and Blackwell's divergent viewpoints may have led to both institutions' growth but later led to the women's persistent enmity.[15]

In fall 1866, Mary Safford entered Dr. Lozier's school where the faculty was nearly equally divided between genders and included professors of anatomy, surgery, chemistry, physiology and hygiene, obstetrics, medical jurisprudence, theory and practice as well as materia medica and toxicology.[16][17] Tuition and fees for the year were $115 with an additional $10 diploma fee for seniors.[18] Admission requirements included a certificate of moral character and only a rudimentary knowledge of science and Latin.[19]

Mary was at the right place and time to gain a thorough medical education. She could attend the school's lectures and also clinics at Bellevue Hospital, the Ophthalmic Hospital and the Eye and Ear Infirmary.[20] One classmate was Mrs. Isabel, "Bella," Hayes Chapin Barrows whose many accomplishments included her working part-time as Secretary of State Seward's stenographer. Her 1891 eulogy for Mary attested to their fast friendship:

"The first time I saw Mary Safford was in New York twenty-five years ago…sitting on the edge of a desk with her feet in the chair was a bright, eager little woman, quizzing her classmates on materia medica 'What is the composition of Dover's powder?' was the question on her lips as I entered the door. Her musical voice, her intelligent face, her great head set upon a frame too slight for the precious burden, her gentle winning manner at once attracted the attention and captivated the hearer. From that day we were friends…"[21]

Mary's medical school preceptor was Henry Millard, MD.[22] Having both allopathic and homeopathic training, he appreciated the two therapy systems and probably taught Mary likewise.[23] The curriculum was much like that of modern medical schools, and the anatomy text was *Gray's Anatomy.*[24] Anatomical dissections were requisite in the first two years, and upper level students diagnosed and presented cases to professors.[25] The school had its own dispensary for students' acquiring diagnostic, prognostic and presentational skills---the hands-on experience for proper medical practice.[26] Optional work at Bellevue Hospital allowed additional exposure to autopsies and surgeries, but male students made life difficult:

"In the late 1860s, a group of thirty women homeopathic medical students went to Bellevue Hospital for their clinical training. The women faced such hostility from male professors and students that they carried switchblade knives to fend off their persecutors…One day, they were greeted by hundreds of male students who blocked their entrance, pelted them with chewed balls of paper, and laughed and shouted at them. Dr. Lozier, as president of the college, organized a large public meeting with Henry Ward Beecher and Horace Greeley (editor of the *New York Tribune*), who denounced the boorish behavior of the male medical students. After considerable media attention supporting the women, the mayor of New York agreed to send a police force to 'protect the ladies in their right,' thereby enabling them to obtain a full medical education."[27]

With powerful supporters like Beecher and Greeley backing them against Bellevue's obnoxious men, the women's victory was predictable. The image of thirty potentially hoop-skirted women, some as small as 4'4" tall, armed with switchblade knives in defense against hundreds of heckling men armed with spitballs would have been memorable. One can only imagine the male students' vowing never again to bring spitballs to a knife fight.

Despite living in New York City, Mary still considered Cairo home and returned there for Christmas 1866.[28] She sent presents then, for she received a significant thank you note about a month later:

"HEADQUARTERS ARMIES OF THE UNITED STATES

Washington, Jan. 21, 1867

My dear Miss Safford:

I owe you an apology for not earlier acknowledging the beautiful token of remembrance which you were so kind as to send me about a month ago. The box containing it came duly to hand and supposing it to be a box of cigars, a present which I often get, it was sent to the house where I have several dozen boxes just like it, though with different contents. I supposed that a letter would come along through the mail announcing who had favored me, as is usually the case. But no letter came and the matter was forgotten until last evening I had occasion to open a fresh box of cigars, and accidentally opened the one you sent me, and then found your letter and beautiful present. It was the first I knew of your return from Europe. I was indeed glad to her from you and shall also prize most highly both your letter and the cigar holder which I shall preserve in remembrance of the donor.

I had hoped ere this to have visited Europe. The unsettled condition of our country, politicall (sic), has however prevented me doing so up to this time.

Remember me kindly to your brother and Mrs. Safford. Mrs. Grant and the children also join me in this and in desiring to be remembered to you.

Yours truly,

U. S. Grant"[29]

Undoubtedly, many of Dr. Lozier's students had personal opinions on women's rights, but she further inspired the women by contributing much of her considerable medical practice income to this cause.[30] Through her, Mary Safford could access a host of 19th century reformers including Stanton, Susan B. Anthony, Henry Ward Beecher, Horace Greeley, Julia Ward Howe, and Lucretia Mott.[31] Mary was active in the Illinois' women's rights movement during her medical school years, as her name was among, "Illinois Advocates of Suffrage," and she attended an 1867 Illinois lecture series presented by Dr. Lozier's friend Susan B. Anthony.[32][33] A summer 1868 Chicago convention lead to an Illinois' association for universal suffrage, and Mary was among, "the large number of representative men and women who have from the first identified," as suffrage supporters."[34] In September 1869, the same group led by Mary Livermore, named Dr. Safford its representative to the Berlin Woman's Industrial Congress.[35]

Mary's senior year ended in March 1869. Commencement at New York Historical Society Hall began with addresses on, "Woman's Education," followed by Dr. Lozier's speech on the school's progress and announcement of graduates' names.[36] Mary Safford gave a reputedly warmly received valedictory address, but, unfortunately, no transcript of it survives.[37] The *New York Times* somewhat disparagingly reported Mrs. Stanton's speech on woman suffrage.[38] Mary's hometown paper recognized her achievement:

"Miss Mary Safford of this city, graduated at the New York Medical College for females, on the 23d instant, delivering the valedictory address of the graduating class...'

'It seems to be the ruling purpose of Miss Safford's life to minister to the sick and the afflicted, and that she may do this more efficiently than before, we doubt not, is the motive for her present course. Hundreds and thousands of the sick and wounded soldiers of the Mississippi valley, who filled the hospitals at Cairo, Memphis, Vicksburg, Nashville, Mound City and other points will recall her kind visits and ministrations..."[39]

The reporter's wildly enthusiastic exaggeration of Mary's feats aside, Cairo could be proud of the Saffords. U.S. Grant became President just prior to her graduation and a month later named A. P. K. Safford as Arizona's Third Territorial Governor, a position he kept until Grant left office in 1877.[40] [41]

Mary pursued European post-graduate study, but before leaving, she visited John Greenleaf Whittier who wrote:

"I have just had a visit from Miss Dr. Safford a graduate of N.Y. Medical College, and on her way to Germany for a year. She is to be specifically a surgeon: and says she can cut up one's mortal frame, without tremor of her delicate hand or long fringed eyelid. Her brother is Gov of Arizona, and she is going there on her return expecting to have plenty of gun shot wounds and knife stabs among the pioneers and "Greasers," for her experiments."[42]

His description of Mary's expectations of Arizona's patients sounded like the OK Corral gunfight's aftermath. Any further relationship between Mary and Whittier is unknown, and she may have met him via introduction by mutual friend and fellow abolitionist Dr. Lozier.[43] Mary also attended Howard University Law School's graduation in Washington.[44] Her letter from New York to the *National Anti-Slavery Standard* described the progress made by freed blacks in the short time since they were, "chattels, bought and sold for a price!" In a long newspaper column, she poured forth admiration for these remarkably eloquent, intelligent black men who transformed themselves from illiterates into functioning lawyers.

While in Washington, she participated in a homeopathic, "proving."[45] Now called a homeopathic pathogenetic trial, a proving is:

"A pre-defined number of repeated doses of the homeopathic remedy are given to healthy volunteers until symptoms are experienced. These are collated by observers and distinctive symptoms common to multiple participants (which are most likely to be related to the medicine) are identified. According to the central homeopathic principle that 'like cures like,' the remedy may have the potential to treat these specific characteristic symptoms."[46]

The experimental substance to be proved was, "chewed coca leaves," said to be:

"Now in general use by the Indians, as a narcotizing beverage."[47]

The human guinea pig homeopaths took a variety of coca dosages and reported symptoms ranging from none to one person's hallucinating, "most wonderful visions," and comparing it to cannabis.[48] Dr. Safford's several reports after chewing coca included:

"Aversion to concentration of thought upon any one thing."

"Frontal headache; next above the eyebrows; not constant; increased by elevating the head and turning the eyes up."

"An intense gnawing, hungry sensation, at the pit of the stomach."

"A desire to urinate frequently, with increased flow of urine."

"A dull severe pain in left leg from hip-joint to knee."

"A weak, trembling sensation in legs."

"Flashes of heat up the back, and burning across abdomen, in flashes."

"All symptoms ameliorated by being in open air."[49]

The event discovered new uses for medical coca including treatment for, "mental and physical lack of will to do anything," and, "sleeplessness with desire to work."[50]

Mary returned to Cairo May 1st and a week later headed to Hot Springs, Arkansas, for rest:

"…We are apprehensive that this lady owes her physical prostration to an overworked brain. Of a nervous temperament anyhow, she has imposed mental labors upon herself, which very few indeed would have the energy and self reliance to undertake."[51]

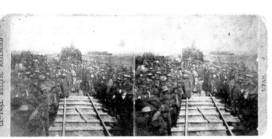

"Last Rail Laid at Promontory Point, May 10th, 1869." Stereoscopic view. Alfred A. Hart, Albumen silver print, 1869. Courtesy J. Paul Getty Museum's Open Content program.

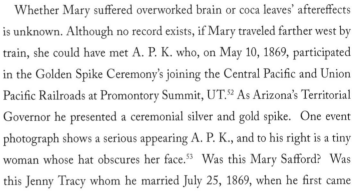

Whether Mary suffered overworked brain or coca leaves' aftereffects is unknown. Although no record exists, if Mary traveled farther west by train, she could have met A. P. K. who, on May 10, 1869, participated in the Golden Spike Ceremony's joining the Central Pacific and Union Pacific Railroads at Promontory Summit, UT.[52] As Arizona's Territorial Governor he presented a ceremonial silver and gold spike. One event photograph shows a serious appearing A. P. K., and to his right is a tiny woman whose hat obscures her face.[53] Was this Mary Safford? Was this Jenny Tracy whom he married July 25, 1869, when he first came to Tucson, Arizona Territory?[54] Only history knows. A month later, at the Cairo bank, Alfred Safford exhibited several small silver spikes manufactured from the same metal used to produce Arizona's ceremonial spike.[55]

To further her education through post-graduate training in Vienna, Mary braved seasickness once again in crossing the Atlantic, and she wrote to the Marshes in Florence in October 1869:

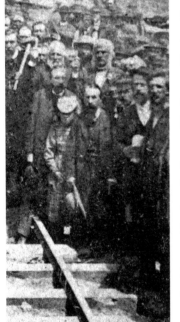

Detail of prior stereoscopic view. Man holding hat is A.P.K Safford with small woman. Alfred A.Hart Albumen silver print, 1869. Courtesy J. Paul Getty Museum's Open Content program.

"I have been here since the early part of July. I was fortunate in finding an apartment in the hospital and in meeting with no barriers opposed to the accomplishment of my object. You can imagine what a rich field of labor and observation I find here free to select that which most interests me, among a population of nearly three thousand sick which this hospital contains.'

'A very dear friend who graduated with me last spring, Mrs. Barrows from Washington, has just joined me and I am very happy in having a companion so earnest and desirous as myself to profit by the rich advantages to be had here."[56]

Mary's letter to a medical journal told of her Viennese reception:

"…Armed with letters of introduction from the highest authorities, medical and others, with diploma in hand, I appeared before one of the professional fraternity in Vienna. When I had made known my wishes, and extended my hand with the documents therein…he said, I do not care to read your letters; all I wish to know is, that have come to learn of us. You are at liberty to profit by all of the interests of my wards."[57]

The good doctor arranged for Mary and Bella to be, "internes."[58] Although Paris was the favorite post-graduate city for many women allopaths, Mary and Bella's first choice for study was central Vienna's immense hospital, the Allegemeine Krankenhaus.[59] Later, Mary recounted her reasons for choosing Viennese post-graduate training:

"It has many advantages over other Universities. Its great hospital is within one enclosure, and all lectures are given in it, so that no time is lost… Its vast material is used ad libitum for clinical purposes. And here, I believe as in no other University, are private lectures for the benefit of native and foreign M. D.'s (sic), who wish to go over certain subjects more rapidly than can be done in the regular course for students...'

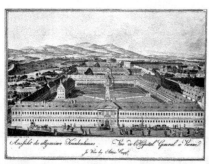

Allegemeines Krankenhaus, Vienna's immense general hospital as it appeared in 1784.

'These courses last from four to six weeks…The price of these private classes varies from 10 to 20 guldens. (A gulden is about 50 cents.)'

'… Foreign, as well as native students, rent furnished rooms, and live at restaurants. An occasional foreigner is fortunate, as I was, in securing lodgings in the hospital, where he has the advantage of being called at night to any operations of importance…One can live plainly and comfortably for $30 per month."[60]

The women roomed together as recounted by Bella Barrows:

"For a year we occupied the same large, sunny room in Vienna, where we were students together in the university, the first women who were ever allowed to matriculate there."[61]

Mary's friend Kate Doggett reported the hospital's enormity:

"… I began to form an idea of the size of the establishment, for our direction read, 'Dr. Mary Safford, seventh court, twenty-seventh staircase.' I learned afterwards there were nineteen of these courts, and that the various buildings had more than three thousand patients."[62]

All of Vienna's obstetrical work occurred at one location divided into a midwives' section for uncomplicated births and a physicians' section for all others.[63] This was the ideal site for study of obstetrics and gynecology, and Mary was constantly occupied, seeing enough procedures to cover an ordinary lifetime. In a letter to *New Covenant* the next year she wrote of her typical day:

"It is seven o'clock in the morning, and so dark that the glimmering gas lights guide me through the many courts and to the wards which I first visit at this early hour. I enter a long room, a flickering oil lamp burns over the door...'

'We are now in a ward where all minor surgical cases are received; primarius and assistants, each carries a lighted wax taper, and the visit begins with a close inquiry into the case, symptoms asked for, wounds examined. The medicine to be given is written upon the tablet at the head of each bed, which bears name, age, day of entrance, disease, and when the case is a critical one the condition of the pulse, temperature and respiration, as well as the food of each patient, whether requested or prescribed. We visit five rooms corresponding in size and arrangement to the one first entered, one is occupied by women… most perfect order prevails in the different wards, regular as clock work system in the entire hospital of 3,000 patients...'

'At ten o'clock I enter the surgical department… The seats rise steeply from the floor to the ceiling…under the large double window that throws its abundant light upon the operating table…The first hour is spent with the ambulance, as outside patients who come in to be treated, or for advice, are called; and we see during that time much that is practical, and that must come into the every day practice of every physician---tumors of all kinds, sprains fractures and dislocations, and then follows operations until twelve o'clock…The professor is a most thorough gentleman… I took an operative course from his first assistant, where all operations, surgical, are made upon the cadaver…eating becomes a secondary consideration, we will go directly from surgery to a course upon electricity…'

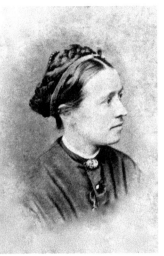

Mary Jane Safford, Vienna, Austria, May 20, 1870. Courtesy Tarpon Springs Area Historical Society- 013.0001.0188.

'In this our electric course…the professor diagnoses the new cases and his assistant plies the poles to those previously examined. I am becoming more and more strengthened in my belief that properly applied there is a healing power in the subtle element…'

'At one o'clock we enter the lecture room of the professor of obstetrics, thronged with students. Last year the total number of births in the Lying-in ward were four thousand one hundred and fifty-five, and my notebook for this year closes, with a record of one hundred and fifty operations witnessed…'

'The first assistant of the world renowned pathologist Prof. Rokitensky (sic), lectures daily between four and five o'clock, which all that is abnormal and pathological in connection with the autopsies of the day is shown and explained. Then follows topographical anatomy from six to eight o'clock, with illustrations upon the cadavers …"[64]

The University of Vienna's faculty allowed the women's full participation in all medical matters, and the fifteen hundred Viennese male medical students were utterly courteous.[65] Among Mary Safford's private teachers were Drs. Braun and Rokitansky.[66] Obstetrics and Gynecology Professor Carl Braun edited a gynecology journal, invented several medical instruments and published a gynecology textbook.[67][68] Pathologist Dr. Karl Rokitansky devised the, "Rokitansky Evisceration," a classic autopsy dissection technique, wrote several handbooks on it, and performed a remarkable 30,000 autopsies.[69] When Mary matriculated, 66-year old Dr. Rokitansky was one of Europe's leading pathology teachers, and he allowed her seeing as many autopsies as she desired—quite a bargain for $10 in 1869.

Mary observed and treated obstetrical complications ranging from prolapsed umbilical cords to the delivery of two hemi-cephalous monsters.[70] She performed the operation of fetal decapitation, an unfortunate necessity of that age for instances of fetal intrauterine death.[71] Dr. Braun was expert in the procedure, as he invented the, "Schlusselhaken," or key-hook to remove the fetal head in situations where delivery was impossible but removal of fetal remnants imperative.[72]

Years later, Bella noted her friend's work in Vienna:

"No man in the university put in so many hours a day of solid work. Once a week for a little while she allowed herself the relaxation…of a game of whist. Rarely she went to the opera or a concert. But, as a rule, she was in lectures or studying from six in the morning till eleven at night. Her life was abstemious and simple…Never did I see an adult human being subsist on so little. Though never vigorous, she was almost never sick but month after month kept up this steady plod."[73]

Mary corroborated this in her correspondence to the Marshes:

"My ambition is unlimited to understand thoroughly the work I have begun and the profession I have chosen and now that our opportunities are daily broadening I feel that perseverance will accomplish it-- My health has steadily strengthened since my body and mind have been so busily and profitably occupied.'

'As yet I have not found the time to call upon Mr. Jay and family to whom I brought a pleasant letter of introduction from Gen. Grant."[74]

By October 1869, "Gen. Grant," was President Grant, and, "Mr. Jay," was the U.S. Envoy John Jay in Vienna.[75] Mary must have been highly preoccupied to miss that visit.

The years may have dimmed Bella's memory of Mary's health in Vienna, but her ascetic lifestyle had consequences, as reported:

"Dr. Safford was twice sent for to perform craniotomy, but unhappily, was suffering from severe angina, which confined her to her room. We are glad to see…that she has entirely recovered, and has entered upon her regular duties again…"[76]

Despite her hectic hospital schedule, Mary maintained a keen interest in women's rights as reported by fellow advocate Chicagoan Kate Doggett.[77] After receiving Kate's introduction to Viennese feminist Madame Auguste von Littrow-Bischoff, Mary called on her often and participated in her active social circle. Madame von Littrow was an author, friend of Florence Nightingale and introduced Mary to many of Vienna's royals, wealthy, and cultural elite. [78] Von Littrow wrote a biography of famed Austrian poet Franz Grillparzer whose 80th birthday party Mary attended in early 1871.[79][80] He jokingly asked Professor Rokitansky to dissect his head to determine what caused his deafness. Mary's report of the poet's death a year later lacked any report of such an investigation.[81]

For both medical and non-medical periodicals, Mary wrote a variety of articles on her Viennese studies and women's rights work experiences. In 1870, for Susan B. Anthony's suffrage newspaper *The Revolution,* Mary reported, "Sights in Vienna," about relaxing in Paradise Garden, listening to an all-woman musical octet, and reading a letter of, "Madam Muhlback."[82] Mary also wrote of the *Tages Presse,* a new German language paper with a women's section to which she sent copies of *The Revolution* to share American women's movement news.[83] Probably, Kate Doggett or Madame von Littrow introduced Mary to the Viennese Woman's Association that she frequented and even addressed in a woman's rights speech delivered in German.[84][85] Although named an Illinois delegate to the Berlin's Women's Industrial Congress, Mary did not attend.

In a March 6, 1870, letter to Clara Barton in Geneva, Switzerland, Mary wrote of, "dear mother Gage," referring to a fellow woman's rights worker.[86] Mary's letter to Miss Barton inquired of her recovery from poor health and spoke of Switzerland that Mary hoped to visit in August. Mary also wrote to Consul Marsh in October 1869 of her desire to see the mountains again:

"Nothing could give me more pleasure than to meet you and Mrs. Marsh during my stay in Europe. I should like to anticipate a month or two of rest in the mountains next summer, but if I remain well, and adequate to the work shall not afford the time since the opportunities especially clinical are gold here during vacation." [87]

By June 1870, Mary's hard work pace took its toll, and she wrote of her need for rest:

"In the midst of summer, almost a year since I came. I am weary; my brain at times addled, and yet I can not break away from the charm of the work. I shall try to go to some quiet nook near here for August, and then back to work yet another year."[88]

Her exact vacation site is unknown, but record exists of a most unusual phenomenon a, "Miss S.," supposedly experienced in summer 1870 when Gorham Blake, a man important in Mary's future, claimed telepathic communication.[89] He wrote to the English Society of Psychical Research, an organization formed in an era when science tried to explain the world in terms' challenging both the traditional religious and spiritual worlds.[90] Reports of paranormal activity including visions, telepathy, and other such activity increased in the Western world concurrent with the rise of Spiritualism. Gorham Blake described, "Miss S.'s," August 1870 event:

"In the year 1870 I was in Cambridge, Massachusetts, near Boston, and had an occasional correspondence with Miss S., an American, then residing in Europe. I received a letter from her, dated Murzzuschlag, August 6th, 1870, in which she says: 'Yesterday I sat alone in my room, arranging my herbarium, till I was very tired, but there was such a fascination in the work that I did not seem able to break the spell and leave it; but of a sudden someone touched my shoulder with such force that I immediately turned. You were as plainly to be seen as if in the body, and I said, "Why, Mr. Blake, are you really here?" and directed by you I laid aside my work and went to the woods. I do not know that my mind was upon you at the time. I tried to trace the influence to a concentration of thought upon you, but failed to do it. Whether it was your letter, your spirit, or my imagination, certainly it was a reality to me.' I wrote for more particulars. She answered: 'Vienna, Austria, 23rd October, 1870. In explanation of your coming to me, I heard your voice, or a voice, speak my name. I turned, and you stood near me. I arose as if it were a reality, and as I turned again you were gone; and yet before I did that it seemed many minutes, for I said, "Is it you?" and you replied, "Do you not know me?" and then you said, "I have come because you are tired, for you to go to the woods and rest yourself," and, as I told you, I obeyed the summons, and wished that I could have a tangible evidence of your companionship.' My diary does not record any dream or thought of Miss S. on August 5th, 1870. I was at home, and quiet, and under good conditions for such a visit as that described by Miss S."[91]

Sixty miles southwest of Vienna, Murzzuschlag is a resort town and restful nook. Given the times, locations, the herbarium as a homeopath might own, and Gorham Blake's authorship, "Miss S.," was probably Mary Safford. He may have confabulated the event, but a restful walk in Austria's mountainside woods on a warm summer day sounds like good therapy for an overworked and over-stimulated mind before returning to the hospital's non-stop activity.

In winter 1870, Vienna suffered a major outbreak of puerperal fever, an infection seen in women just after giving birth:

"From Vienna. Puerperal Fever.—Dr. Mary Safford writes from Vienna, that puerperal fever rages in the lying-in asylum, and in spite of the varied forms which it assumes, there is but one method of treatment—leeches applied to the distended abdomen, followed in many cases by cold water applications, Laudanum, Quinine, Tannin, and they pass away without any apparent beneficial result from anything given. Great precaution has been used in regard to ventilation and cleanliness; but all has seemed of no avail. There is one singular thing connected with this epidemic: not a woman who has given birth to her child in the street, or outside of the hospital, and been brought in after being confined, has been attacked by the puerperal fever. There is much less close observation of the disease than there should be for the advancement of science; such a scourge deserves to be met boldly, and the origin sought for diligently."[92]

Mary's critically reporting the outbreak probably stirred an ideological hornet's nest grown insidiously for the prior 20 years. In 1847, Dr. Braun's predecessor Dr. Ignaz Semmelweiss postulated puerperal fever's cause was doctors' inadequate hand washing between fever victims' autopsies and new obstetrical patients' examinations.[93] Unfortunately, Braun vociferously criticized Semmelweis.[94] Braun believed proper room ventilation the only necessary prophylaxis against puerperal fever and convinced authorities to install an expensive ventilating system in the hospital's maternity section.[95] Semmelweis' ideas eventually led to the germ theory of disease transmission favored today. Braun realized if mere hand washing solved the infection problem he would look foolish and be blamed for unnecessary costs. Given the notoriety of such an important intradepartmental feud and Rokitansky's support of Semmelweis, Mary would have known of it.[96] Whether Braun knew of Mary's writing to an American journal about the epidemic is unknown, but, soon, she was off his service. Another woman physician wrote of Braun's later opinion of Mary:

"Professor Spathe and Carl Braun only of the University professors refuse women admittance to their lectures and clinics…A few years since, Professor Braun admitted to his lectures and clinics Dr. Mary J. Safford, now of Boston, and, it is said, she was so eminently clever, so successful and skillful, as to have alarmed this dear old Professor as to his laurels; and though he admitted she was wonderful, incomparable, and that he had nothing but the greatest admiration for her and her ability, yet since then he has refused admission to all lady applicants to his lectures and clinics."[97]

Dr. Braun's effusive language contradicts his actions and suggests he found teaching Dr. Safford a challenge he dared not repeat. Possibly, she butted heads with him once too often, suffered, "angina," at inconvenient times, or her women's rights promotion annoyed him.

Accompanying Mary Safford's puerperal fever article in the homeopathic journal was a note:

"Among the 1,500 medical students, there are between 30 and 40 Americans studying in Vienna, among them five Homeopaths. Profs. Oppolzer and Skoda take Misses Safford and Barrows under their protecting wing, and make space for them by their side. Oppolzer still believes in the old therapeutics; Skoda gives hardly any medicine. Vienna is not a good school in which to strengthen one's faith in the use of drugs.'

'By order of the Faculty, ladies are now admitted to the full course of studies, and to the honors and rights of the university."[98]

Dr. Safford's new mentors were two of the faculty's respected elder statesmen. Supporter of Semmelweis, Professor Skoda was graduated from the University of Vienna in 1831 and was known for astute physical diagnosis with use of that new instrument the stethoscope.[99] [100] His reluctance to use drug therapy was legend, preferring such treatments as cold-water baths for fevers. As a homeopath, Mary generally treated patients with ingested remedies and seemed disappointed at Viennese physicians' reluctance to do so.[101] Skoda's use of nutrition and hydrotherapy may have inspired her later advocating diet and exercise to achieve good health.[102] However, even he realized medicine based solely on physical diagnosis was becoming passé and on his retirement stated:

"Now the microscope and chemistry may take their turn!"[103]

Mary's other mentor was 61-year-old Professor Johannes von Oppolzer whose therapy was equally simple, as every one of his remedies contained white sugar.[104] She found him endearing despite being, "a little tottering and feeble."[105]

At Dr. Skoda's retirement in early spring 1871, Mary joined students and professors outside his home for presentation of an elegantly wrapped written commendation signed by 2500 appreciative students.[106] In assuming Skoda's patients, Oppolzer contracted exanthematous typhus and died within weeks.[107] Mary's touching letter to *New Covenant* told of his always providing her a place at his side during lectures while saying, "give way to the little American."[108] Mary did not attend his funeral, as just a few days before his death she left Vienna for Breslau, Germany (now Wroclaw, Poland). There she found an altogether different medical educational opportunity as the first woman to study at its university, entering with trepidation and finding relief upon acceptance:

"Having been two years, nearly, in Vienna without meeting with an obstacle to impede the progress of my studies, I almost feared the attempt to break new paths, not trodden before by the feet of women. I faced, however, the realities of asking admittance to the University here, and to my joy I met with a kind and generous reception...The professors are comparatively young, and as industrious as intelligent. Prof. Woldeyer (sic), the pathologist and microscopist, with whom I work and whose autopsies I attend, has made for himself an early and deserved reputation by his discoveries and writings.'

'In Vienna I was interrogated the first day of the term by at least a score of students as to where and what I had studied, but here they manifest as little curiosity in regard to my presence, as if they had always had women students in their midst...it is a pleasant memory ...the universal kindness that I have everywhere met with, from the medical faculty, as well as from students."[109]

A German correspondent to *The Woman's Journal* described Mary's first few months in Breslau:

"...She has been present by invitation at the weekly meetings of the Scientific Association of Breslau, and received the congratulation of many as the first woman who had listened to their discussions.'

'With Professor Waldeyer of the University she is studying Pathology and Pathological Microscopy, and we hear that she diagnoses the various specimens of tumors laid before her with a skill that astonishes the Professor.'

'In Prof. Spiegelberg's department she hears his lectures upon Obstetrics and Gynaecology and attends his clinics... she is a guest in the family of one of the most noted Gynaecologists in North Germany, a private student in his office."[110]

Prof. Heinrich Wilhelm Gottfried von Waldeyer-Hartz was a famous anatomist credited with introducing the terms, "neuron," "chromosome," and, "plasma cell," as well as for whom Waldeyer's Ring, the annular area of pharyngeal lymphoid tissue, is named.[111] [112] After teaching Mary Safford he refused teaching any additional women students.[113] Perhaps he and Dr. Braun found teaching her equally challenging.

Mary's other mentor, Obstetrics Professor Otto Spiegelberg founded the journal *Archiv fur Gynakologie* and later authored a midwifery textbook.[114] The Gynaecological Society of Boston respected Spiegelberg's work, and included his publication in their library.[115] At their August 1871 meeting, the organization's Secretary presented a paper by Breslau physicians Dr. William Alexander Freund and Dr. Ludwig Joseph on, "Uretero-uterine Fistula."[116] The journal described the paper as, "translated by Mary Safford, an American Medical Student at Breslau."

Mary wrote of her initial Breslau medical studies:

"I have attended lectures upon Surgery, the only woman among four hundred students, witnessing not only all operations that were made, but taking, with a class composed of all nations, a surgical operative course, where I made upon the cadaver all operations."[117]

Shortly after Mary moved to Breslau, she wrote fellow student and American physician Dr. James Jackson Putnam in Vienna about visiting Mrs. Ellen Washburn Freund, wife of Dr. Max Freund, brother to, "her," Dr. Freund.[118] [119] Mary's Dr. Freund was William Alexander Freund, the man for whom she translated the fistula paper read to the Boston gynecologists.[120] Dr. Putnam's brother Charles Pickering Putnam, MD, also trained in Vienna in 1869 and married Ellen's sister Lucy in 1888.[121] [122] [123] Possibly, the Washburn/Freund/ Putnam connection gave Mary entry to Breslau's medical world. Reputedly, during her four months in Breslau, she lived with Dr. William Freund's family and accompanied him to surgery and autopsies.[124] [125]

To American women's rights workers, Mary recounted her European educational experiences and compared the Europeans' good manners with the American medical students' boorish ones:

"I have gained a wonderfully rich experience in women's disease. I have been received as guest into the family of a very skillful gynaecologist, who has an immense private clinic, the most important of which he has kindly permitted me to examine…and, the most invaluable of all experience, he has allowed me to operate myself. I have made one of the most important operations that is made—the removing of an ovarial tumor—and my pen lacks in expression to tell you how I rejoice to find myself adequate to the work. The doctor complimented me very highly upon my ovariatomy. He said he had never seen one operate with such perfect coolness; there was no trembling of the hand, and no unsteadiness of action. I understood the work before me, and did it with an interest that must be felt to be appreciated.'

'Not until we are educated together till our opportunities are the same as those of men, till we prove to the world that we accomplished the same in acquiring our diploma, shall we be recognized by the faculty and the world as physicians…"[126]

Dr. Freund's faith in Mary's abilities was justified, and Mary described an ovariotomy (now called an oophorectomy, removal of an ovary) in a paper entitled, "Case of Ovariotomy by Prof. Freund, of Breslau," presented at a Gynecological Society of Boston meeting January 2, 1872, about 3 months after her return from Europe.[127] As she was barred from meeting attendance due to her gender, Dr. A. L. Norris of East Cambridge submitted the paper, and it was read on his behalf.[128] The all male allopathic society's Corresponding Membership rolls included both Drs. Spiegelberg and Freund.[129] Mary's paper was only begrudgingly allowed presentation accompanied by numerous derogatory comments on women physicians' abilities and the illegality of the society's allowing a work, "possibly written by a woman," although discussed as though she was merely the translator. Society members fearing the American Medical Association whose Code of Ethics precluded recognition of female doctors, allowed reading of the work only with the proviso that doing so did not constitute their approving women's medical practice. These gallant gentlemen feared treading politically thin ice in acknowledging a woman's potentially writing about medicine let alone practicing it.

Never once in the paper does Mary state she was the operative surgeon, but from her intimate knowledge of the case's aspects she must have been. The article provided a comprehensive medical history of a patient who eventually required removal of a large ovarian cyst after trans-abdominal needle drainage failed its resolution and, in fact, led to peritonitis, an inflammation of the abdominal cavity. Mary's clearly detailed description of the patient's pre-, peri- and post-operative clinical course showed her complete comprehension of it and intimate involvement in the patient's care. Her supposed reason for reporting the case was to include acute peritonitis following inadequately drained ovarian cyst fluid as a new indication for emergency surgery, much as one might operate to drain an abscess or pleural effusion.[130] Never did the good doctors of Boston's Gynaecological Society refer to Mary as Dr. Safford, only as Miss Safford, and eventually they incorporated the paper into the society's, "Proceedings," but left it to their journal editor's discretion as to publication beyond a mere abstract. The entire paper's online availability over 140 years later in the *Journal of the Gynaecological Society of Boston* shows the editor's decision.

Dr. Safford was finally putting her education to work and operating on real patients who both remained alive and improved. When she wrote, "How They Treat American Women Medical Students in Germany—A Lesson For Bellevue," Mary must have felt sweet revenge for treatment she and her classmates received in New York:

"He has permitted me to make several important operations, and to-day I have made one an ovariotomy, which, you know, is the most difficult, as well as dangerous of all operations. I received the warm congratulations of the physicians who assisted me, and from Dr. F., who gave me the operation to make, the cheering words that no one could have done it better."[131]

One unnamed, open-minded, kindly German Professor, probably Dr. Freund, who recognized Mary Safford's abilities, wrote to her later, as she quoted:

"I wish I could have each Semestre a lady scholar like you…And now I realize that your sex is just as competent to grasp scientific truth as mine, and henceforth my influence shall be given to remove the hindrances and prejudices which now shut them out from the fields of intellectual labor. All doors open to us, must be open to them, which lead to spheres of activity and usefulness…you have enriched me with an experience for which I shall ever be grateful."[132]

Her successful ovariotomy, first ever performed by a woman, was a milestone in women's medical educational history. If anything had gone awry with the procedure or post-operative course, the male medical establishment would have blamed the problem on the surgeon's inferior gender and not the patient's circumstances. While most women's rights advocates held meetings, gave speeches and printed preachy newspapers,' "sermons to the choir," Mary Safford's tangible act firmly demonstrated woman's equal abilities. This pioneering success of a, "first experiment," the first successful ovariotomy performed by a woman, opened the door to women's medical educational opportunities just a crack that allowed future generations of women physicians' passage. News of the surgery spread to a wide audience, and Kate Doggett wrote of her own trepidation had the patient's outcome been different:

"God bless the brave woman! Her hand did not tremble, but mine did, and my heart beat hard and fast as I thought—had she failed? For a man failure in a first experiment would have been of little consequence, except to the victim…but had Mary Safford failed there would have been no second trial for many a day for her, perhaps for no other woman; so knowing what hopes hung upon her knife, her hand was strong for her heroic work."[133]

Mary was ambivalent about returning to the U.S., as European opportunities and courtesy contrasted with the American male allopathic medical establishment's bigotry and disrespect of women physicians. However, after four months in Breslau, Mary began her return to America.[134] Stopping in Paris that was just emerging from the Franco-Prussian war's devastation, she visited Clara Barton who noted Mary's planned departure for America was to be on September 26th.[135] Possibly, in London she received the sad news of A.P.K.'s year-old son Frank Alfred Safford's death on August 28th.[136] One newspaper reported Mary's intending establishing a women's hospital in Washington, but any indecisiveness on a future practice locale changed quickly with a Chicago event that occurred the day her ship docked in New York City.[137]

9 REESTABLISHING AMERICAN LIFE

Arizona Citizen reported Mary Safford's New York City arrival:

"Her frail form was sadly broken down when she arrived in this city on the 8th of October, after a voyage during which she could scarcely raise her head for illness. But badly as she needed rest, she hastened to Chicago, saying to a friend, 'I had intended going to Chicago in her prosperity, and now that she is in distress I can not stay away. I may be able to do some good as a physician; but at any rate...I can cook food for the starving if nothing more.' "[1]

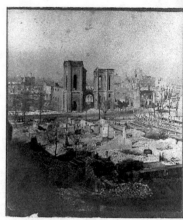

Chicago fire's aftermath, scene looking northwest from a Michigan Avenue hotel, 1871. Library of Congress Prints and Photographs Division, Stereograph cards, 2016651829.

The distress was the Great Chicago Fire. In summer and early autumn 1871, the drought-stricken and windy Midwest's raging firestorms burned thousands of acres and killed hundreds. As Mary Safford's boat docked in New York, Chicago's DeKoven Street fire alarm sounded, as a series of wooden shanties burned. Despite numerous early October fires, one act of bovine urban terrorism has persisted as the great fire's proposed ignition source and led to years of speculation about Mrs. O'Leary's cow's motives. Resolution of this controversy is beyond this book's scope.

Intense heat incinerated theoretically, "fireproof," stone and brick buildings. Chicagoans even half a mile away were nearly roasted alive or blinded by smoke and flying cinders, but the worst came the next day when the City Water-Works burned. After 36 hours, the flames died as the wind direction changed. The fire killed about 300, left 100,000 or around one third of the population homeless, burnt an area approximately four miles long and three-fourths mile wide including about 17,500 buildings, and destroyed over $222 million in property.[2] Even the Chicago Historical Society's original copy of Lincoln's Emancipation Proclamation burned.

The Chicagoans' initial response was shell shock. Fortunately, U.S. Army Lt. General Philip Sheridan had Chicago headquarters and used military supplies and personnel to restore order.[3] Within weeks, volunteers and donated supplies poured into the city while Chicago area women mobilized to the great task of caring for the needy.

Mary Safford appeared on this Pompeii-like scene and probably helped in any way possible. As a physician, she could handle victims' extensive burns and injuries or perhaps assist with numerous premature deliveries' resulting from pregnant women's hurried flights from the blaze. After ten days of drinking river water, many Chicagoans developed gastroenteritis, and smoke inhalation was common. Reputedly, ordinarily antagonistic allopathic and homeopathic physicians worked together harmoniously treating fire victims, but it is unknown if Dr. Safford, whose medical skills were as yet unknown to Chicago's established physicians, was allowed to practice medicine or merely cook dinners.[4]

Chicago quickly rebounded, and Mary rented medical office space at 798 Wabash Avenue, the address from which she wrote Cairo's Benevolent Society ladies in December 1871.[5] Seeing a fund raising opportunity, the women recruited her speaking, and the newspaper promoted her lecture at Cairo's Athenaeum on December 30th. The talk netted the benevolent ladies $145 and prompted the paper's praise for Mary's lecture style albeit neglecting mentioning her subject.[6][7]

Three days later, she reprised her speech in Shawneetown.[8] Two months later, she spoke in La Salle, Illinois, and the newspaper described her as, "…still young, petite, rather handsome…"[9] At a Terre Haute, Indiana, ladies' school she lectured on, "Dress and Ornament," and the town's newspaper reported her as an, "accomplished young physician," and her lecture as amusing and to the point.[10] Mary was over 40 years old, but her small stature belied her age.

As well as commencing medical practice and joining the lecture circuit, Mary began volunteer part-time teaching as lecturer on Physiology and Hygiene at Evanston College for Ladies.[11][12] Frances Willard was President of the new women's college affiliated with Northwestern University. Compared to the prior year's lecturer's contract, Mary Safford's read:

"1872. Miss Mary J. Safford M. D. accepts same conditions – only she pays her own fare!"[13]

Later known for her involvement with the Woman's Christian Temperance Union, Miss Willard wrote of Mary Safford's participation on the college faculty:

"Lectures on the care of health are given by Dr. Mary J. Safford, the well-known Chicago physician. Common sense applied to dress is one of the problems in the solution of which we earnestly solicit the co-operation of our patrons."[14]

Mary may have acquired this job through friendship with Mary Livermore or her associate Jane Currie Hoge, a college founder and board member.[15] Dr. Safford could acquire patients from her position, but teaching young ladies' hygiene classes would seem tame to one who aspired performing complicated gynecological surgery. Her medical practice was growing, but she needed greater association with medical peers. For several years she wrote for Chicago homeopathic chemist/pharmacist C. S. Halsey's journal *Medical Investigator* that suffered significantly in the fire.[16][17] Flames destroyed much of Chicago's medical infrastructure including many doctors' offices, pharmacies, publishing houses and several hospitals. Thus, as Mary first established her practice, Chicago's medical community was in great disarray with doctors' having little time to tuck her under their professional wings.

Despite all this, Chicago's homeopaths welcomed Mary with election to membership in the Illinois Homeopathic Medical Association at their 18th annual meeting in May 1872.[18] She received appointment to the IHMA's Committee on Diseases of Women and became a delegate to the annual American Institute of Homoeopathy (AIH) meeting held in Washington the following week.[19] Although never on Chicago's homeopathic Hahnemann Medical School faculty, Mary associated with its more prominent members such as Dr. Ludlam, the school's founder, dean, gynecologist, and professor of physiology and pathology.[20] He openly advocated women's admission to the AIH and likely chose Mary as delegate to the national meeting for that purpose.[21] Her IHMA membership provided yet another portal to the woman's rights network through the organization's secretary Dr. J. S. Mitchell whose sister Ellen Mitchell Mitchell was active in the women's movement as was her sister-in-law astronomer Maria Mitchell, Vassar College's first president.[22][23]

Mary and nine prominent male homeopaths visited Washington for the AIH's 25th Annual Meeting led by Bostonian Dr. Israel Tisdale Talbot.[24] On May 23rd, the physicians assembled in the White House East Room where Dr. Talbot addressed President Grant who gave a short, noncommittal speech about homeopathy.[25] He must have been delighted to find Mary Safford among his guests.

Back in Chicago, Cook County's Homeopathic Medical Society met June 5th and discussed a case of the kidney disorder Bright's disease missed by several other physicians due to the patient's unusual initial presentation.[26] Mary's astute diagnosis just before the patient's death attracted local doctors' notice and secured her election to the society.[27] That summer a letter to a Cairo paper noted Dr. Safford's growing, paying medical practice and large number of patients' filling her waiting room.[28]

Homeopathy society meetings were informative but limited to medicine. With her interest in natural science including geology, Mary likely sought broader exposure to current non-medical scientific thought. In August, the American Association for the Advancement of Science (AAAS) held its 21st annual meeting in Dubuque, Iowa, and elected her to membership.[29] Perhaps Chicago friend Kate Doggett sponsored her.[30] Even today the AAAS has lectures on diverse and esoteric scientific topics, many with far reaching political consequences. In addition to political contacts, the organization provided a grand spot for women's connections. In 1850, Maria Mitchell was the first woman AAAS member, and at least 30 other women joined by 1872.[31] Mary maintained membership through 1875, dropped out, then rejoined in 1882 but never addressed a meeting.

Outwardly, Mary had the perfect situation. Chicago improved daily and offered a variety of cultural activities. Family was easily accessible by train. Her years of medical training led to a successful office practice and growing reputation for medical expertise. Connections with local, state, and national medical and scientific organizations were useful, but without hospital staff privileges, she could not perform gynecologic surgery.

Although written records of Mary Safford's religious affiliations don't exist, she wrote for the Universalist newspaper *New Covenant* and had Universalist friends such as Mary A. Livermore. In her 1868 article, "After the Battle of Fort Donelson," she said of Mary Safford, "I had known her for some time as a Universalist…"[32] In August 1872, notice of the Oak Park, Illinois, Unity Church's dedication appeared in *New Covenant*.[33] The Reverend A. H. Sweetser was pastor, Reverend J. S. Dennis read the scripture, and Rev. Dr. Ryder gave the dedicatory sermon. A newspaper announcement of a September 25, 1872, event that possibly occurred there read in part:

"Last night, by the Rev. Dr. Ryder, a lady well known in this city for her medical and scientific attainments, Dr. Mary J. Safford, was married to a highly esteemed and wealthy gentleman of Boston, Mr. Gorham Blake. The affair was exceedingly quiet, being known only to a few of the most intimate friends of both…The residence of Mr. and Mrs. Blake will be at Dorchester, Boston, where Mrs. Blake will divide her time between 'beholding the bright countenance of truth in the quiet and still air of delightful studies,' and such practice of her preferred profession as leisure will permit. They left last night for their new home…"[34]

The record of their marriage is clear, but why did 40-year-old Mary wed 43-year-old Gorham?[35] Where did they meet? What common interests motivated her Chicago exit to start anew in Boston? Leaving family and friends, why did she marry so seemingly precipitously? Did he marry her for her money or she for his prominent Boston family name and a chance to live and practice medicine in progressive Boston? His story may provide a few clues.

Born in 1829, Gorham was second son of Boston Brahmins James and Polly Clapp Blake.[36] In January 1840, Gorham's mother died as did Grandfather Thomas Blake soon after.[37] Five years later, Gorham's father married his widowed older sister-in-law Catherine Clapp Harris who, with her 3-year old daughter Mary, joined the family in Newton.[38][39] Thus, Gorham's family dynamics changed considerably in his early years.

Before their mother's death, Gorham and his brother Jim attended the elite Chauncy-Hall School.[40] However, no record exists of their subsequent education beyond Jim's studying at Boston engineering firm Blake & Darracott.[41] The company belonged to his father's younger and far more successful brother, chemist, civil engineer and metallurgist John Harrison Blake.[42] In his youth, adventurous Uncle John eschewed a Harvard education to favor individually studying chemistry before entering the chemical manufacturing business and exploring remote parts of South America. Lacking college tuition or possibly inspired by Uncle John's example of success via independent study, Gorham supposedly began adult life as a, "supercargo," on an East India merchant ship in 1848.[43] Later in life, Gorham Blake wrote about this trip:

"The year 1850 found me exploring the Island of Sumatra...I was stricken down exhausted with symptoms of sunstroke and fever...a wild, savage, naked, native Malay appeared, directed my clothes to be removed, then commenced manipulating and making passes from my head to feet, during which I felt his great magnetic (mesmeric) power, was put to sleep and within an hour awoke free from pain and refreshed. It astonished me and set me to investigating 'animal magnetism.' "[44]

Despite this exotic backdrop, Newton's 1850 Federal Census mundanely listed, "Goram," Blake at home and occupation as, "seaman," although apparently he did travel to Sumatra that year.[45 46] In 1852, he and cousin Francis Wheeler Blake reached San Francisco on the ship, "Constitution," from Panama.[47 48] Almost immediately, Gorham found work as an express agent in Placerville, California, and was subsequently a gold dust buyer, mine owner, assayer and minter of gold coins.[49 50] A. P. K. Safford was then

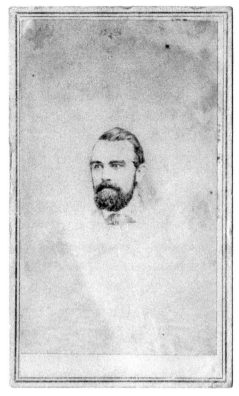

Gorham Blake, Mary Safford's husband, 1872-1879. William L. Clements Library, University of Michigan.

mining just northeast of Sacramento, and possibly the two met or at least knew of each other there as A. P. K. was a California legislator.[51] The 1860 Census listed cousins F. W. and G. Blake's living together in Grass Valley, California, and Gorham's worth at $250,000.[52] In a June 1862 letter, Gorham wrote of A.P. K. in Humboldt County:

"We here found Mr. Safford of Placer Co. and having no better chance accepted his invitation to occupy a portion of his tent..."[53]

Gorham liked paleontology. As a resident member of the California Academy of the Natural Sciences, he collected and donated to the California Geological Survey numerous fossils he found in the Humboldt County district, and two were named for him.[54 55] Nearly concurrently, Mary Safford viewed fossils in Scotland with Professor McChesney, but in this pre-internet era Mary and Gorham were ignorant of their mutual enthusiasm for paleontology. She was fascinated by it and possibly by McChesney while Gorham's interests included geology, mining, and exploration of the paranormal world as it related to science and the works of geologist and Harvard Professor William Denton.[56 57] Perhaps on Gorham's return to Boston he attended one of Denton's lectures on psychometry.[58] Denton's psychometer was one who, theoretically, through touching an object, could know its origin and identify anyone who previously handled it. In an 1890 letter to his sister, Gorham boasted comprehending fossils' prior living forms through touching their mineralized remnants. He also claimed performing experiments with telepathic communication to his mining partner who was:

"...so sceptical (sic) about magnetism and kindred subjects that I refrained from talking with him about it, and he was not aware that I was experimenting, which made the tests more satisfactory to me."[59]

Gorham's true occupation is unknown, but, by the end of December 1868, he was bankrupt.[60][61] Miners had either great fortune or lack of it, and, apparently, he was no different. By 1870, he returned to Boston to live with his 71-year-old father.[62] Gorham's successful sibling Jim had a family, was a bank trustee, gas works superintendent and Worchester's mayor.[63][64] On December 16, 1870, 42-year old Jim stopped by the gas works to check a repair, but an accidently open valve filled the building with gas that, when ignited by a lantern, blew the place to kingdom come.[65] Unitarian Rev. Edward Everett Hale officiated at Jim's funeral.[66] Later, Gorham's letter to his sister noted his chatting with their dead brother several times through a medium.

Gorham's restless lifestyle contrasted with that of his seemingly stable, responsible older brother. However, Jim's death revealed a large unpaid debt to Uncle John Blake, and John's son Dr. Clarence Blake took cousin Gorham to court to collect.[67] Possibly, Gorham was Jim's will's executor and had not repaid the loan from the estate. Otolaryngologist Clarence had worked with Alexander Graham Bell on developing the telephone and studied medicine in Vienna just before Mary Safford did.[68][69] Possibly, she knew of him. In October 1872, a few weeks after Gorham married her, the Massachusetts Supreme Court ruled against him, and the debt repayment was due in full.[70] Given the original loan's timing, did Jim use the money for repayment of Gorham's creditors, or was Jim covertly as financially irresponsible or unlucky as his brother? Did Gorham's marriage to Mary Safford help alleviate some of this debt? Did she even know of it when she married him?

Little is known of Mary and Gorham's early married life, but, initially, they moved to his ill father's home at

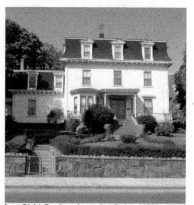

James Blake's Dorchester home where Gorham and Mary Safford-Blake lived on first arriving in Boston in 1872. Photo by Earl Taylor, Dorchester Historical Society.

5 Percival Street, Dorchester.[71] His three-story, Italianate/Mansard type house was between Percival and Adams Streets, and, possibly, the couple moved in to care for him. An 1872 Boston City Directory listed Gorham's work address at an iron foundry business.[72]

Shortly after arriving, Mary spoke at Boston's Second Radical Club.[73] This forum for theological and religious questions evolved to cover scientific and educational topics with reading of papers and subsequent debates.[74] Many club members belonged to the Free Religious Association, "an ultraliberal faction of the Unitarian Church interested in scientific theism, and the complete separation of church and state."[75] The organization was said to bring, "contemporary scientific concepts to bear on Unitarian thought..."[76] FRA member Mary participated at Second Radical Club discussions as noted in FRA publication *The Index*.[77] In mid-November, Reverend Dr. Bartol's debate on the topic, "The Prayer Gauge," was prompted by Professor Tyndall's idea of scientifically testing the power of prayer. Boston's intellectual luminaries heard Mary speak:

"Dr. Mary Safford Blake told of a mother who lost successively seven children by consumption. She had prayed for them all unsuccessfully. She had needed to learn that the laws she was neglecting in teaching them to dress tightly and observe fashionable, unhealthy habits, were wrecking their possibilities."[78]

Although she previously lectured on prudent dressing, this comment was Mary Safford-Blake's first Boston volley in a later, fervent dress reform campaign.

On November 9th, Mary visited Boston's venerable woman physician and rights activist Dr. Harriot Kesia Hunt, one of the first women practicing medicine in America. It was Dr. Hunt's 66th birthday, and Mary's writing reflected reverence for the woman whose autobiography *Glances and Glimpses* Mary had read and reread. She was Mary's role model:

"Her words, 'The soul grows strong with struggles, and acquires bravery by conquering obstacles,' had reached my ear long ago, and I had gone forth, and walked in ways made less thorny, because she had trod them before me."[79]

Depending upon when she left Dr. Hunt's Boston house, Mary may have had difficulty returning home. The city currently suffered the Great Epizootic, a horse flu epidemic.[80] Horses moved people, goods and vehicles such as police and fire wagons, and with the equine illness, any movement either ceased or required human effort. On the bright side, Mary had fewer road apples to dodge on her walk home. However, that Saturday had few bright sides beyond the glow of the conflagration just starting at a building near Boston's bay.[81] Neither Mrs. O'Leary nor her cow visited Boston on November 9th, but that evening the Great Boston Fire of 1872 erupted. Horse flu greatly hindered the fire department and forced men's pulling the fire equipment. Eventually, about 60 acres, 100 homes, and 776 commercial buildings burned, but only 30 deaths were reported.[82][83] Unlike Chicago that lacked a great number of venerable old buildings, Boston lost historic treasures including Trinity Church and part of the Old South Church.[84] Gorham Blake's foundry business address was within the map line of destruction, but his and Mary's Dorchester home was safe.[85] Unlike the shell-shocked Chicagoans, Bostonians responded by organizing relief committees within days.

Mary probably helped with humanitarian efforts after the fire, but even if not, she commenced medical practice shortly after her Boston arrival. In a January 1873 letter to *New England Medical Gazette's* editor Dr. I. T. Talbot, writer Elizabeth Stuart Phelps promoted establishing a homeopathic medical school in Boston:

"Look at our own Dr. Mary J. Safford, who has just entered the homoeopathic profession in this city, after more than six years of devotion to her preparatory studies, most of it in the hospitals and colleges of the continent, and after an unusually brilliant private practice in Chicago. Perhaps the successful management of a case of ovariotomy may have been considered a masculine prerogative; but it can never be again, since this little woman (scarcely up to my shoulder!) brought her 'feminine nerve' and 'feminine intellect' to bear upon the operation."[86]

Unfortunately, Mary's, "brilliant," Chicago practice precluded her utilizing her significant surgical skills. Later, to the New England Women's Club she recounted her exclusion from Chicago and New York hospital practice due to her gender.[87] All this was about to change.

With both allopathic and homeopathic degrees, Dr. Talbot also studied in Europe and was considered a highly competent surgeon.[88][89] In the early 1870s, the allopathic Massachusetts Medical Society heard he practiced homeopathy and immediately dismissed him and other prominent homeopaths.[90] Fearing the AMA's censure and expulsion of them, allopathic surgeons refused operating on homeopaths' patients. Thus, homeopathic surgeons like Drs. Talbot and Safford received numerous referrals. "Homeopathic surgery," seemed incongruous with homeopathic treatment principles of minute drug dosages, but operations were identical. Only post-operative medical care differed.

The same journal with Ms. Phelps' letter to editor Talbot contained:

"Mary J. Safford, MD...will devote herself to the medical and surgical diseases of women. She is perhaps the only woman living who has performed the operation of ovariotomy, and who would shrink from no task in the profession, however difficult. Her office is at 3 Boylston Place, daily except Tuesdays, from 11 to 2 o'clock. She will be one of the associate editors of the Gazette."[91]

Dr. Talbot had even higher aspirations for Mary. The Boston University School of Medicine (BUSM) was soon opening as a coeducational homeopathic institution.[92] The New England Female Medical College opened in 1848 but closed when debt and the Boston fire left the school in financial straits. Since college administrative infrastructure was otherwise intact, the institution welcomed affiliation with Boston University. Simultaneously, Dr. Talbot and the prominent homeopaths expelled by the Massachusetts Medical Society planned a new homeopathic medical school and became BUSM's faculty and administrators.[93] [94] Also, Talbot was personal physician of Isaac Rich who lived up to his name and endowed Boston University with ten million dollars.[95] In March 1873, following further fundraising by the homeopaths and Boston University, the Homoeopathic Association of Boston University began designing the coeducational medical school.[96] The organization's executive committee consisted of Talbot, prominent Massachusetts legislator David Thayer, MD, Mercy B. Jackson, MD, J. H. Woodbury, MD, Conrad Wesselhoeft, MD, and Mary J. Safford-Blake, MD.[97] A July preliminary announcement listed Mary as, "professor of disease of women."[98] Pediatrician Dr. Mercy B. Jackson and anatomist Dr. Caroline E. Hastings were the only other women faculty members when classes began in November 1873.[99]

Before school opened, the *New England Medical Gazette's* associate editor wasted no time appearing in print under the name Mary J. Safford, MD, sans Blake, with two back-to-back articles.[100] The first entitled, "Pruritis," was four pages of unabashed, thoroughly professional discussion on causes and treatment of vulvar and vaginal itching. Her second piece reported a poor woman who, after giving birth the prior year, had her uterus veritably turn inside out after delivery, remaining in the vagina, a condition known as complete inversion. Mary called the patient's allopathic physicians worthless in both diagnosis and treatment. After initial homeopathic remedies proved unsuccessful, the patient's cure came via a device Mary described:

"Being convinced that reinversion of the organ could not be accomplished merely by pressure of the air bags, and never having seen, in Europe or America, any instrument that seemed suited to such an operation, one was invented for the purpose by Mr. Gorham Blake and myself."[101]

This was the only time Mary reported any collaborative effort with Gorham. Even though she was married for eight months by the article's publication date, she did not identify him as her husband or use her married name as author. In her editorial capacity, Mary translated a German gynecology article to provide current European medical ideas to her American audience.[102] She also relayed practical medical information to the lay public via letters to various editors:

"SURE TEST OF DEATH. Dr. Mary J. Stafford (sic) writes, under the above head, a note to the *Boston Transcript*, in which it is asserted, on the authority of Dr. Magnus of Germany, that 'the surest test of death is to tie a string snugly around a finger or toe; if the subject be not dead, the member thus tied becomes red, and grows constantly deeper and darker colored, until it is tinged a blue red from the end to the point where it is ligated. Comparative experiments on the living body and on the cadaver have in every instance proved this satisfactorily.' "[103]

In 1873, Dr. Safford-Blake became affiliated either through the medical school or on a charitable basis with the Cullis Consumptive Home, an 80-bed tuberculosis treatment facility founded in 1864 to care for indigent consumptives in the disease's final throes.[104][105] Since both tuberculosis' cause and cure were unknown, such homes were necessary, but nothing further is known of Mary's activity there.

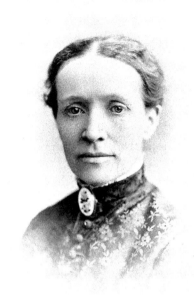

Mary Jane Safford. Courtesy Boston University School of Medicine Alumni Medical Library.

While Mary had a full social and professional life in early 1873, other events may have distracted her. Brother A.P.K. divorced wife Jenny through an act of the Arizona Territorial Legislature's placing him as Governor in the unique situation of decreeing his own divorce.[106] Concurrently, Joel Matteson's Springfield, Illinois, palatial mansion and nearly all its contents burned, and three days later Matteson died in Chicago.[107] Additionally, America encountered rough economic straits later called the Financial Panic of 1873.[108] Suffering massive unemployment, financial upheaval, lowered wages, and fiscal scandal, the depression was second only to that of the 1930s. Whether Mary or Gorham suffered from this is unknown, but at least she had marketable skills.

Aside from assisting Mary in designing the medical instrument, little is known of Gorham's activities during their marriage. As in most of his adult life, he changed occupations and now was sole agent for Tilghman's Sand Blast, purveyor of equipment for industrial and artistic purposes.[109] Essentially, he was a salesman serving the company's distribution offices in Boston, New York, and Chicago. Possibly, after twenty years' adventure and freedom from conventional living, he found settling into a stable domestic life difficult. Both he and Mary had specific niches in Boston, but aside from their only child of a medical instrument, their lives did not appear to overlap.

In June 1873, Mary attended the Cleveland AIH meeting and resumed medical politicking she began in Chicago.[110] She was named to the AIH Bureau of Obstetrics and the Board of Censors, the first woman to hold an AIH office. Since Chicago's Dr. Ludlam and Boston's Dr. Woodbury were bureau members, Dr. Safford-Blake was hobnobbing with the brightest stars in the homeopathic gynecologic galaxy. She presented a paper entitled, "Inversion of the Uterus," a polished, more thorough account of her May 1873 *New England Medical Gazette* report and described the instrument she and Gorham devised but gave him no credit.[111] Her paper and presentation received rave reviews in the next months' national homeopathic medical journals.[112] By now, Mary had met most of the important men and a few intrepid women in her field and joined discussions on a collegial rather than token level.

That summer, Mary focused her attention on another project. In April, the New York women's organization Sorosis hatched the idea of forming a national women's rights group to be comprised of all reform and rights minded women whose coordinated strength far outweighed individual efforts in the women's rights arena.[113] Their topics of interest included several near and dear to Mary's heart including woman's higher education, dress reform, and woman in surgery and medicine. The overwhelmingly positive initial response to the inquiry for interest among America's elite women led to a September 1873, "Call," for an October Congress of Women. Promoters' names read like roll call for famous 19th century women. "Mary J. Safford, MD," appeared along with Mary A. Livermore, Frances Willard,

Julia Ward Howe, Elizabeth Cady Stanton, Prof. Maria Mitchell, Kate Doggett, Mrs. F. J. M. Whitcomb and over a hundred others who proposed calling themselves the Association for the Advancement of Women. This was possibly a play on the name American Association for the Advancement of Science, an organization to which several of the Call's signers including Mary Safford belonged. President Mary Livermore led the First Congress in New York in October 1873 with Dr. Mary Safford-Blake among 27 Executive Committee members. The next year she was among its Vice-Presidents. Although she made no presentation at this first meeting, numerous others' works ranged from Rev. Celia Burleigh's and Abba G. Woolson's, "The Relation of Woman to Her Dress," to Elizabeth Cady Stanton's, "The Co-Education of the Sexes."[114] Mary likely heard those along with lectures on temperance, suffrage, women professors, and one on, "Social Aspects of the Readmission of Women into the Medical Profession," by allopathic Dr. Mary Putnam Jacobi.[115] Fortunately, the allopathic vs. homeopathic controversy had not visibly spread to the AAW. Subsequent meetings provided continued networking opportunities for Mary who remained active at least through 1886.[116]

As if Mary wasn't busy enough, Salem's Essex Institute elected her to membership in October 1873.[117] Through merging of Essex County's Historical and Natural History Societies, the institute was a repository for numerous historical and natural history publications and objects.[118] Mary may have joined to access their library and collection of over 30,000 items, but notices of her regular correspondence in ensuing years showed her deeper involvement. Gorham Blake was not a member of this or the AAAS.

In November 1873, with a 26-member faculty, Dean I. T. Talbot presided at opening exercises of the Boston University School of Medicine.[119] Although involved in designing the new school's curriculum, Mary may not have taught immediately, as her subjects were more appropriate for upperclassmen.[120] Admission standards for the coeducational, three-year school were high, requiring either a bachelor-of-arts degree or passage of an entrance exam.[121] Dr. Safford-Blake wrote to Chicago homeopaths of her experience:

"Boston News: --Dear Investigator: ... I must first tell you of our infantile, but vigorous college...you can well imagine my pleasure and surprise to know that at 9 o'clock, the appointed morning hour for the first lecture, at the tap of the bell, students were in order, and professor at his post, and since that time everything has moved off like clock-work. With dispensary rooms to arrange, and a dispensary to open; with a spacious amphitheater under way; with many changes to institute in the college building, you can well understand that busy work has been going on behind the scenes...the Boston University School of Medicine was built a few years since for the New England Woman's Medical College, in which a school exclusively for women has been carried on until now. It is situated opposite the City Hospital on an open space of ground, a generous slice of which is being negotiated for as the site of the new Homoeopathic Hospital, to establish which a fund of $100,000, you will remember, was raised some two years ago or more, through the efforts of a Fair...'

'At the expiration of ten years from the time Mr. Rich endowed the Boston university, it will come in possession of over a million of dollars, and it is doubtless well that there is a few years interim before becoming fully possessed of it, so that each department will accustom itself to the virtue of economy... The Faculty of the College is, I think, known to you. If any of the brethren of the heroic school should hint in the gentle manner characteristic of them, that it is composed of ignoramuses, you can tell them that in so doing they are heaping ignominy upon one of their cherished Alma-maters, for several possess parchments stamped with Harvard's 'well done, good and faithful servant.'

The majority, I think, have studied in foreign universities, and a number took their degrees there. Each seems to approach the work assigned him, determined to do his best for the advancement of the students, seventy of whom have matriculated this term. That which is still called an experiment here, but which in Chicago has long since proven a success, co-education and co-operation in medical studies and work, goes on as one should expect it to where professors and students are high–toned men and women…You will see by this that our three years' course means work. I should like to enter into the details of our course, but if I tell you all I know this time, you will not desire to hear from me again, and so I will close… ever yours sincerely, Mary J Safford Blake. Jan. 6, '74"[122]

Two months later, a listing under, "Special Notices," in the women's rights publication *The Woman's Journal*, read:

"Dr. Mary J. Safford-Blake. Residence and office No. 16 Boylston Place. Office hours 11-2. Tuesdays excepted."[123]

Just as a physician might relocate today, Mary probably sought better space or lower rent, but, in moving, she left Gorham. Her new fashionable address was at the end of a short alleyway off busy Boylston Street and a short distance from Boston Common. As well as having a popular medical practice, she gained a coveted Massachusetts Homeopathic Medical Society membership in spring 1874.[124] Also, Boston's, "Business Woman's Mutual Benefit Association," a health and life insurance group, named Mary one of its vice-presidents.[125] To further occupy her time, Mary launched a staunch dress reform crusade.

10 THE DRESS REFORM CRUSADER

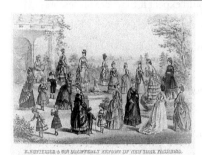

Assorted 1870 fashionable women's dresses in E. Butterick & Company's quarterly report. Library of Congress Prints and Photographs Division, 200467234.

Beneath the lovely dresses lurked the diabolical corset. Corset ad, 1860–80. Library of Congress Prints and Photographs Division, 2002696098

Through her travels, Mary Safford-Blake viewed fashions unimaginable to ordinary Americans. The freedom of movement offered by harem women's loose garments sharply contrasted with 19th century Western women's ridiculously constrictive clothing with its steel ribbed corsets, large bustles, and long, heavy, dirt-catching skirts.

Beginning in January 1873, lay periodical *Herald of Health* published three long articles entitled, "Ornament and Dress," by Dr. Mary J. Safford (sans Blake).[1] The first gave a world-view of clothing styles and body decorations. From her memories of British Museum specimens, Mary compared the skull deformities inflicted on African children and the bone-crushing foot binding of aristocratic Chinese girls to the follies of Americans' corseted martyrdom. The second article addressed American women's upbringing to be delicate, weak creatures starved for proper exercise and health by a negligent educational system. Mary's sarcastically toned narrative contained examples of fashion foibles' leading girls to a dissipated life, as their style choices implied membership in the world's oldest profession. The final article explained how various military uniforms determined European battle outcomes. She felt Germans prevailed in the Franco-Prussian War specifically for, "more practical and healthful," attire and summarized with a battle cry:

"The women of America to-day are situated much as soldiers of the empire were; they have outlived the social tactics of feudal times, and are now called forth to fight the battle of life as responsible, earnest individuals.'

'Shall they meet these responsibilities with a burden of clothing excelling in weight the armor of the knights of old. Shall they be bound at every joint, fettered at every limb, compressed about the vital organs, not by one leathern girdle, but by a multitude of tightly adjusted bands and bones; shall they carry upon their trailing garments the filth and rain of the streets; or shall they go forth under the new dispensation so dressed as to meet the demands of an active life, freed from the tyranny of fashion that dictates without reason to soul and body?"[2]

Her fiery rhetoric must have touched raw nerves in women who lived within fashions' bounds but were too timid to free themselves from its tyranny. Mary helped reignite the war on absurd fashion and even aimed her weapons at its very fabric by including caveats on poisonous green and magenta dyed cloth.[3] She summarized her proposals for change:

"It seems to me that our first study in dress should be, in regard to the style and material selected; first, what is healthful; second, what is becoming, and third, what is fashionable.'

'As the French Revolution swept away the fantastically absurd costumes of men, so would an American revolution—a revolution of ideas and of education—relieve us from this bondage of dress, so illy becoming our day and generation."[4]

Mary's reform ideas commenced with fashion but proposed curing a panoply of social ills. She continued:

"Give to women high aims and ennobling aspirations, educate them to a purpose as men are educated, instead of making them parasites, of teaching them to live on the growth and vigor of other lives, make them self-supporting.'

'Elevate marriage to the rank of a divine institution, instead of making it a degrading contract, a moneyed matter, a means of support to women."[5]

Appearing less than nine months after her marriage, Mary's words don't sound like those of a happy newlywed. She was then 41 years old, and years of self-reliance may have precluded her offering compromises necessary to live amicably with a man. Perhaps she had an epiphany about Gorham Blake's true character.

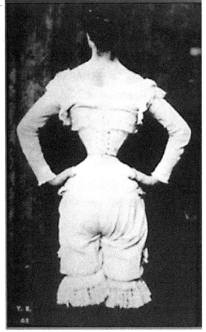

Years of, "corset training," sometimes commencing in early childhood, led to the highly prized, "wasp waist." Victoria and Albert Museum, London.

In fall 1873, Mary heard Abba Goold Woolson's lecture on, "The Relation of Woman to Her Dress," at the AAW's New York meeting.[6] After Elizabeth Stuart Phelps' lecture, "Dress Reform," the New England Woman's Club established a committee on the subject chaired by Mrs. Woolson with consultants Dr. Mary J. Safford-Blake and Dr. and Mrs. Dio Lewis.[7] The following winter and spring, Abba Woolson and Doctors Safford-Blake, Haynes, Hastings and Jackson presented a free lecture series entitled, "Dress, As It Affects the Health of Women."[8] Dr. Safford-Blake presented the first lecture at the Arlington Street Unitarian Church vestry on February 25, 1874, a day of blinding snowstorm.[9] Prominent allopathic physician, abolitionist, and proponent of women's medical practice Dr. Henry I. Bowditch introduced her to the packed audience of prominent women and four men. A report noted her dressing as she advocated and her candor:

"...no masculine agitator would for one moment dare to use the boldness of description and of advice on the subject of ladies' attire which will be found in this lecture...She understands the subject as only a woman can; as a thoroughly trained physician she has studied it in all its physiological and hygienic bearings; and she evinces throughout a proper regard to the demands of taste, the customs and conveniences of society and to the feminine nature.'

'Dr. Blake states that considerable progress has been made in maturing recommendations as to the material, arrangement and style of female clothing, having regard particularly to health and convenience... whole subject handled with wit, propriety, intelligence and vigorous thoughtfulness."[10]

Mary's topics included ills caused by temperature disparity from one body part to another, constrictive corsets' displacing internal organs, absurd clothing

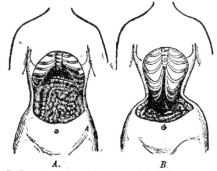

A. lbs of large curve; the lungs large my; the liver, stomach and bow-their normal position; all with nt room.

B. The ribs bent almost to angles lungs contracted; the liver, stomac intestines forced down into the p crowding the womb seriously.

Nature versus Corsets, Illustrated.

Corset effects on the body. "Golden Thoughts on Chastity and Procreation," John William Gibson, Toronto, ON, 1903, p. 107. Library of Congress Prints and Photographs Division, 2002716762.

weight, necessity of exercise, the dangers of wearing, " false hair," "cosmetic poisons," long skirts' leading to mud-bedraggled hems, and the:

"…décolleté dress of the salon…historically one of the relics of the period of lust, when women were shut out of the kingdom of thought and were linked with men only in bonds of sensuality."[11]

She recycled her story of the evening at the German professor's home where his wife graciously entertained while unapologetically wearing her unaltered fourteen-year-old wedding dress. Mary concluded by emphatically advocating reforms including suitably warm undergarments, suspension of all clothing weight from the shoulders, suspension of stockings from a vest or union suit, leggings for winter, thick and wide-soled, low and broad-heeled shoes year around, clothing to be constructed of sturdy, washable cloth, and no hat veils, especially spotted ones that caused blindness.[12]

Later that year, Mrs. Woolson published the lectures' transcripts with a notice of the dress committee's store's offering, "reform," garments at 25 Winter Street, room 15, over Chandler's dry-goods store. A later writer attributed a quote to Mary's lecture though not in Ms. Woolson's transcript:

"As regards jewels, if they must be worn, to show them to the best advantage, follow the example of the Apache squaws, and hang them on the nose."[13]

The 1870s dress reformers felt that changing undergarment structure without drastically changing clothing's outward appearance would avoid pitfalls that led to the earlier Bloomer movement's failure. Apparently, Mary practiced what she preached but still suffered the slings and arrows of outraged detractors when, reputedly, in response to her appearance, she was harassed by a, "…hooting mob of loafers and small boys."[14]

Dress reform promotion surfaced at the Second Radical Club two months later:

"Mrs. A. G. Woolson read a paper full of earnest and beautiful thought, on 'Dress Reform,' before the Second Radical Club, last Monday evening. Dr. Bartol, Mrs. Zina Fay Peirce, Mrs. Mary Safford Blake, Miss Hotchkiss and others followed in an interesting discussion."[15]

Melusina Fay Peirce wrote on co-operative housekeeping and in 1868 organized a group of 40 households, rented an appropriately equipped building in Harvard Square, and embarked on what resulted in an unsuccessful three-year experiment in shared household tasks' including charging the participants' husbands for services rendered.[16] Such exposure to Zina may not have helped Mary's relations with Gorham. Also, Mary's participation at the club's events and constant dress reform promotion may have made her a target of writer Sherwood Bonner's scandalous and satirical poem, "The Radical Club." This parodied Edgar Allen Poe's, "The Raven," and appeared in the *Boston Sunday Times* May 1875.[17] These stanzas reflected Mary's views well:

"Then a lively little charmer, noted as a dress reformer,

Because that mystic garment called a chemiloon she wore,

Said she had no "views" of Jesus, and therefore would not tease us,

But that she thought 'twould please us to look her figure o'er,

For she wore no bustles anywhere; and corsets she felt sure

Should squeeze her nevermore.'

'This pretty little pigeon, said of course the true religion

Demanded ease of body before the mind could soar;

But that no emancipation could come unto our nation

Until the aggregation of the clothes that women wore

Were suspended from the shoulder, and smooth with many a gore

Plain behind and plain before!"[18]

Even years later, Dr. Safford-Blake's dress reform comments at Second Radical Club meetings were considered memorable:

"Dr. Mary Safford Blake was a lively member, sternly convinced that humanity's destiny hinged upon woman's corsets, and seldom popping into the discussion without mention of feminine raiment as 'rags' and 'duds.' 'Why do we women sit here today in wet rags while every man is dry?' she asked, indignantly…"[19]

Mary bore the dress reform crusade's banner everywhere including it in her medical writing wherever possible and reporting it in the *New England Medical Gazette*.[20] Under the name Mary I. (sic) Safford-Blake, MD, a letter to the *North American Journal of Homeopathy* appeared as the article, "Lac Defloratum."[21] She described refusing treating a patient's pains until the woman dressed more prudently. Upon this occurring, Mary tried various homeopathic remedies without response until she dispensed extreme dilutions of Lac Defloratum presented upon small pellets. Mary attributed the woman's return to vigorous health to infinitesimally small doses of Lac Defloratum. And just what was this magical substance? Answer: skimmed cows' milk.[22] Perhaps the change in dress was helpful after all.

Mary's dress reform pieces continued appearing in lay literature, and her allegorical piece entitled, "How a Daughter was Educated," was in the *Herald of Health*.[23] She related the maudlin travails of a young brother and sister whose formerly wealthy parents' deaths left the siblings penniless, destitute, and, in the daughter's case, devoid of hope for her lack of self-supporting skills and poor clothing choices. Mary summed the girl's sad educational deficit and hapless lot in a sentence that foreshadowed a theme Mary enlarged in her later book *Health and Strength for Girls*:

"If my body had only been considered of some importance as well as my soul, I might then have had health and strength upon which to rely now in this time of need, and then I could do---something."[24]

June 9-12, 1874, the AIH annual meeting was in Niagara Falls, New York, and Dr. Mary Safford-Blake was to have served on the Board of Censors.[25] The meeting's transactions included her paper's recounting her Viennese puerperal fever outbreak experiences.[26] Later reports noted her not attending or serving on the Board of Censors due to, "failing health."[27] It is curious that despite illness' preventing her AIH meeting attendance, a miraculous recovery allowed her active participation in one of the most publicized 1874 dress reform events. *The New York Times* reported Boston's June

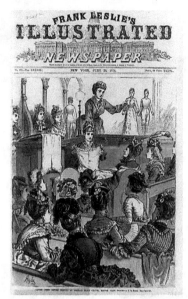

'Ladies' Dress Reform Meeting at Freeman Place Chapel,'
Frank Leslie's Illustrated, 20 Jun 1874, wood engraving
after sketch by E. R. Morse. Library of Congress Prints and
Photographs Division, 90705405.

10th Dress Reform Convention:

"For some time the more daring spirits of the 'club' have been studying and experimenting in variations, more or less radical, from the established rules of costume. A few days since the 'club' held a meeting at Freeman Place Chapel, for the exhibition of inventions in ladies' clothing calculated to give the wearers more freedom of action and less physical discomfort.'

'After brief introductory remarks by the President, the ladies who had garments to exhibit were called upon. Mrs. B., a physician of no little local repute and social standing, exhibited several garments which, she said, she had found better adapted to her own wants than the ordinary female costume..."[28]

The nationally circulated *Frank Leslie's Illustrated* further reported:

"...No living models were exhibited by way of illustrating the advantages of the proposed reforms, as was said to have been done at the recent convention held in San Francisco, but large dolls were used as lay-figures on which to display the improved gowns and underwear."[29]

News of the San Francisco event's live underwear models must have sold far more papers in 1874. The following November's *Herald of Health* reported the event and Mary's long letter regarding undergarment designs including those of Mrs. Crane's chemiloons, a united chemise and pantaloon.[30] Mary wrote of the chemiloon elsewhere with alternate names of chemile, chemilette, chemette, get-in, under-all and union-garment.[31] Its purpose was total body temperature equalization Mary thought necessary for health. She revealed personally wearing a similar undergarment and invented a novel construction for it using commercial patterns she altered to her own specifications. Of course, here also, Mary railed against corsets and wasp waists while lamenting patented designs' causing high prices for healthful dress.

Mary expanded her dress reform message through advertising testimonials to various dress reform products such as the LGS or, "Ladies' Garment Suspenders." The ad's illustration showed two simple over the shoulder straps attached to a skirt's waistband, and supporting dialog read:

"Suspending skirts about the waist is and ever has been a greater curse to the human family than the use of both Rum and Tobacco. The remedy for this former is the 'L. G. S.' To cure or prevent the latter, never put anything strong or nasty into the mouth."[32]

In September 1874, Mary took her message west to the Illinois Industrial University, precursor to the University of Illinois at Champaign, IL.[33] She either previously knew or then met fellow dress reform advocate Louisa Catherine Allen, the school's home economist and teacher of domestic science and physical education.[34] *Daily Illini's* report of Mary's visit failed mentioning her lecture topic, but Mary later recounted speaking extemporaneously on dress reform there.[35]

Perhaps on this visit Mary encountered Professor of Geology and Zoology Don Carlos Taft.[36] His vast paleontological and mineral collection would have intrigued her.[37] Also, Taft was deeply involved in developing the university's natural history museum with its many collections that included a herbarium that might interest a homeopath.[38] Affectionately known as, "Darn Careless Taft," he acquired his professorship in 1872 and replaced John Wesley Powell who had been elected to Professorship but left the university for one of his Colorado River voyages' ending in Arizona Territory, home of A. P. K. Safford.[39] [40] In March 1875, approximately six months after Mary's university visit, A. P. K. sought and received in Pima County, Arizona Territory, guardianship for 7-year old, "orphan," Leandro Taft, born in Sonora, Mexico, son of Carlos Taft.[41] In the guardianship papers A. P. K. swore to, "properly educate, rear and instruct," Leandro who a few years later joined Mary's Boston household.

On this same trip, Mary visited southern Illinois schools including one in Cairo where she saw a new instruction method:

"A recent interesting feature connected with public schools in Cairo, Ill., is the introduction of telegraphy. All communication in the classes between pupils and teachers, is carried on by means of the telegraph, and in this way every ear becomes skilled in reading its language.'

'Ten years since there was not a free public school for the numerous colored population of Cairo. Now there is a high school, an intermediate and primary department, under the judicious and intelligent instruction of colored women teachers. Formerly these hundreds of children were considered stupid, unteachable, 'niggers.' Now, no one can look into their bright faces and listen to their ready recitations, without acknowledging their intelligence, and without believing that the day is not far distant when the accident of race and color will be lost sight of in our schools. When, side by side, each will be taught by competent teachers, be they white or colored."[42]

Although currently concentrating on dress reform, Mary maintained strong opinions on racial equality and hoped for integration that did not materialize in her lifetime. She remained in Illinois for the AAW's October Chicago event. Topics included dress reform with a private women's reform clothing exhibit as reported:

"Dr. Mary Blake exhibited several undergarments, fashioned after the kind she herself wore, and which were especially well adapted for female physicians, being quickly put on and off."[43]

Mary and dressmaker Olivia Flynt presented detailed information:

"Mary Safford Blake discussed the advantages of the chemiloon before a mixed audience at the Second Woman's Congress in Chicago; it was a discourse notable for its frankness. 'I will say legs,' she declared, 'whenever I mean legs.' Loud applause greeted both the chemiloon and Blake's candor. Her speech, coupled with the exhortations of others, triggered genuine demand."[44]

Mary gave her usual anti-corset talk, but women who tried dressing sans corsets complained of an, "all gone," sensation due to their weak abdominal musculature's inability to constrain internal organs. An audience member's solution to this dilemma provided tabloid fodder:

"Here Mrs. Vibbard of Massachusetts, spoke, and said that those who took off their corsets and suffered with the all-gone feeling should make their husband manipulate their bodies until they felt strong and a reaction took place. Some unkind member asked what those women were to do who had no husbands to rub them down, but her question was not answered. It was evident that there was the rub."[45]

At this same Chicago meeting, Mary lectured on, "Our Inheritance with Reference to Prenatal Influences," a topic she expounded upon through speeches and pen the next year. The AAW elected astronomer and Vassar College President Dr. Maria Mitchell President for 1875 and Dr. Mary Safford-Blake one of several Vice-Presidents.[46]

On return to Boston from her three-week western sojourn, Mary visited the then six-year old Cornell University.[47] After meeting with its first President Andrew White and Professor Burt Green Wilder, she was optimistic for the school's future although her report lacked description of Wilder's unique lecture style recounted elsewhere:

"White imposed on him the duty of giving annually an obligatory course of lectures on physiology and hygiene to the freshman class. In later times the course dwindled to a single lecture in sex hygiene, in which his dramatic demonstrations caused many an auditor to faint."[48]

The main events of Mary's dress reform efforts now past, she continued lecturing, writing, and teaching dress reform for years.[49][50] At least one individual did not appreciate her campaign. BUSM student Frances Janney wrote home in May 1875:

"Take Dr. Blake for instance. She may do an immense amount of good, but she talks of 'dress reform' continually and makes herself disagreeable to many thereby. She goes at the men and tells them its their faults that women dress as they do. What if it is, it does no good to hurl it at them in that way. And besides she goes to the other extreme... Really, it seems Dr. Blake's object to make women as much like men as possible."[51]

Janney even criticized Mary's appearance:

"...simply ridiculous on the rostrum! Her dress is so short that you can almost see the tops of her shoes and such shoes! Run down at the heels, big enough for a woman twice her size, and not even dusted."[52]

Likely, Mary wasn't pondering shoe dust as she began her new lecture series.

11 FURTHER NORTHERN LIFE

Although never ceasing dress reform promotion, Mary's new topic was, "Prenatal Influence," and the *Herald of Health* printed her AAW paper verbatim.[1] She invited the audience's imagining outside influences' changing a microscopic germ cell's potential for differentiation into an adult form. Included were Darwin's thoughts, plant and animal genetics, and Francis Galton's eugenics. She followed with examples of developmental idiosyncrasies before embarking on outside forces' causing intellectual and mental aberrations. Mary then provided examples of famous artists' familial traits before she discussed parental prenatal impressions on offspring:

"As the sculptor models the plastic clay into an ideal form, giving his best thought to its conception and creation so may the parent, directed by love divine, in harmony of spirit and holiness of purpose, influence the embryotic germ as his will directs. We may have the clean offspring of a holy marriage, or the child of lust..."[2]

Mary compared parental sensory impressions on a fetus to a, "photographer's impression left upon the negative, which awaits only the proper conditions for development."[3] As far as she was concerned, all of a child's intrauterine and later maturation hinged upon the parents' prior experiences. She preached the evils of alcohol abuse, provided examples of its ill effects and thought it caused inherent alcoholism and mental illness in offspring. She also railed against tobacco, tea, coffee and spices as gateway substances' leading to, "the desire for stronger irritants."[4] She concluded with a cheery message on happy households' breeding superior children.

Later, in a manner possibly suggesting personal sexual repression, she spoke disparagingly on, "hereditary sensuality:"

"It would indeed seem a miracle of saving grace if children begotten in hot-beds of licentiousness, and sired perhaps by inebriate fathers, should not be branded by the lusts of the flesh; children with such precocious animal passions show a prurient curiosity in regard to their own sexual organs and those of other children and of animals. Unless all this can be stopped the worst possible results may be anticipated." [5]

Her broad lecture topics suited a variety of audiences including one Mary felt truly needed it—young women. As house physician for the girls' Lasell Seminary, she taught physiology and hygiene in 1874-75.[6][7] Lasell's numerous ads in church and lay publications touted Dr. Mary Safford-Blake's instruction. A letter to *Herald of Health* reported:

"...The school is very fortunate in having Dr. Blake in charge of that department. She knows just what's wanted for our girls, and just how to supply it. The day will come when it will not be thought a matter of course that our young women who have graduated at a school should be sickly, feeble bodies, and without physical capital with which to begin the more serious duties of womanhood."[8]

She spoke on health intermittently at Lasell in Auburndale, Massachusetts, for years, and today it is four-year degree granting, coeducational Lasell College that prides itself on pioneering women's physical education.

In May and June 1875, Mary lectured both young women and their teachers over several days at Boston's Gannett Institute, another progressive girls' school.[9] Illinois Industrial University Professor Louisa Allen attended and recorded verbatim, likely stenographic, notes on the talks, "The Womb and Menstruation," "The Beginnings of Life," and, "Food and Nutrition." Mary began her first lecture by calling books on reproduction aimed at young people mere treatises on anatomy and physiology, full of large words and impractical technical explanations of little interest to their audience. Through a very lengthy discussion, she delicately described human anatomy including the reproductive system using accurate, clear wording and did not mince words when discussing puberty and dangers of masturbation:

"… it is a fearful evil, found in high places as well as low and because it does exist very largely through ignorance. It must be spoken of, so that every woman, girl may know how to help herself and others. I refer to self abuse…very soon the poor suffer (sic) finds that she has no control over her will and gives herself up to practices that very soon undermine her health and if continued in very long the brain too becomes affected and insanity, idiocy or what is even more terrible than either she seeks companions who take advantage of her."[10]

With equal candor, Dr. Safford-Blake introduced concepts of menarche, ovulation, female genital anatomy, normal and abnormal menstruation, menopause and, of course, dress reform.

In presenting her lecture on embryonic and newborn growth and development, Mary compared analogous processes in other animals including kangaroos, viviparous fish, whales, catfish, toads and hens. She carefully described human pregnancy and fetal development, how to deliver a baby with practical points on cutting the umbilical cord and delivering the placenta, then reiterated her prenatal influence lecture tailored for her younger audience. Mary followed with caveats against stimulating substances including tobacco. Apparently, she spoke from experience in her advice on picking a marriage partner:

"…two lives so soon to be blended in one ought to ascertain by the mutual and most unreserved interchange of thought, the opinions desired and feelings of the other upon all the vital topics pertaining to the interests of both…'

'Two individuals should strive in every way to know each other in temperament and in disposition. There should be a harmonious sympathy in the opinions and tastes of the two persons although the perfect blending of thought can only come with time. There never can be, and there never should be a giving up and a loss of individuality on the part of either man or woman. Each strong and true in his own way is the needed counterpart of the other.'

'Wealth takes to itself wings, position is fleeting, health is precarious, so that the only thing that may and can and should abide to all eternity, with husband and wife is love.'

'It is a truth that every young girl and woman should cherish in her heart that if marriage does not come as a divine gift to elevate and strengthen the soul in growth that she is far better without it. I am glad to know that the stigma of old maid does not brand women now as useless."[11]

Mary finished with a diatribe against abortion that she called a growing evil, equal to murder, dangerous to the mother, and explained that life began at conception and not in the 4th month, as was the impression then.

Her food and nutrition talk mirrored modern dietary ideas somewhat.[12] She advised against ingesting pepper, highly seasoned foods, pastries, white flour, very cold drinks and overeating in general then launched a long description of humans' digestion times for various meats.

Louisa Allen's notes on Mary's presentation entitled "Generation," suggest it was directed at an older audience, as she used much anatomical detail and medical terminology. An accompanying reading list was more suitable for sex education teachers than adolescent girls.

Albeit known more for her teaching and dress reform positions than as an ardent suffragist, Mary was one. In April 1874, she wrote a scathing article about Glastonbury, Connecticut's, taxing authorities' mistreating the Smith sisters.[13]

The women's refusal to pay unfairly levied property taxes led to the town's confiscating their assets in a case that became a cause célèbre for woman suffrage. Mary was not a property owner yet, but she empathized through political action via the world of public education. In December 1874, Democrats endorsed and Republicans nominated Mary to represent Ward 16 on the Boston School Committee. On her election she was one of its very first serving female members.[14] She worked actively but lost election the next year.[15]

Although Mary was childless, her interest in early childhood education led to her becoming one of numerous vice-presidents of the American Froebel Union that promoted kindergartens.[16] Near the Kindergarten Movement's start, Mary traveled to Florence, Massachusetts, where she may have consulted with radical abolitionist Samuel Hill's Nonotuck Silk Company about materials for reform underclothing.[17] Possibly, she came specifically to meet Hill, founder in 1876 of the Hill Institute, one of the U.S.' first kindergartens, then and now, free to every Florence child. Started in his home, Hill's class moved to Cosmian Hall built by Florence's Free Congregational Society that Hill founded.[18] Impressed by the organization's Sunday school session, Mary wrote of an imaginary such class though not specifically naming Hill in, "The Ideal Sunday School."[19] Her model kindergarten taught science and theories of Darwin, Spencer and Huxley but did not cover traditional Christian doctrine, the Bible, or even mention God. She supposedly helped Dr. William P. Wilson and a Mr. Hyde in establishing Boston's charity kindergartens in 1876.[20]

Of course, Mary still actively practiced medicine, taught at BUSM and was named to BU's, "Faculty of the School of All Sciences."[21] Her subjects included, "Menstruation as a natural function and its deviations; hysteria; ovarian physiology and pathology; ovarian tumors, their diagnosis and treatment; diseases of the uterine ligaments; diseases of the mammae."[22] With the immense amount of pathology and complicated physiology of these systems, Mary's lecture subjects were huge even in the 1870s. Reputedly, her course's 3½-hour examination consisted of 36 essay questions, daunting to both students and the teacher's grading.[23] Also, Mary was preceptor to four women students one being fellow AAW director and friend Fidelia Whitcomb who later joined her in medical practice.[24][25]

When first in Boston, Mary undoubtedly faced the same frustrations at gender discrimination's barring her from Chicago's hospitals, for a working surgeon needs staff privileges and operating room access. Boston's women worked too long and hard promoting the coeducational medical school to tolerate the affiliated hospital's precluding women physicians.[26] By the mid-1870s, Mary received staff appointment to the Massachusetts Homeopathic Hospital where she practiced until 1885. She joined the hospital's Medical Board in 1884.[27]

Making the most of referrals, Mary reported memorable cases including that of a 47-old woman with years of indigestion, pain, irritability, insomnia and, "rectal tumor," with origins' confounding all prior physicians. Mary's operative description:

"...By slow degrees and with great care, which was especially needed, owing to the haemorrhoids, the entire hand was introduced into the rectum, and circumscribed the tumor, which proved to be a detached, solid ball. It was removed whole, not without considerable haemorrhage, and was about the size of a childs head at the sixth month of pregnancy. Another, the size and somewhat the shape of a goose egg was removed, as well as several lesser ones.'

'But whence came these solid, stone like balls? For several years, owing to her dyspeptic tendencies and to constipation, she had been in the habit of eating magnesia... and by continuous accretion, the result was what had been found."[28]

In the spirit of making lemonade of lemons, Mary made a magazine article of magnesia. One has to admire a woman

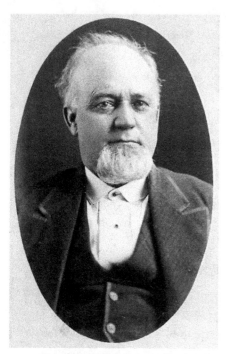

Alfred Boardman Safford, 1870s. Courtesy Cairo, IL, Public Library.

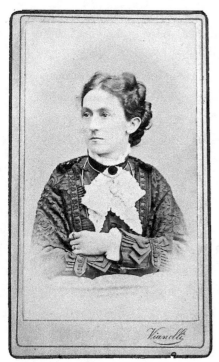

Anna Candee Safford, wife of A. B. Safford, circa 1880s.
Courtesy Cairo, IL, Public Library.

who radiates propriety while simultaneously extracting stone balls from a rectum.

Her schedule left little time for rest, but, in summer 1875, she traveled west with brothers A.P.K. and Alfred, his wife Anna, and Chicago's Universalist Reverend J. S. Dennis and his wife.[29]

Ever observing women's dress mode, Mary documented it and other Salt Lake City sights in a long letter to the *Woman's Journal.* With a play on William Cullen Bryant's poem, "The Battle-Field," with line, "Truth crushed to earth, shall rise again," Mary described the Mormon women's new fashion worldliness' leading Mormon Leader Brigham Young to cringe and regret encouraging Utah's railroad development:

"Since the railroad has brought the Saints into direct communication with the outside world, Brigham has found an unconquerable enemy in milliners and dressmakers. For many years the Mormon women were dressed in plain homespun and home-made material; in the language of the poet, Brigham will now have to exclaim that, 'Fashion crushed to earth will rise again and you cannot stop her.' " [30]

Although not meeting Young, Mary attended Mormon Tabernacle services and had frank discussions with Mormon women including one among his 55 wives called the, "poet of Salt Lake." During a service Mary attended, Young's daughter (one of his 58 children) read an essay on trials of the, "Latter Day Saints."[31][32] Mary discussed polygamy with Emmeline B. Woodward Harris Whitney Wells, editor of the Mormon *Woman's Exponent.*[33] Entering pleural marriage several times, she was Utah's vice president for the National Woman Suffrage Association. Mary reported her as very intelligent and her, "free and frank conversation," about polygamy:

"...I could never have conceived it possible for women to believe in the rightfulness of polygamy...But, they said, 'The greater the cross here, the surer the crown hereafter.' " [34]

Apparently, Emmeline was not completely convincing of polygamy's charms, and Mary researched further at an afternoon Tabernacle lecture on marriage given by Elder Orson Pratt, Quorum of the Original 12 Apostles of the Mormon Church member. She recounted his talk:

"They look upon marriage as a living ordinance...for all eternity...The dead, in ages past or in times modern, who neglected their opportunities here, can be married by proxy...The most entangled family relationship is formed by means of this close and most unnatural intermarriage. A mother and her daughters sometimes become the wives of one man. Baptism, as well as marriage and child-bearing, is effected by proxy..."[35]

She only obliquely referred to Pratt's comments on polyandry where a woman takes more than one husband and dismissed his remarks as, "too distasteful to repeat." Pleural marriage's whole premise must have played mental havoc with Mary Safford's thoughts on prenatal influence. She observed the Mormon women:

"The martyr spirit was deeply impressed upon the countenances of the large majority of women, whom I saw in the Tabernacle. There was no light of joy in their faces. They are the same material which has often been found in all ages and brought under the spell of religious fanaticism. They are ready to be burned at the stake, if need be, for their souls' salvation."[36]

Following Elder Pratt's lecture, Mary called upon his ex-wife Sarah who abhorred polygamy.[37] She married Orson in 1836, and, reputedly, while he was away on a mission trip to England in 1841-42, Mormonism's famous founder Joseph Smith propositioned her to be, "his spiritual wife."[38] Her reputation suffered for her refusal. A controversial series of events led to Orson's becoming an avid polygamist and Sarah's excommunication in 1874.[39] In response to Mary's desiring further publication of the woman's sad story, Sarah's sensational interview appeared in a subsequent *New York Herald* expose.[40] For all Mary's recounting polygamy's restricting Mormon women's rights, she still found hope after meeting a woman graduate of Philadelphia Medical College who had an active practice and contemplated establishing a medical college in Salt Lake City. Mary conceded the Mormons had transformed a desert into a bountiful garden but repudiated their lifestyle:

"...the evils arising from the seeds of immorality in the relations of the sexes which they have sown, will bear fruits of lust long after the system they have inaugurated is dead, and are, it seems to me, far in excess of the good they have done."[41]

Mary and the Illinoisans subsequently traveled by stagecoach across Nevada to California. Her lengthy letter to the *Woman's Journal* detailed women's issues including occupations, settlers' hardships, temperance, all levels of education including university and medical, gender pay equality, Kindergarten Movement (or lack thereof), suffrage and dress reform.[42] She described travel through southern California's more desolate parts but was pleasantly surprised to find women's tending ranches and following the day's progressive movements. After a Los Angeles stop, the group traveled by stage to San Francisco.[43] Mary saw Yosemite but chose reporting recent human activities rather than the valley's appearance. At San Francisco, she wrote of touring the:

"Club Rooms of the 'Pioneer Fathers,' which, in their appointments, are every way complete. There are spacious, elegantly furnished parlors; there is a large and well selected library; there are amusement rooms and the walls are adorned with portraits, in oil, of prominent members...'

'No one entering the State later than 1870 is entitled to membership. We did not need to be told that the pioneer mothers are not members of the society, or frequenters of the club-rooms..."[44]

Presumably, A. P. K. provided Mary's entrée to the Pioneer Fathers' Club Rooms. She met a variety of San Franciscans and toured establishments including a women's engraving firm, public schools and the six-year old University of California that had admitted women since 1870. Another highlight was, "Lotta's Fountain," before its September 1875 dedication.[45] To promote temperance, Mary wrote of the extravagant, expensive and ornate sculpture:

"A veteran Californian said to me: 'Many a man has been induced to drink whisky, who would have drank water, could it have been procured without asking for it at a bar.' "[46]

Mary's other destinations are unknown, but after spending the time and money to travel several thousand miles, she likely saw as much as possible before heading east for the annual AAW meeting in Syracuse, New York, where she was elected a Director.[47] Several months later, she addressed a full meeting of the New England Woman's Club with, "Travels in the East," highlighting parts of her 1860s Grand Tour.[48] In a partially veiled dress reform talk, she detailed Middle-Eastern women's loose clothing and their perceiving Americans' crinolines as an exoskeleton. She recalled the, "Mohammedan temple," with its excluding women's entrance (let alone their entry into Heaven) and recounted her own having accidently touched, "a Mohammedan book, found she had committed a serious offense—a 'Christian dog' not being allowed to pollute so holy a thing."[49]

Divorce papers Mary's lawyer Charles Pratt served on Gorham three years later in Loudsville, Georgia, where he was mining gold, referenced his deserting Mary on May 1, 1876.[50] That August, Gorham's father died at Cambridge, and, soon after, Gorham sailed to Scotland.[51][52] If he and Mary ever met again is unknown. Given Mary's outside activities, the couple's disparate interests, and Gorham's unsettled tendencies, the result was predictable. Perhaps she indulged in numerous pursuits as diversion from an unworkable marriage. Perhaps he retreated because of her pursuits. Concurrently with Gorham's desertion, Mary was president of the Universalist Moral Education Association, an organization that member Edward Hinckley stated:

"...is to educate men and women up to a standard where none but a perfect union could be made. Touching upon the free love doctrines, the speaker urged the largest freedom and purest love, but called no man free who did not hold his passions in the most perfect control."[53]

Other members of this group included A. Bronson Alcott, Lucinda Chandler, Abba Woolson, Caroline Severance, Mary Livermore and others who strived for, "social purity," under the heading of, "free love." Critical medical student Frances Janney's fears of Mary Safford-Blake's, "...traveling toward that terrible free love...she has readings of that sort at her house," were probably justified.[54]

Mary could preach a choice in marriage partners to her young students, but she hadn't chosen wisely herself. Later communications between Gorham and his sister Mary Clapp Young and between her and Gorham's second wife Mary Ann Gordon Blake after his death showed his vast abilities to misrepresent himself. In an 1890 letter to his sister, Gorham offered questionable medical advice and wrote:

"... I took my papers as M.D. about 13 years ago...'

'Just now, aside from my business as a mining engineer, and physician I am much interested in Psychometry..."[55]

A thorough search of 1870-1880s medical school student listings revealed no Gorham Blake among students or graduates. Just as he claimed ability to determine a fossil's origin by handling it, so, too, he claimed special medical powers. He wrote of being a, "psychometric healer," in his letter to a journal that investigated such phenomenon:

"...I had strong magnetic power, which, to cure disease, must emanate from a pure source. To comply with the necessary conditions, I gave up the use of tobacco and all stimulating food and drink, and commenced a diet of plain nourishing food, with plenty of exercise on horseback, and sleep. I soon found my magnetism sought for by invalids for headache, rheumatism, neuralgia, and other disease..."[56]

Gorham's letter to his sister also described his, "medical," practice and partnering with second wife Mary Ann to cure patients merely through contemplating or touching them. If Gorham's sister didn't already think him deranged, she may have upon his reporting recently conversing with physician Dr. Benjamin Rush, a Declaration of Independence signer.

Later, to sister-in-law Mary Young, Gorham's widow Mary Ann Gordon Blake wrote of his penury at their 1885 marriage and destitution on his demise.[57] She also recounted his readily borrowing money and making questionable mining investments but spoke of him in endearing terms:

"I cannot rest till my darling husband's debts are paid even to the last farthing if it is possible for me to do it. I know he had a sanguine temperament and made some mistakes like all the rest of us. But no one had a kinder heart or more generous nature than he."[58]

As for Gorham's final thoughts on Mary Safford, his widow wrote:

"... of the former marriage very little, I felt it was a sad remembrance & never referred to it...Whether he still cherished her memory I never knew."[59]

From all appearances, Gorham Blake was either mentally ill or a con man. Mary's earning potential as physician and possible loneliness as a 40-year old spinster made her a prime mark for a fascinating and penniless con artist. He could weave stories of his worldly adventures' surpassing her real ones and mislead on his life's success. Possibly, the only genuine thing about him was his prominent family name. Mary now understood and was likely relieved at his departure.

In May 1876, the United States Centennial Exhibition opened in Philadelphia's Fairmount Park, and Mary's invention was there. Lacking further description beyond, "surgical instrument, Medicine, Surgery, Prosthesis," the item was in the, "Women's Pavilion."[60] It is unknown if she patented this item--possibly her 1873 uterine prolapse treatment device.[61] Additionally, Philadelphia hosted the 1876 American and World Homeopathic Conventions in late June.[62] Along with BUSM's Drs. Woodbury and Jackson, the program listed Mary among the program's, "Debaters on Obstetrics and Gynecology," tasked with discussing submitted papers. Whether Mary even attended is debatable, as on July 14, 1876, she wrote to former New England Women's Club President Caroline Severance from the East Gloucester house of famed feminist and writer Elizabeth Stuart Phelps:

"I left not nearly two weeks since just in that condition where one straw more would have finished me. I had planned to find rest in visiting the Centennial but my better judgment came to my rescue and instead, I put work one side and went to Nantucket, with two friends..."[63]

Before reaching Phelps' cottage, Mary and her friends rented a Martha's Vineyard house and visited Nantucket that she called a, "Sleepy Hollow," with its very old inhabitants and, "average of twenty-five women to one man."[64] Mary's letter continued:

"I can't conceive of surroundings more heavenly I write you suspended in a hammock on the piazza of Miss Phelps 'oyster shell cottage.' The sea comes within 40 feet of her door and rocks high and rugged reaching to its brink tell of the throes of the ages. Reaching as far as the eye can to is the blue expanse of sea… Dotting the horizon, half concealed and half revealed by a gentle mist, are vessels so indistinct that they may well pass for phantom ships."[65]

Mary signed her name Mary J. S., including neither the initial, "B," nor the name Blake.

In October, the AAW met in Philadelphia with Mary as a Director and on the, "Committee on Reform."[66] While

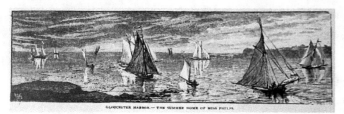

View from Elizabeth Stuart Phelps' Gloucester, Massachusetts, summer cottage. Gilman, Arthur, Poets' Homes: Pen and Pencil Sketches of American Poets and Their Homes, Boston, D. Lothrop, 1879, p. 103.

attempting investigating the conditions of America's incarcerated women and girls, the committee was disappointed that few places would share facts on care of, "Magdalens" (reformed prostitutes), unwed mothers, erring, tempted and destitute girls. Mary continued medical practice, teaching, and, in May 1877, was re-elected president of Boston's Unitarian Moral Education Association for, "personal righteousness."[67] The group now issued leaflets, lectured, and attempted manipulating legislation on what were considered socially evil acts while appealing to police to appoint matrons to station houses to oversee women prisoners' care. She was said to preside over the MEA with:

"… wisdom, dignity, and grace, calling women 'pioneers for the removal of the chief causes of immorality.' "[68]

Like many women of her day, Mary belonged to multiple overlapping reform organizations. In 1878, her election as Boston's First Liberal League Vice-President provided her pulpit to protest pornography.[69] Also, she supported the Women's Educational and Industrial Union or WEIU from its inception.[70] Begun in June 1877 by an 1865 graduate of Mary's medical alma mater, the nonsectarian WEIU promoted sisterhood among all classes of women by providing educational, employment, spiritual, social, and medical services.[71] On the, "Committee of Hygiene and Physical Culture," Life Member Mary provided health lectures and a free clinic.[72] She reprised one of her first WEIU talks, "Some Elements of Success," six years later at Boston University.[73][74]

As BUSM's 1877 summer vacation began, Mary attended Essex Institute's Field Meeting at Boxford and practiced what she preached about exercise while joining fellow institute members for a day's fun and group discussion on diminution of forests.[75] On July 26th, Alfred and Anna Safford were in Burlington, Vermont, with Mary while visiting Cousin Emerson Oels Safford and paternal Aunt Lydia Safford Wilson:

"Mr. Safford went on a visit to his native State. He seemed in perfect health…He drove with an aged relative to the beautiful cemetery in Burlington. She said to him while driving, do you not have a dread of death? No, he replied, it is inevitable, and comes in the order of nature, and when it calls me, I shall be ready and willing to meet it."[76]

Hopefully, he was serious, as Mary's letter to Anna's brother H. H. Candee described the evening's events:

"He had been joyous all day, planning, as usual, for the happiness of others…We were gone perhaps an hour…and were told that Alfred had fallen in apoplexy, and was in a near drug store…We found him sitting in a chair, a Dr. and many around him doing all they could. He recognized us, and spoke indistinctly. We got him into a hack and to the house, and on a lounge—got his feet into hot mustard water, and the Dr. asked him if he could not drink some water, and he said 'I'll try,' and that was the last he spoke. He began to breathe heavily, could not swallow, and in less than an hour he fell peacefully, without a struggle into the sleep of Death."[77]

A.P.K., having recently finished his Territorial governorship, wrote to Anna:

> "Tucson Aug 9 1877
>
> My Dear Sister Anna
>
> I do not know where to direct letters to you have been sending them to Cairo but will now send to Marys address I have just received Marys letter of 27 giving me particulars of dear brothers death I know it is wicked to mourn for him for he is better off than to remain in this world of sorrow but no one ever had such a brother and it seems as though my heart would break If I can do any thing that will smooth your pathway of life it will be my greatest pleasure to do it You was an angel of light to him and have ever been a loving sister to Mary and I and anything I can do for you will be a great pleasure
>
> I hope to see you all soon
> I am too sad to write Lvg yours
> A P K Safford"[78]

Alfred's, "apoplexy," was probably a cerebrovascular accident or stroke. Anna's brother H. H. Candee went east almost immediately by train to accompany her to Blue Island, Illinois, for Alfred's burial there.[79][80] Mary's devotion to Alfred made it likely she joined them. Condolence messages poured in to Anna, and, possibly, she was the one who assembled them in a handmade scrapbook now housed at Cairo's Public Library.

A letter from Jessie Willcox gave insight to Mary's condition:

"…Little Dr. tries to be brave under her double sorrow, I wish I could bear some of it for her…"[81]

Earlier in the same note, Jessie referenced, "my two years with Dr.," and BUSM records show she was Mary's medical student.[82] Perhaps, "double sorrow," referred to the deaths of both Alfred and her marriage.

Two months later, Mary attended a Chicago meeting of an AAW offshoot organization, and again lectured on dress reform.[83] Immediately afterwards, she spoke in Cairo on "Inheritance Mental and Physical," and the $0.25/person donations went to the town's library.[84] She possibly helped Anna with executrix duties, as the women collaborated to sell 1000 acres of Mississippi River land Alfred left them.[85]   Several years later, Anna provided funds and land, along with Mary's donations, for the construction of Cairo's A. B. Safford Memorial Library, a huge Queen Anne style, red stone structure with well appointed interior and even a Tiffany clock.[86] Cairo's library still occupies the building, home to some of the Saffords' original effects. Mary supported it even before Alfred died, and in response to Cairo's young women's soliciting her guidance in choosing library statuary, she suggested busts of Shakespeare, German scientist Alexander von Humboldt, Ben Franklin and abolitionist Charles Sumner.[87] Surprisingly, she suggested no woman.

Autumn 1877, A. P. K. visited Cairo possibly to help with estate settlement and then traveled by train with Anna to Boston.[88] Mary likely welcomed the company, as she had additional sorrow when in December, friend, fellow homeopath, BUSM faculty member, and dress reformer Dr. Mercy Jackson died of, "softening of the brain."[89] Mary persevered with dress reform lectures and spoke twice at the Lowell Unitarian vestry on March 7, 1878.[90] By now, she could probably give the talk in her sleep.

The next summer, Mary visited her friend and former student Dr. Fidelia Whitcomb in Nunda, NY, where she ran

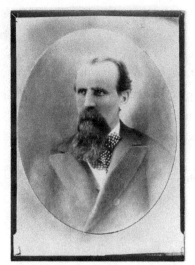

A.P.K. Safford, 1870s. Courtesy Coppola Family.

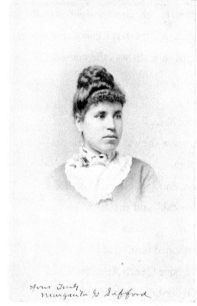

Margarita Grijalva Safford, A.P.K.'s second wife and mother of his daughter, also named Margarita, circa 1879. Arizona Historical Society AHS13756.

an active homeopathic medical practice.[91] Concurrently, A. P. K. and Anna Safford toured several eastern, "principal watering places," including fashionable seaside resort Long Branch, NJ, where U.S. Grant had a summer cottage.[92] As the Grants were on their world tour, they were not home to greet A. P. K. whose territorial governorship ended when Grant left office.[93] Perhaps A. P. K. and Anna joined Mary for an eastern tour, but no record exists.

A. P. K. probably missed his annual governor's salary and used his political contacts to embark on business adventures that ultimately reunited him and Mary. He became a director and vice president of newly organized Southern Pacific Railroad and with fellow director Charles Hudson began Safford & Hudson Bank in Tucson and Tombstone.[94][95][96] A. P. K. was president of two spectacularly successful Tombstone mining companies that deposited their silver in his bank.[97][98] He was among original purchasers of the town's development site, and one thoroughfare is still named Safford Street. He acquired additional venture capital in New York and Philadelphia where one of his associates was Hamilton Disston, son of a wealthy saw manufacturer.[99][100] Having covered all bases in hopes of acquiring a fortune, A. P. K. then married young Mexican Margarita Grijalva on December 11, 1878.[101]

Concurrently, Mary lived a contrasting eastern urban life. Her participation in the New England Women's Club's 1879 conference on cooperative housekeeping and division of labor included her advocating communal living practices reminiscent of Zina Peirce's known to Mary from the Second Radical Club.[102] However, as Peirce concentrated on the organizational aspects of household reform, Mary added the icing to the progressive cake by suggesting women use the spare time gained through efficiency to self-improve through education.

Known for delivery of inspirational speeches, Mary was chosen for the BUSM faculty's response to class valedictorian John Preston Sutherland's graduation address on March 5, 1879. Gathering at Tremont Temple, the thirty-five doctoral candidates sat within a veritable greenhouse of flowers. Dr. I. T. Talbot's lengthy address included news of the school's switching to a four-year program the next year. Professor Mary J. Safford-Blake's speech included the following thoughts:

"The science of homoeopathy has shared the fate of all progressive ideas; its growth has been slow but sure wherever intelligence has paved the way for it. The New World has not had the precedence of centuries to overcome in accepting new truths, and hence the strength and growing vigor of homoeopathy to-day in America. Its blindest, and as a consequence bitterest, opponents are compelled to acknowledge the great good it has done in one direction, at least, namely, that of ameliorating heroic doses in the old school."

"I am glad to see not only how the theories of our school have modified those of the old but that homoeopathy seems to inspire a broader and more generous spirit of humanity into the medical world. I am glad to know, for instance, that if you were called to counsel or aid a brother physician, you would not hesitate to respond to his urgent need till you had ascertained to what medical society he belonged, and then refuse to help him, when life might be at stake, because the views of your society did not accord with the regulations of his. You will go forth wherever your skill is required. You will be tolerant to the intelligent opinions of all who may differ from you. You will endeavor always to ground your judgments upon the sure foundations of intelligence."

"When once dedicated to the study of medicine, if you would progress your whole life will be that of the student. Nor must it be forgotten that the close relation between medicine and the other sciences compels a physician who would attain the highest levels to keep pace with the march of all scientific truth."

"Not only science, but philanthropy, must have a close place in your mind and heart."

"There are many unsolved problems in the care of the unfortunate—those diseased morally, mentally, and physically— which the physician, by the nature of his education, is best fitted to solve. There are social questions, vital as life itself, with which he can deal best for the greatest good of humanity. Perhaps the most striking and yet the most obscure of these questions is that of heredity, upon which, as evolution teaches us, the future progress or decay of races depends."

"When the record of public health tells us that out of one thousand children born in Boston, two hundred and seventy-five die under one year of age, and more than eighty-six in one thousand under five years of age, we are brought to a realization of the dangers that encompass us. This startling death-rate among the innocents must strike terror to the hearts of those able to command their surroundings, as well as those subjected to the privations of poverty; for Back-Bay mansions offer up almost as many victims, in proportion to their numbers, as the tenements at South Cove."

"The responsibility of the physician, then, in the household, to help remove all health-depressing and disease-developing conditions, cannot be overestimated. The purity of the water supply...The selection, preparation, and administration of food...The dangers from faulty drainage...The great questions of ventilation, light, and sunshine...The question of dress, as much as any other, a question for the physician.....And then comes the good gospel of cleanliness,---when to bathe, how to bathe, and why to bathe."

"The physician knows as no one else knows the importance of well-balanced nerves and muscles. Hence his duty to prescribe understandingly proper exercise and proper rest. Does the physician's duty cease in the house and with his patients? Far from it. To him must be largely entrusted the care and intelligent oversight of the public health. Where is the intelligence of the physician to-day more needed than in seeking in our public schools the causes which so largely undermine the vigor of our children? Whose duties and responsibilities are greater towards the unfortunate class deprived of their reason?"

"These are vital, moral questions, ever presenting themselves for his discussion and settlement. To these the physician must give his attention in order to add the weight of his approval or denial."

"I have pointed to the heights toward which your profession may lead you. May your life conduct you to those heights, led by these ambitious and high examples, accompanied by pure and sustaining friendships, and by many worthy deeds, until at last you reach the company of those gifted with the noble title----Good Physician."[103]

In October 1879, Mary had a very special houseguest. Vivacious Margarita Grijalva Safford was over 30 years younger than 51-year old A. P. K. who had educated her, married her and brought her east on his business ventures.[104][105] From all indications and despite their age disparity, A. P. K. and Margarita's joyful marriage was the kind Mary had desired. Pregnant Margarita's charmingly teasing letter's salutation of, "Querido viejito," meaning, "Dear Little Old Man," suggested the 20-year-old's love for her much older husband.[106] He joined her in Boston, and on October 11th their baby arrived.[107][108] A. P. K. wrote:

"When our little daughter was born she feared I would prefer a boy but was soon assured that a girl was quite as acceptable she named her Mary after my sister…"[109]

The baby was healthy, but, postpartum, Margarita was not:

"For much of the time during her three months of constant illness, the physician would not allow her husband to see her. But, her condition not improving, at last his supreme affection for her broke all the barriers of physicians, and he brought her to where he could daily minister to her wants and be with her. As death neared, her reason evidently returned, to the unutterable joy of her husband, and she spoke to him of her love and of her desire to have him near…"[110]

On January 7, 1880, young Margarita died in New York City.[111] Two days later, the funeral proceeded to Woodlawn Cemetery with ten pallbearers' including two past governors of Arizona Territory, two Congressmen, and A.P.K.'s friend and business partner Hamilton Disston. Although her obituary gave cause of death as consumption, now known as tuberculosis, another account of postpartum events noted:

"Soon after the puerperal fever set in, her mind wandered and for weeks she was delirious, knowing no one; and finally an attack of 'quick consumption' hurried her to the grave."[112]

Of course, in 1880, no antibiotics were available to treat either puerperal fever or tuberculosis, and an otherwise healthy woman, if exhausted from labor and delivery, could contract either. Even with today's hygienic obstetrical techniques, occasional fatalities from postpartum infections occur. The ultimate outcome of Margarita's demise was Mary's abrupt entrance into surrogate motherhood. A. P. K. made one little change before presenting his daughter to her aunt:

"…I changed the name to Margarita as I preferred to have her bear her mother's name that was so dear to me in life."[113]

Dr. Mary Safford aka Aunt Mary was then in prime position to actually implement her espoused efficient household hints. Two months later, A. P. K. conveyed his ward Leandro to Mary who abruptly had charge of a newborn and a preteen boy—a true challenge to her progressive idealistic household's efficiency.[114] It is unknown if she voluntarily cared for the children or if the responsibility was merely thrust upon her. She likely employed a wet nurse for Margarita. A reference Mary provided her Gannett Institute students was Dr. George Naphey's *Physical Life of Woman*, a compendium of instructions for women of all ages with a chapter on practical advice for newborn care. Much of the book's advice is still valid today, but several topics including, "Effect of Anger on the Milk," how to apply a puppy to the breast to treat nipple inversion, and, "Men as Wet Nurses," might raise a few eyebrows.[115] Mary was as well prepared for a newborn's care as any new parent. News of her precipitous journey into motherhood pleased 88-year old Aunt Lydia Safford Wilson in Burlington, Vermont, who wrote of her desire to see Mary and Margarita.[116] Although it is unknown if they ever visited Auntie Lydia, it was certainly possible, as the retired schoolteacher lived until 1890.[117]

Relocating 12-year old Leandro from the Mexican border area to 48-year old Mary's Boston home must have posed significant cultural challenges for them both. Leandro had been a good student in Tucson's school, and Mary sent him to Boston public school.[118] In 1882, Mary and Leandro attended the Montreal AAAS meeting where he could meet the days' famous scientists.[119] Event highlights included physician Sir William Osler's speech on, "Demonstration of the Bacillus of Tuberculosis," and several papers by Alexander Graham Bell.[120] Also, Leandro could have heard Bell's friend and Mary's ex-husband's cousin Dr. Clarence J. Blake speak on a rousing topic regarding the eardrum.[121]

An assistant teacher in Leandro's Tucson school was industrious Ignacio Bonillas whom A. P. K. hired as secretary.[122] Reputedly, in fall 1880, A.P.K. financed 22-year old Ignacio's mining engineering studies at MIT where he received his degree in 1884.[123] [124] [125] His younger sister Soledad also attended Tucson's school, and A. P. K. was said to have assisted with her eastern education.[126] [127] While matriculating in Boston, possibly, both Bonillas siblings stayed with Mary who had moved her home and office to 308 Columbus Avenue.[128] [129] In the only Boston home she ever owned, she had two household servants who undoubtedly helped supervise the young people while Mary maintained her medical practice and social schedules. Her BUSM teaching expanded to include hematologic topics, and she still lectured elsewhere while continuing her WEIU work.[130] [131] Her occasional short medical articles included one entitled, "Artificial Alimentation."[132] Later biographer Elizabeth B. Sammons said of Mary's household:

"Her home in Boston was a model of a well-managed household. It has been said that literary and professional women fail in domestic life. To this Dr. Safford was a brilliant contradiction...'

'Her home in Boston was a centre of attraction to the progressive element of the city, for she was an ardent worker in the cause of equal rights for women and other progressive movements, and many famous leaders were often her guests. Her home was also the refuge for hundreds with whom she came in contact while practicing her profession, or whose needs were made known to her by others..."[133]

Perhaps she hosted some of these women when the AAW held its October 1880 Woman's Congress in Boston. At one evening's session, Professor Rachel L. Bodley of Philadelphia's Women's Medical College spoke on, "Scholarships for Women," followed by a lively discussion:

"Dr. Safford desired that the help extended to women should not prevent the offer of similar assistance to men..."[134]

While Mary promoted women's rights, she spoke from an egalitarian viewpoint, emphasizing that woman's equal rights and opportunities should not result in men's losing theirs. Perhaps having two generous brothers tempered her opinions. Mary then presented her lecture, "On Physical Culture in the Home." One listener's description:

"This paper...being given without notes, was very direct in its effect upon the audience. Her simple naïveté of manner, good sense, and great sincerity, won the audience to her opinions, and to her earnest enthusiasm for the better physical training of the young."[135]

Mary's speaking extemporaneously impressed many, but such ability arose from thorough knowledge and passion for her topics. She truly believed in dress reform, diet and exercise for health, and pushed her message at every available opportunity.

Excessive activity disrupted Mary's immune system during the Civil War and when she suffered Roman Fever. Similarly, she caught pneumonia in winter 1881.[136] Conceding her limitations, she sent regrets for her inability to comply with a now long forgotten request made by friend, woman's rights advocate and medical school classmate Dr. Mary Holywell Everett. Fortunately, Dr. Safford recovered and resumed work by speaking at Loring Moody's Boston Institute of Heredity along with Elizabeth Cady Stanton, Parker Pillsbury, Matilda Joslin Gage and others.[137] Dr. Safford's later proposal to study the potential physical, mental and moral deficiencies of offspring of consanguineous marriages may have related to work within that organization.[138] Results of such an investigation are unknown but could have extended from her prenatal influence work and been useful for her later temperance lectures.

June's AIH meeting was at Brighton Beach, New York, and Mary was appointed a Committee of Legislation member.[139][140] This highly time consuming activity required her monitoring municipal and state governments' relations with homeopaths, their civil service activities, and following laws' affecting homeopaths.

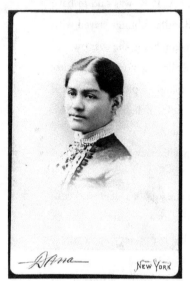

Soledad Bonillas de Safford, A. P. K. Safford's third wife, New York City, 1885. Arizona Historical Society AHS228.

On September 10, 1881, in Tucson, 53-year old widower A. P. K. Safford married 21-year old Soledad M. Bonillas, sister of his assistant Ignacio.[141] The couple left immediately for San Francisco followed by several months in New York City.[142]

Hopefully, A. P. K. was truly in love with her, but perhaps he envisioned Soledad as mother for Margarita and Leandro. For two years, Mary cared for them, but now she was almost 50 with an active medical practice and diverse outside interests. A. P. K. liked children, and with a new wife and money, he likely desired settling down. If he even saw Margarita in her first two years is unknown, but Mary's letter from Boston on November 18th suggested they met at Thanksgiving:

> "Dear Brother,
>
> I enclose a letter Baby has just written, folded, stamped for you. You will doubtless be able to distinguish the dog monkey and bird. Poor little heart is quite hoarse today. I dread the night for her because she is much worse then. She can't go out because of a drizzling rain but she amuses herself in sweet ways with fish and her toys. We can't be too thankful for a house through which she can roam when she is shut in. Hope the Parsons will come with you for Thanksgiving.
>
> Yours Mary"[143]

Accompanying the letter, on a piece of Mary's office stationery, was a freeform, abstract, line drawing by 2-year old artist Margarita. This was Mary's sole letter among Margarita Safford's effects on her 1963 death at age 83.[144] Obviously, Mary was glad her Boston house allowed the child's exercise, but drizzly, cold Boston was not A. P. K.'s preferred site to unite his family. He and his friend Hamilton Disston had already commenced planning new homes in Florida.

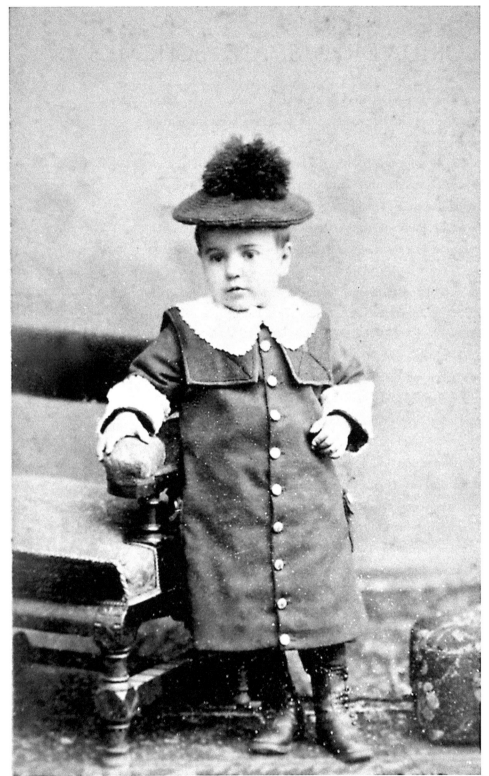

Margarita Safford (1879-1963), A. P. K. Safford's daughter, age 3, circa 1882. Courtesy Tarpon Springs Area Historical Society-2002.009.0190.

12 FLORIDA DREAMS AND SCHEMES

Although Florida achieved statehood in 1845, Indian wars, insect infestation, alligators, heavy taxation, and poor transportation options hindered development, but:

"...there were farseeing people who never lost sight of the fact that in the middle of winter, when the whole of the Northern States of America were lying under the deepest snow and not a green thing to be seen, this State of Florida, far away in the South, was growing every kind of vegetable and fruit out in the open air with the utmost profusion, and with very little trouble to the producer."[1]

A. P. K. Safford and Hamilton Disston were among those, "farseeing people." Partly with Tombstone's silver fortune funds, the men planned a vast new enterprise. Florida's legislature had encouraged development through an act requiring the state's guaranteeing interest payments on bonds issued by companies' building transport lines. Things hadn't gone well, and development ceased as the state neared bankruptcy. On June 1, 1881, Disston and a capitalist group agreed to pay Florida's Internal Improvement Fund's Board of Trustees

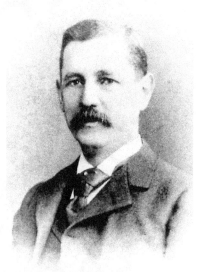

Hamilton Disston. FL Memory Archives/FL Photographic Collection, Rc02832.

$1,000,000 for 4,000,000 acres of Florida land in what was eventually known as the Disston Purchase. Three weeks later, A.P.K., Disston, and W. C. Parsons arrived to examine the acreage.[2] Disston's group formed an associated venture for an even grander Florida land reclamation project with A. P. K. as its managing director.[3] The men were literally the ones referenced in old jokes about being up to one's ears in alligators when merely trying to drain the swamp. Grand plans had hatched since the sorry day Disston was one of Margarita Safford's pallbearers. Later, A. P. K. wrote:

"Disston...is my partner in all my Florida interests, as he was in all my mining interests in Arizona, and is of course, one of the best friends I have in the world."[4]

Although possibly aware of Disston Purchase proceedings, Mary continued her frenetic Boston life. Her BUSM student Dr. Anna Howard Shaw wrote of her:

"I was in Boston three nights a week, and during these nights subject to sick calls at any hour. My favorite associates were Dr. Caroline Hastings, our professor of anatomy, and little Dr. Mary Safford, a mite of a woman with an indomitable soul. Dr. Safford was especially prominent in philanthropic work in Massachusetts, and it was said of her that at any hour of the day or night she could be found working in the slums of Boston."[5]

Possibly, one of those slums was the birthplace of a baby Mary called Gladys Safford.[6] According to a letter from Anna Safford to Mary Ann Bickerdyke, Gladys was, "a little adopted girl for M's company three years younger," and, reputedly, born in Massachusetts December 1882.[7][8]

Besides Mary's many obligations and care of now three children, she wrote a highly technical treatise on cervical laceration treatment.[9] On reviewing this, modern day gynecologist Dr. Deborah Trehy noted some of Mary's points remain valid albeit she worked without benefit of modern technology.[10] Gynecologic care improved because pioneers like Dr. Safford shared their knowledge.

Reform work continued, and at Massachusetts' Women's Christian Temperance Union's annual meeting, Mary gave a spirited tirade on alcohol's physiological dangers to the nervous system leading to:

"… the drunkard in the gutter, the most pitiful sight that the eye of mortal can rest upon."[11]

Her lengthy diatribe against evil alcohol advocated its prohibition and drunkards' loss of citizenship. Exhausting activities may have sidetracked Mary's own nervous system even without alcohol's help. Boston's bedlam tired her with its seemingly non-stop bustle on dress reform and other fronts, and she sought a healthier climate for her family.[12] In 1882, about 9500 acres of western Floridian Disston Purchase land ripe for development became available through A. P. K.'s Lake Butler Villa Company.[13] With Mary's help, a quiet, largely unpopulated corner of peninsular Florida was about to undergo an extreme metamorphosis.

Long before Disston's purchase, ancient peoples occupied central western Florida. In the 1890s, anthropologist Frank Hamilton Cushing led by Leandro Safford excavated the, "Safford Mound," a large, archaic peoples' burial site on the Anclote River that empties in the Gulf of Mexico.[14] French and Spanish explorers superseded the natives, but the area was sparsely populated by the latter 19th century. In 1867, two Meyer brothers started farms, and after both fellows died of yellow fever, their widows persevered in the wilds complete with howling wolves.[15] Born in 1878, Meyers' descendant Robert Pent wrote of family hardships including 20-mile boat trips for supplies.[16] In 1875, South Carolinians A. W. Ormond and daughter Mary arrived, and, soon after, Bahamian Joshua Boyer married her.[17] Supposedly, around 1880, Mary Boyer saw tarpon fish rise in the town's springs and named the place Tarpon Springs.[18]

Although life there was tough, the area's beautiful tall pines, Spanish moss and winding bayous attracted Hudson River landscape painter George Inness, Sr., who, in 1877, built his home and studio near tranquil Tarpon Springs.[19] His painting solitude was short-lived, as others were discovering the region's beauty, fresh water springs, abundant wildlife, fertile soil, and both fresh and saltwater fishing opportunities. In 1882, those, "others," set on development were Disston Purchase principals.[20] Boyer's stable quickly transformed into a hotel called, "The Long House," and within the year, A. P. K.'s family and friends were onsite.[21] Soon, the Tropical Hotel rose followed by the Tarpon Springs Hotel of lumber, "cut, marked and shipped from Atlantic City, N. J., where Mr. Disston had sawmill interests."[22]

In winter of 1882-3, Mary Safford could not maintain both her frenzied pace and her health. Even traveling to and within Florida was arduous as described in the later obituary of Elizabeth Ingalls Sage who accompanied Mary from Boston to Tarpon Springs that winter:

"…In company with Mr. and Mrs. W. C. Parsons and Dr. Mary Safford, Miss Sage came as far as the railroad could bring them. Then the party hired a wagon into which they put their belongings, which included two babies, Margarita and Gladys Safford…and drove across the country for seventy miles. There were no roads…"[23]

Mary, Margarita, and Gladys arrived in unincorporated Tarpon Springs to spend the latter part of winter of 1883.[24] Likely, they left Leandro behind, as he was graduated from Boston's English High School that spring.[25] Perhaps Mary experienced a breakdown that required her really resting. Words from her May 1883 article entitled, "Nervous Prostration," suggest it:

'Since I have been in Florida this winter, my attention has been frequently called to the marked and rapid improvement that an entire change of scene and habit brings to those suffering from nervous prostration.'

'Those who seek health through recourse to natural means, must go somewhere, and do something that will compel an out of door life.'

'On this Gulf coast of Florida, from which I now write, there has not been a day since February, in which we could not live out of doors, and bask in sunshine, and breathe the balmiest air, sweet with the healing fragrance of the pine.'

'In order to counteract the high pressure life of the nineteenth century we must learn how to rest.'

'The closer our communion with nature during our vacation seasons the better will be the results, spiritually, as well as physically."[26]

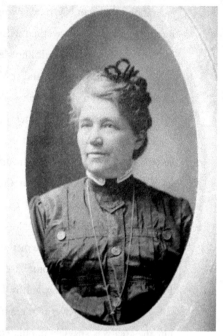

Lily McCrady Styles, the Saffords' housekeeper from New York City who moved with them to Florida. Courtesy Lily's granddaughter Betty Hammock of Largo, Florida.

She sounded like a woman refreshed, or was she simply planting propaganda seeds for future Florida development? Her friend and former student Dr. Fidelia Whitcomb from Nunda, NY, joined her for rest.[27] Mary knew European health spas, and possibly by utilizing A. P. K.'s land and partnering with Fidelia, she considered emulating Dresden's health cottage system.[28] Perhaps both women were aware of Richardson's 1876 address, "Hygeia: A City of Health," with its imaginary model city designed with the ultimate in healthful conditions.[29]

Although his health utopia lacked a site, perhaps Mary had one in mind when she wrote of Tarpon Springs' wonders in spring 1883:

"We seem at last to have struck the real, 'Fountain of truth,' if what 'they say' is true. There is a spring near here, the water of which is a deep blue color, and quite tasteless. An elderly man has been very badly crippled with rheumatism for several years. He was induced to go and bathe in and drink the water. In a surprisingly short time he found his before-stiffened limbs now supple with an agility belonging to youth. Not only that; his previously bald head became covered with a luxuriant growth of brown hair, and the fringe of gray hair, all that was left of the original growth, was also restored to its natural color. He now still lives to tell this wonderful tale, and there are living witnesses to support him in it.'

'While I write, this last day of winter, I look from my open window upon the perfected foliage of early summer. There are twelve varieties of wild flowers on my table before me. The thermometer ranges about 68-70 degrees. There is always a cool breeze coming inland from the Gulf. We have no mosquitoes, and flies are very amenable to treatment, if one gets accustomed to their idiosyncrasies. Fever and ague are rarely contracted on this west coast. I don't see how graveyards are ever started here especially in localities where doctors are unknown."[30]

Mary's, "fountain of truth," was running a bit dry. Possibly, she had potential ulterior motives for extolling the area's wonders. In May 1883, Francis Willard's WCTU house organ *Union Signal* had the following:

"Dr. Mary Safford, sister of ex-Gov Safford of Arizona, has taken 200 acres of land near Tarpew (sic), Florida, where she intends to plant a colony. She has an idea of establishing a sanitarium in that colony, to which invalids will likely be attracted from all parts of the States. Dr. Safford is an energetic, shrewd and brilliant woman, highly cultured, and exceedingly able in her profession." [31]

Also, Fidelia purchased 40 acres bordering what eventually became Tarpon Springs' Whitcomb Bayou.[32] The two women homeopaths predated by two years allopathic Dr. Van Bibber's *Journal of the American Medical Association* report of Pinellas Peninsula's being the, "healthiest spot in the world."[33] Both he and the women failed disclosing their ownership of significant properties in regions they respectively touted, but, with both homeopathic and allopathic blessings, Florida appeared the ultimate health resort site.[34]

Mary Safford had grand designs for Tarpon Springs but took time to be kind to A. P. K.'s housekeeper Lily Styles' son Louis, then a small boy whose granddaughter Betty Hammock related the following story:

"My grandmother Lily was born in Scotland in 1852 and came to New York around 1859. She married James Styles and had a son Louis on Long Island, December 2, 1878. James died leaving her without support so she became a housekeeper. She apparently met Mr. Safford in New York, but I don't know what year or if he was married to Soledad yet. The Saffords took her and Louis to Florida. He was lonely on arriving in Florida. He'd sit on the woodpile and cry because he had no playmates. Dr. Safford was said to have taken a shine to him, spoiled him and frequently would let him sit on the stairs in the house and play with her basket of yarn."[35]

Tarpon Springs' initial promotional literature's author is unknown, but advertisements held glowing, apt topological, hydrological (including a hint that the fountain of youth was near), botanical and zoological descriptions while praising the region's virtues for recreation, amusement, accessibility, and for:

"...the invalid in search of health and the emigrant seeking a new home...The aroma of the pine and the purity of the air, with the opportunity for outdoor sports and pleasure, causes the invalid to forget his disease, and daily he finds his lungs expanding and healing, his strength increased, his appetite improved, his spirits exhilarated, and a new life and new hope is opened to him.'

'The first-class steamer 'Gov. Safford' is now being built at Wilmington, Delaware, to run from Cedar Key to Tarpon Springs and other ports along the coast. She will commence running on the line Nov. 15, 1884, and will make the trip in full view of the Florida coast, and in comparative still water from Cedar Key to Tarpon Springs, in six hours. Passengers can go in Pullman cars from all parts of the United States to Cedar Key. A good hack line runs between Tarpon Springs and Tampa, 25 miles distant, and it is expected that steamboat communication will also be established between Tarpon Springs and Tampa, the coming winter. A railroad is also projected that will no doubt be built to Tarpon Springs within a year, and a telegraph line is now in course of construction. There are two hotels already built at Tarpon Springs—the 'Tarpon' and the 'Tropical,'—and another is in course of construction; rates of fare or price at $2.00 to $3.00 per day.'

'... it is destined to become the most famous Winter resort in the State of Florida."[36]

The nascent town's advertisement proclaimed further information would be, "cheerfully given," at A. P. K.'s New York address.

Following her rest, Mary returned to Boston to tackle more of what she came to Florida to escape. In October 1883, she addressed a Boston WCTU meeting and joined its school committee. [37]

After years of mentoring teenage girls, Mary wrote what was initially a series of health essays in the 1883 *Chautauqua*

Annual.[38] In early 1884, she and co-author Mary E. Allen, Superintendent of the Boston Ladies and Children's Gymnasium, combined the articles in their book *Health and Strength for Girls*, a guide for mothers and daughters whose health was jeopardized by what the two Marys considered the age's evils—improper dress, bad diet, and inactivity.[39] The first pages of Dr. Safford's half of the 88-page book recounted a 13-year old bookish society girl's dissipated life and that of her befuddled mother. Mary presented her usual dress reform tirade in a chapter entitled, "How She Was Dressed," followed by an equally ardent condemnation of the socialite's eating habits in, "What She Ate." Mary advocated soup's benefits and gave snack food caveats:

"…I rather you would give candies the go-by along with the peppers and limes, and get your positive sweets and sours from fruits…"[40]

The subjects of preparing soup and protests against pepper appeared in Mary Safford's contribution to the 1886 *Woman Suffrage Cookbook*, a foremost suffragists' favorite recipes compilation. Mary's essay followed most of the more mundane offerings, and others who submitted recipes might have been a bit miffed after reading Mary's:

"Protest Against Pepper. Soups, and Their Value'

'I send this protest for the WOMAN SUFFRAGE COOKBOOK, viz.:

That pepper, especially black pepper, be omitted from every receipt given. It is an abomination to the sense of every normal stomach. If one is so abnormally constituted as to desire it, it can be added ad libitum, and thus give those who cannot endure it, a chance to eat many a dish that would, without the pepper, be palatable and wholesome. There is nothing more grateful, especially in cold weather, and after fatigue, than well-prepared, nourishing soups; but at hotels, in boarding-houses, and often in private homes, they are made so unpalatable and injurious by pepper that no right-minded person would think of giving them to children, nor of eating them themselves."[41]

Perhaps Mary suffered from gastric reflux and thought everyone else did, too. In concluding her part of *Health and Strength for Girls*, Mary Safford wrote of her own reaction to her young patient's unexpected enthusiasm for reform:

"How could I help spending another hour with her, trusting to her enthusiasm to waken other girls! How could I help telling her of the cooking schools, and of the Women's Laboratory where domestic chemistry is taught—what the things we eat are made of, what are put into them to cheapen and render them unfit; and of the Women's Physiological Society, and that there are opportunities for women to learn about the best methods of heating and ventilating houses, even how the sewerage pipes should be arranged to keep our dwellings free from hurtful gases, and what materials every housekeeper should keep and use to avoid bad odors in the house. I told her, too, of art rooms and art-lectures where the principles and illustrations bore straight upon making home beautiful."[42]

The latter part of the book contained Mary E. Allen's far less entertaining recommendations for properly therapeutic exercise. Favorable book reviews called it, "…as readable as a romance."[43]

Mary's mentioning, "art rooms," and, "art lectures," may have related to the WEIU's Committee on Art and Literature meetings over which she presided starting in January 1884.[44] She wrote of sculptress Annie Conway Damer a few years earlier, and visits to European art museums and artists' studios may have sparked Mary's interest.[45] In 1889, she donated art works to the WEIU.[46] Her art collection's remnants are now gone as are the, "books of engravings and sketches," she bequeathed in her will.[47] An article's extolling Mary's qualifications for lecturing at Lasell noted her, "wide culture in science and art…"[48]

Mary had no time to return to Tarpon Springs the winter of 1883-4. She spoke at WEIU's memorial for member, friend, and fellow gynecologist Dr. Arvilla Haynes who died of pneumonia January 3, 1884.[49][50] Mary remained on the hospital's attending staff and served at BUSM's Dispensary Association's free clinic.[51] In April, she attended a homeopathic meeting, and, in May, gave a WEIU Social Festival address.[52][53] She even wrote another of her unique and memorable medical case reports with this year's offering entitled, "An Extraordinary Case of Constipation."[54] Mary cured the months' long constipation of a 16-year old girl who eventually passed, "pailfuls of faecal matter."

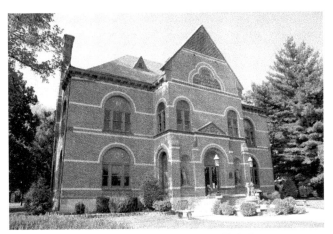

A. B. Safford Memorial Library, Cairo, IL, built 1883. Photo by Michael R. Coachman.

Mary's 1884 summer activities are unclear, and, surprisingly, the Cairo papers did not record her attending the July 19th grand opening of Cairo's Safford Memorial Library donated by Anna in memory of Alfred. Perhaps the idea of transporting two little girls to Cairo's stifling heat deterred her attendance. Also, A. P. K. and Soledad failed attending but traveled west that summer to San Francisco, settling real estate transactions before visiting Tucson.[55][56] Tarpon Springs' *Gulf Coast Herald* noted his travels:

"The Governor will remain in Arizona for a couple of weeks longer, after which he will... return to his Florida home arriving there in the fall. His health is not good, and he sought the Pacific Coast hoping for its improvement."[57]

A. P. K.'s seeking health in California was a bit hypocritical, as Florida was supposedly, "the healthiest spot on earth." Although not on passenger lists with A. P. K. and Soledad, Mary possibly ventured west that summer, too. She purchased Pima County, Arizona Territorial bonds dated July and August 1884.[58] Did A. P. K. buy them in Mary's name but in her absence? Three months earlier she bought 200 acres of Tarpon Springs land from A. P. K.'s Lake Butler Villa Company for $2500 and soon had the land surveyed and platted for a subdivision.[59][60] Was this in preparation for her envisioned health colony?

Tarpon Springs' 1884 winter weather had been lovely, and life was good according to a series of articles Fidelia Whitcomb wrote to her hometown Nunda, New York, newspaper.[61] Although not yet migrating with the seasons like Fidelia, Mary followed Tarpon's activities and, in October 1884, wrote from Boston to *Gulf Coast Herald* editor Lucie Buckner:

" I am much interested in Mr. Webster's Meteorlogical (sic) Summary. It is such information as that, that assure northerners that a summer, as well as a winter home may be comfortable in Florida. I am glad to note the progress that is being made in Tarpon, if each one strives to do his part to make it a centre of brotherly love and of intellectual and moral growth, it may be a second Eden..."[62]

The *Herald* started June 1884 and began reporting weekly weather in September when temperatures averaged 82.7 degrees high and 75 degrees low, the high being only slightly lower than current averages. Krakatoa's massive volcanic eruption of 1883 supposedly produced 1884's weak global cooling, and one would wonder if a volcanic eruption on the other side of the earth encouraged Florida land sales by cooling that summer's climate.[63] In the same issue the paper's editor boasted:

"The roaches have not carried off the printing office yet."[64]

According to *Herald* editor Lucie Buckner, A. P. K. Safford enticed her and husband Joseph to move to Tarpon Springs specifically to publish the paper as real estate propaganda. Her desire to establish a real newspaper and not just a Chamber of Commerce mouthpiece led to verbal war through the paper, and after a series of unpleasant events including questionable circumstances surrounding Joseph's October 1884 drowning, Lucie took matters onto her own printing press and described a less complimentary but possibly more realistic view of Tarpon Springs:

"Do not be fooled by the bright promises held out by this company. They will tell you there is plenty of employment and room for all. I tell you this is not so. There is room, hundreds of acres of barren land, on which no man, unused to the climate and soil can make a living. Land held at exorbitant prices...beautiful as a poet's dream...But in their very beauty lies their danger, for here malaria lurks...As for employment, for every man needed, a dozen stand ready.'

'To business men many inducements are held out. False every one...Lots advertised at reasonable rates, are held at four times their value."[65]

Just prior to Editor Buckner's spewing vitriol, Mary and family reunited with A. P. K. and Soledad in Tarpon Springs where Lucie recently reported numerous town improvements.[66] By now, through the Lake Butler Villa Company, Disston had financed the elegant, three-story, 50-room Tarpon Springs Hotel.[67]

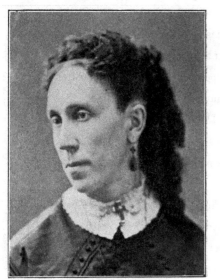

MRS. DR. F. J. M. WHITCOMB

Dr. Fidelia Jane Merrick Whitcomb, friend and practice partner of Dr. Mary Safford. Hand, H. Wells, A Centennial History of the Town of Nunda, Rochester Herald Press, 1908, p. 400.

Beginning with November 1884's issues of the *Nunda News,* Dr. Whitcomb advertised her new medical practice:

"F. J. M. Whitcomb, MD

Dr. Whitcomb's Office, Tarpon

Springs, Hillsboro Co., Florida"[68]

Possibly, Mary's student Fidelia practiced medicine during Tarpon Springs' prior winter, but, in 1884, she commenced what was probably Florida's first medical practice by a trained woman physician.[69] Whether Mary formally practicing medicine in winter of 1882-3 or 1884-5 is unknown although she likely gladly cared for those in need.

From all appearances, Whitcomb and Safford associates were greatly responsible for initially populating Tarpon Springs during the 1880s boom years. Fidelia attracted Universalists from Bradford, Pennsylvania.[70] Her brother-in-law Samuel Pierce Whitcomb sold his book and variety store there to run the Tarpon Springs Hotel a few years later.[71][72] He likely knew Bradford's *Diminutive News* publisher George Truax who started the *Tarpon Truth* newspaper.[73] Supplier of meteorological reports to the *Gulf Coast Herald* and eventual Tarpon drug store owner C. D. Webster was Bradford's city engineer, and his brother Philip ran a Florida citrus grove in winters.[74][75] Bradford watchmaker and postmaster Wilbur DeGolier became Tarpon Springs' first mayor in 1887.[76] Bradford's florists Walter and Amelia Meres ran Tarpon's modest Tropical Hotel and provided flowers for town events.[77][78]

Also, Fidelia's Nunda, New York, area friends and family bought Tarpon property. Among them were Seymour and son C. B. Thornton who became a famed horticulturalist for whom the "Thornton," a hybrid citrus fruit was named and is now called a tangelo.[79] [80] [81] Fidelia's son Merrick enthusiastically supported Tarpon Springs' growth, and as a citrus grower and Agent for the Sale and Improvement of Lands, he gloated to his Harvard Class Secretary in 1885:

"…I yielded to the prospective charms of a Florida Orange Grove, and came to this extremity of the 'Sunny South.'… While you are shivering before your grate, we are enjoying the sweet odor of new-opened orange blossoms. In fact, I am so well satisfied that I can with clear conscience advise all lovers of eternal springtime to visit me."[82]

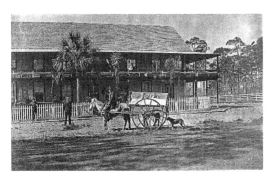

One of Dr. Mary Safford's patients arrives at the Tropical Hotel.
On reverse, in Dr. Safford's handwriting is, "Native man, dog, colt cart, child, wife inside sick who came 40 miles to consult me and rode his horse as seen in picture House the Tropical." Courtesy Coppola family.

Just as their parents relocated with friends and family from Vermont to Illinois 50 years earlier, A. P. K. and Mary Safford helped build Tarpon Springs with a familiar flock's migration. Cairo and Blue Island, IL, people purchased property and even worked for the land company.[83] Alfred Safford's first brother-in-law, "W. H." Massey was a Disston land agent and erected what Lucie Buckner called a, "pretty little cottage on his place adjoining Gov. Safford's." [84] [85] His sister Emily Elizabeth Massey from Blue Island also built a two-story house near the Saffords in 1885.[86] The town's mid-1880s title abstracts reveal a vigorous real estate market, and though documents show Mary's land purchase, no records of her constructing anything exist. Mary wrote of her 1884-5 Florida seasonal life:

"It is astonishing how little one accomplishes in a climate like this…I have had my little brood under my wing in a little cottage or a four roomed shell with my helpmate and companion Mrs. Martin a competent, intelligent Cape Cod woman—widow---and we have been very comfortable indeed. We have a charming location overlooking the bayou an arm of the Gulf whose winding picturesque way leads us by sail or row boat three miles to the broad open sea…'

'My brothers cottage is near us. We dine with them and I take our simple…fare for the children with them morning and evening—They…the black eyed Margarita and the blue eyed Gladys are just as brown as the sunshine can make them rosy, plump and happy the day long—digging in the sand setting out miniature orange groves building chip houses always playing harmoniously together and always more than repaying for their every day care in the joy they give me in return.'

'…The perfect immunity here from all forms of childrens diseases more than compensates for the lack of the flesh pots of dear old Boston—our little colony of two houses, two years ago has grown to forty and more in prospect of a Railroad at our door before very many months, we feel that our hardest pioneer work is done. The weather this season has been influenced more or less by the severe changes in the north but it cannot be said that we have suffered very severely from the cold since we have not had a frost that has blighted the most delicate vegetation. My sister Anna, brother Alfreds wife is here this winter …"[87]

Mary had her healthy family, friends, good food, a growing community, exercise opportunities and lived what she preached in health lectures. She reveled in her maternal role and seemed untroubled by lack of reform causes. Mrs. Martin's assistance provided Mary's freedom to travel, as the same letter continued:

"My sister and I have recently returned from a visit to Key West. We had a twenty eight mile ride by stage to Tampa and then a twenty four hours ride per steamer...The climate is equable and must be salubrious or else owing to the unsanitary state of the place perpetual epidemics would prevail.'

'Cigar making is the chief industry of the island one million per day are made. The moral and intellectual status of the City which numbers between sixteen and seventeen thousand inhabitants is what one might expect when a majority of its people are saturated by the filth of that filthiest weed.'

'We shall return to Boston May 1. I wish I could stay until June 1 but some unfinished college work makes it necessary to return to working. I mean to resign my place in the college. It binds me too closely..."[88]

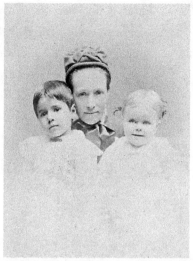

Mary Safford's Family (L-R): Margarita, Mary, Gladys, circa 1884. Courtesy Coppola family.

After resting, Mary returned to Boston and attended a WEIU reception.[89] As a corresponding member of the, "Society for Promoting the Welfare of the Insane," Mary kept her hand in reform work.[90] In early November, she lectured on, "Consumption," at the Parker Memorial Science Class, a Free Religious Association lecture series.[91] Although tuberculosis seems an odd topic for a Sunday school class, Mary likely followed the subject closely, as family and friends died of it. While lecturing on cremation of the dead at the New England Women's Club, she may have recruited clients for her new subscription enterprise.[92] A November 1885 paper listed her among New England Cremation Society's directors and explained the organization's planned non-sectarian chapel beneath which would be a furnace:

"During the religious ceremony the coffin containing the body will be placed upon a platform and lowered into the basement this operation being concealed from the view of the audience by a black curtain. The body is removed from the casket and placed in the receiving chamber of the furnace where it is consumed. The ashes are subsequently withdrawn, placed in an urn and raised by the platform to the chapel. The curtain is then thrown back and the ceremony is concluded. ...Enthusiastic advocates of cremation say that within a few years electricity will be used for the purpose. A wire will be placed at the head and another at the feet, and, presto! the body will be reduced to ashes by the pressure of a button, just as Hell Gate was blown up..."

"A stockholder in the new cremation society will not necessarily be entitled to free incineration. He will have a share of whatever accrues in the way of profits or assessments, but he will have to pay for being burnt like any outsider. If the furnace is kept going by sufficient patronage the cost of a single incineration will not exceed $10."[93]

Business was to commence as capital for chapel construction materialized. Despite (or possibly due to) the irresistible advertisement, the idea didn't catch fire, and the organization fizzled in 1888.[94] However, Mary enthusiastically supported cremation, as she wrote her reasons in an 1889 book of testimonials.[95] Having seen war's horrors and other cultures' burial methods, she desired cremation for herself with spreading of her ashes over her beloved brother Alfred's Blue Island grave.[96] Unfortunately, one does not always get one's wishes.

As winter approached, Mary Safford returned to Florida and commenced a new business venture. The November 1885 *Florida Medical and Surgical Journal* ad read:

"Tarpon Springs Sanitarium. Tarpon Springs, on the west coast of Florida, is situated upon an inlet from the Gulf of

Mexico. After a thorough examination of all portions of the State, this location was selected by Hamilton Disston and ex-Governor Safford as one especially adapted to, and presenting all necessary conditions for a health resort. The land is high and rolling, thickly wooded with aromatic pines, surrounded by the Anclote River, and watered by many miles of beautiful bayous. Malaria is unknown here. The air is remarkably dry, as indicated by the absence of the Florida moss, which is essentially a moisture growth. The Temperature is equable, and the warm air wafted from the Gulf, two miles distant, over the forest of Pines, is peculiarly prophylactic and restorative in all Bronchial and pulmonary diseases.'

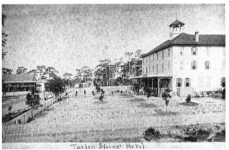

Tarpon Springs Hotel, the town's most imposing structure, circa 1885. Courtesy Tarpon Springs Area Historical Society-2002.009.0165.

'The Tarpon Springs Hotel has been constructed upon the best sanitary principles. It is under the management of Dr. Mary J. Safford, of Boston, and Dr. F. J. Whitcomb, of Aurora, N. Y., both physicians of extensive experience. The appointments are all directed to the attainment of the Maximum Comfort of Invalids. The Rates are Nominal and within the Range of all Health Seekers. Every facility for outdoor pleasure is provided. Sailing, rowing, and fishing offer their attractions. Many patients wintering here in the past two years attest the marvelous benefit that may be derived from this pure air, equable temperature and salubrious climate. Full information may be obtained by addressing Dr. M. J. Safford, Tarpon Springs, Fla."[97]

While practicing medicine together in 1885-6, Mary and Fidelia ran the hotel as a health spa and had a copywriter whose hyperbolic skills matched Mary's.[98] Publications touted the resort's, "large influx of tourists, invalids," and noted the swelled winter population.[99] With verandas on three sides, the hotel was open from fall to spring.[100] For now, Mary's many acres fit for planting invalid cottages remained fallow.

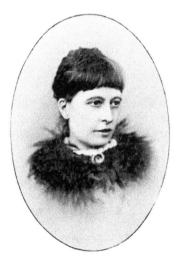

*Ever sincerely yours
Iza Duffus Hardy*

Iza Duffus Hardy. Black, Helen C., Notable Woman Authors of the Day, Glasgow, David Bryce & Son, 1893, p. 198.

In spring of 1886, a most intriguing English writer named Iza Duffus Hardy observed her countrymen's activities in the land of oranges and alligators, thus deriving the name for her book *Oranges and Alligators*. The Saffords showed her a grand time with an Anclote River picnic excursion:

"Our tempting cakes and sandwiches…are washed down by delicious cool draughts of Northern cider, and 'Florida Grape Fruit Juice,' as it is labeled, which turns out to be a most delicious wine, made from the grape-fruit, a wine very like Moselle, but with a peculiar and pleasant flavour all its own.'

'Never was a picnic hour more gaily and harmoniously spent than this in the palmetto woods, in the congenial society of Governor Safford and his family…"[101]

Did temperance advocate Mary know of her brother's beverage choice for guests?

As homeopaths, Mary and Fidelia required various drugs, herbs and medical supplies. C. D. Webster answered the need, and, despite being a civil engineer and not a pharmacist, he opened Tarpon Springs' "Old Reliable Drug Store," in 1886.[102] Of course, an endless supply of foul smelling, sulfurous, "medicinal," spring water was available to those desiring to dip some from below the wooden pagoda on Spring Bayou.

The town also lacked a hospital, and closest city Tampa also lacked significant facilities. Mary had little opportunity to perform gynecologic surgery but practiced general medicine as noted in Robert Pent's memoirs:

"She was small in stature, like her brother, but quick and alert. When I was a boy my parents called upon her to perform a little surgery on my foot which was giving me trouble..."[103]

Although well occupied in Florida, Mary had northern work yet to do. In October, she attended her last Boston AAW meeting and presented a lengthy, passionate speech on, "The Effects of Stimulants and Narcotics Upon the Health and Morals of Women."[104] The polemic was an exuberant expansion of her 1883 *Union Signal* article, "Physiological Effects of Alcoholic Beverages." After experiencing Florida's calmer lifestyle, Boston's chaos may have provoked Mary's words:

"Our modern civilization is based upon high pressure. Our meeting here from distant states and places remote, illustrates this principle. We have been whizzed through space at a speed that would have been considered an impossibility a century ago.'

'There is no actual repose, the brain is ever on the alert to sieze (sic) upon every new impression, and the nervous system never loses its hold upon eternal vigilance."[105]

She continued with a discourse on alcohol's physiological and addictive effects and declared:

"Social wine bibbing has probably made more inebriates than any other one cause."[106]

Did A. P. K.'s grapefruit wine count? In language appropriate for today, she cited prescription drug abuse as addiction's root cause and covered the topic of genetic vulnerability to drugs' and alcohol's effects. For her venerable audience, she expanded the subject to include substances not covered in her prior sermon:

"Tea, which has been classed under the head of narcotic stimulants, has been called the beverage that cheers, but that does not inebriate.'

'If it does not intoxicate to the degrading extent that alcoholic drinks do it nevertheless enslaves, and one who is an habitual tea tippler becomes as dependent upon it and as wretched without it, as the most inveterate drinker without his grog."[107]

Mary's harangue emphasized the equal evils of coffee, opium, morphine, bromide, chloral, ether and cocaine. She provided a long list of male physicians' warnings on tobacco and considered cigarettes worse than cigars or pipes due to the arsenic in their wrappers. Her solutions for ameliorating the situation:

"Reform can only be hoped for by absolutely prohibiting the drug and insisting upon a regular and nourishing diet, bathing judiciously, out of door exercise, cheerful companionship, and what is most essential of all, healthful and happy occupation for mind and body."[108]

Optimistically, Mary lauded many reform organizations' works that, even in 1886, lit the way from dissipation's shadow while she not too subtly promoted gender equality and woman suffrage. The tiny woman's fiery words must have ignited the listeners to her last AAW address. Several weeks later, she briefly rekindled the speech at Boston's Parker Memorial Science Society.[109]

Although gone from the AAW rolls, Mary's name remained on BUSM's notices.[110] She participated in medical school activities until 1888 and reputedly tried resigning three times before BUSM accepted.[111][112] Her Massachusetts Homeopathic Medical Society membership was active at least through 1886, and she resigned from the AIH in 1887.[113][114] A few years after Mary's death, an AIH speaker recognized her contributions in promoting women physicians and said she, "…was an honor to the profession, and was loved and respected by all who knew her."[115]

Exactly when Mary dismantled her Boston household is unknown, but she rented her house to three businessmen.[116] Part of her possessions went to the WEIU:

"…her gift to the Union two years ago of one hundred and ninety-seven volumes, five of which were valuable works of art. The committee have collected all of her books into one case which was also her gift, and had a tablet inscribed with 'The Safford Library,' placed over it in grateful remembrance of her interest in the Union."[117]

The fate of these items is unknown according to personnel of WEIU descendent organization Crittenden Women's Union.

13 THE SNOWBIRD TAKES WING

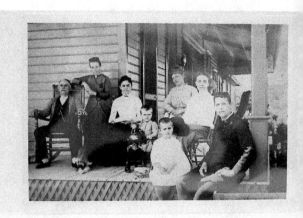

With hectic Boston life's subsiding, Mary's own health may have been fading, as she appeared gaunt in the 1886 family photo to the right. That fall, she, the girls, and governess Miss Elizabeth Burrell Pond arrived in Tarpon Springs just before Fidelia Whitcomb and A. P. K. on the, "Governor Safford."[1][2] Miss Pond taught the girls, now 4 and 7 years, although Tarpon Springs' new schoolhouse opened in early December 1886.[3] A.P.K. and Soledad had added a boathouse on the bayou and enlarged their home with a second story that allowed space for Mary's family.[4]

Safford family and friends on Tarpon Springs home's porch, circa 1886 (L-R): A.P.K., Mary, Soledad, Gladys (with doll), Margarita (with hat on the floor), Lily McCrady Styles (housekeeper), Elizabeth Pond (governess), Leandro Taft Safford.
Arizona Historical Society AHS 17754.

Again, Mary and Fidelia ran the hotel as a seasonal health resort despite a Tampa editor's questioning their supporting themselves financially for Tarpon's being, "distressingly healthy."[5] Like Mary, Fidelia participated in Universalist activities, and both helped found Tarpon's first church, the Universalist Church of the Good Shepherd.[6][7] Also, A. P. K. was among founding members and donated land for it and for Soledad's Catholic Church, the African Methodist Church and the African-American, "Masonic Lodge of St. Safford."[8][9][10][11] By winter 1886-7, the Universalist congregation had fourteen members and preacher Reverend Henry de Lafayette Webster from Oak Park, Illinois. Reputedly, his eye problems forced his leaving the north, and, possibly, he sought health in Tarpon.[12] In March 1887, the new church building's dedication included main speakers A. P. K. and Mary as described by gossip columnist Lucie Buckner, who, by now, had made peace with A. P. K., remarried and was Mrs. George Vannevar.[13] Tarpon's Universalist women's, "Social Workers," began a lecture series that winter as Lucie reported:

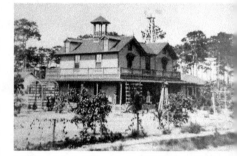

Safford home in Tarpon Springs, FL, circa 1886. Note the windmill in background and Mary Safford at porch corner. Courtesy Tarpon Springs Area Historical Society.

"The leading spirits in this new movement are our President, Dr. Whitcomb, our Directress, Mrs. Webster, Dr. Mary Safford, and Mrs. Johonnot. It is a grand and noble work these ladies are doing... Yesterday Dr. Mary Safford gave us a 'talk' on the 'Education of Women, as the Opportunities Stand To-day'..."[14]

Mary's speech thoroughly covered the subject with emphasis on Boston's kindergartens. Subsequently, she spoke again:

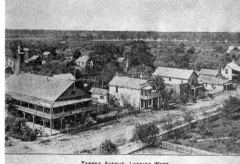

TARPON AVENUE, LOOKING WEST.

Downtown Tarpon Springs, FL, mid-1880s, viewed from top of Tarpon Springs Hotel. Lower left is the Tropical Hotel. Courtesy Tarpon Springs Area Historical Society-2002.009.0042.

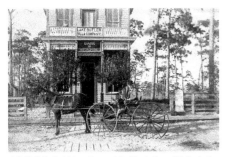

A. P. K. Safford with horse Snap and dog Shep in front of his Bank of Tarpon Springs and Lake Butler Villa Company land office, circa 1885. Courtesy Coppola family.

"We had an afternoon with Clara Barton Thursday, not that she was here in person you know, but Dr. Safford brought her before us vividly, with one of her eloquent word pictures."[15]

On February 12, 1887, the towns' men including A. P. K. and Leandro Safford gathered at the school and incorporated Tarpon Springs as a Hillsborough County town.[16] Of course, the women had no vote.

Also, A.P.K. successfully promoted the Orange Belt Railway's connecting Tarpon Springs to Sanford, Florida, where passengers could transfer to Atlantic Coast Line trains and reach New York in 36 hours.[17] Railroad construction commenced quickly, and Tarpon's first passenger service began in 1888.[18]

As Mary's tendency to overwork lead to her deteriorating health, A.P.K. overdid it, too, and, in spring 1887, he again sought health away from the healthiest place on earth. Lucie confirmed this:

"Governor Safford and his wife left us last Saturday, and although we shall miss them very much we were on some accounts glad to have them leave. The Governor has been ordered absolute rest and that he can not have here…Dr. Mary Safford remains at her brother's cottage and will in degree fill his place. This is the best of news to us not only because she is a superior physician, but because with that gentle but firm hand at the helm we feel that the little craft called Tarpon will sail safely over the summer sea."[19]

Fidelia returned to Nunda, NY, while Mary experienced her first complete Florida summer.[20] 19-year old Leandro kept her company [21] Recently graduated from Massachusetts Institute of Technology, he was now cashier of the Bank of Tarpon Springs started by bank president A. P. K. [22][23][24]

Also, Leandro ran an additional business geared toward more agricultural than political interest:

"MUCK—All persons wanting good dry Muck can obtain the same by applying to L. T. Safford."[25]

Mary continued her informal talks to the, "Social Workers," who met in Saffords' boathouse where she even served homemade, "golden orange marmalade."[26] In July, she entertained columnist Lucie Vannevar who commented on Mary's beautiful new furniture, "that would not be out of place in the parlor of a Vanderbilt…" but was built by a local man.[27]

Tarpon Springs' African-American community provided another audience for Mary's talks on home economy and domestic science:

"Her interest in the negro did not end with the war, but remained undiminished until her work in life was ended. During the years of her residence in Tarpon Springs she went among the colored people, teaching them not only from books, but the art of home-making and home-keeping; showed each his moral responsibilities; exhibited the same anxiety when called to them in sickness that she showed for her white patients. The humblest colored man knew that she would rise from her bed as quickly to go to his sick child as for the most wealthy tourist from the North; and for the greater part of her work among them she labored for no pecuniary reward."[28]

Mary cared for a black child in early June 1887:

"…a little colored boy, a Brown boy in fact, was bitten some two weeks since by a moccasin. Fears were entertained for his life but under the skillful treatment of Dr. Safford he is recovering."[29]

Young Mr. Brown was very lucky, as, occasionally, painful Cottonmouth/water moccasin bites are fatal to children.

The same newspaper column reported a Tarpon Springs man's being stopped and quarantined while traveling. Yellow Fever came to Key West in May 1887, and, on June 4th, Florida declared a prohibition against anyone traveling to or from Key West or places allowing travel to or from there.[30] Dr. John P. Wall was president of the Hillsborough County Board of Health, and, in June, Dr. Safford was appointed to it.[31] As Tarpon Springs' only physician, she could implement measures necessary to prevent the town's involvement in a potential epidemic. Summer passed without an outbreak, but Florida's quarantine on humans' and freight's traveling from endemic Yellow Fever areas remained.[32]

The perceived disease threat waned in later summer, and Mary's interest turned to temperance work. The Hillsborough County Board of Commissioners held a September 30th referendum regarding the county's potentially granting licenses to sell alcohol.[33] Since Tarpon Springs was within the county, the town's men could vote on, "wet," vs. "dry," status. Mary's family served, "Grapefruit juice," to visitors, but she ardently and eloquently promoted temperance, had WCTU connections and seized the podium to promote banning hard liquor sales. In early September, she gave at least two temperance speeches, one at Tampa's Branch's Opera House and another at a large park called the Reservation, as Mrs. Vannevar reported:

"…All the town was there, I trow, to hear our Dr. Mary Safford… the Reservation is beautiful enough to redeem the city…Driving along, we caught glimpses of the bay, for here it is that land and water wed."[34]

And here also mosquitoes congregated, but people were more interested in temperance vote results. Tarpon Springs voted 43 to 6 for, "dry," but overall the county chose remaining, "wet," and the overwhelming determinant was the vote from Tampa's Ybor City Cuban immigrant cigar workers used to imbibing wine since childhood.[35][36] These same workers desired native fruits (with hitchhiking Aedes aegyptii mosquitoes, Yellow Fever's vector), that unscrupulous smugglers' ignoring quarantine, imported from Havana and Key West to Tampa. Concurrently with Mary's lectures, Tampa's first Yellow Fever cases affected Ybor City fruit dealers and their friends. Through the following year, at least 1300 Yellow Fever cases occurred, and one source suggested a roughly 10% mortality rate.[37] Fortunately, and possibly due to Dr. Safford's measures, Yellow Fever bypassed Tarpon Springs.

After A. P. K. and Soledad returned in fall 1887, a Tampa newspaper reported his making the largest donation to the Tampa Relief Fund to help support Yellow Fever victims' families.[38] The names of Tampa's WCTU chapter founders overlap those of the Ladies' Relief Committee members who helped establish the city's Emergency Hospital.[39] Possibly, Mary Safford's WCTU connections spurred her brother's generosity toward Tampa's first hospital that evolved into today's huge Tampa General Hospital.[40]

For an unspecified illness, Dr. Whitcomb, too, sought health outside Tarpon Springs, and, in late summer, visited, Healing Springs, Virginia, where, reputedly, waters ameliorated myriad disorders.[41] George Truax's newspaper *The Tarpon* announced physician and dentist Dr. J. S. McAllister's moving to town in August

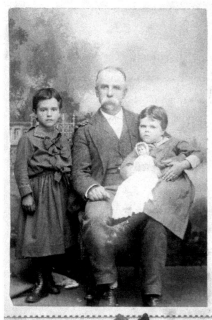

Safford Family (L-R): Margarita, A. P. K., Gladys, 1887. Reverse says, "Dr. J. S. McAllister, Physician, Dentist and Photographer, Tarpon Springs, Florida, Florida Views a Specialty." Courtesy Coppola family.

1887 with his wife the, "photographist," but the extent of his caring for Tarpon's patients is unknown.[42]

Apparently, Dr. Safford practiced medicine alone in western Hillsborough County and even made house calls via boat.[43][44] Mary's real practice challenge came early February 1888:

"SENSATION AT TARPON THIRTY FIVE CITIZENS POISONED BY EATING ICE-CREAM."

"'Tis the old, old story. A festival—ice cream—generous men—fermentation, and cramps…Thirty-five of Tarpon's brightest and best stricken down at one fell blow, and an ice cream festival, and we who stayed at home, and did not eat could smile at the poor victims… The only one who escaped unhurt, the only one of all who ate who walked the street next day with firm and gallant tread, was Dr. Baggett, the great temperance reformer of Dunedin, whose stomach by some strange secret known to temperance reformers, perhaps seems proof against poison. It was a busy night and day. Dr. Safford and Mr. Snyder knew no rest, and neither for that matter, did any in whose house there reposed a victim."[45]

Mary was further occupied in March 1888 when a celebration of the Seneca Falls' Woman's Rights Convention's 40th anniversary occurred in Washington.[46] All of the big name woman's rights workers attended, all, that is, except Dr. Mary Safford. She attended someone far more significant to her in Tarpon Springs, since on April 1, 1888, her close friend and practice partner Fidelia Whitcomb died.[47] Without further details, an obituary noted her, "gradually failing health," and, ten days before her demise, her husband and children gathered for goodbyes. Five years earlier, Mary questioned Tarpon Springs' need for graveyards, but now she and Fidelia's family placed her in Cycadia Cemetery.[48]

Within the month, Mary's friend, mentor and fellow woman's rights worker Dr. Clemence Lozier died in New York.[49] Two months later, Mary's friend Universalist Professor James Johonnot died in Tarpon Springs, too, and was buried near Dr. Whitcomb.[50] His daughter and son-in-law, ornithologist W. E. D. Scott, whose 1886-8 field studies were done in Tarpon Springs, had moved to town where he advertised his, "Special Attention Given in Collecting for Scientific Purposes." [51][52][53] His, "field studies," involved, "sacrificing," numerous birds to acquire specimen skins that eventually resided in the American Museum of Natural History. In his *The Story of a Bird Lover,* Scott wrote of his disgust for marauding tourists' killing birds. Just as biographer Sammons noted Mary's saving animal lives, Scott worked through Tarpon Springs' town council after tourists killed his pet herons. The result was a law forbidding gunfire within a certain distance of town.

Not all was sad that winter, as Mary continued observing nature and reported new species of seed bearing plants, ferns and a butterfly.[54] Also, she attended a young couple's second anniversary party and presented them an alligator-tooth chain to signify their, "tooth anniversary."[55] This comment fits with biographer Sammons' noting Mary's unexpected sense of humor. Also said of her:

"She was a voluminous reader. She read to every one in her household. If any member were engaged in some occupation that made listening possible, a gentle tap would be heard at the door, and book in hand she would enter to share her pleasure; and one of the last and most pleasing tasks of the day, never resigned to others when opportunity permitted, was the reading to her children as they prepared for bed."[56]

Despite later donating much of her personal library to Boston's WEIU, in June 1888, Mary helped create Tarpon Springs' library from a northern visitor's generous gift, and she became a library board member along with Merrick Whitcomb, Lucie Vannevar, Lottie Sammons and others.[57] The Sammons family had connections with the Saffords, as Lottie's father Benjamin was business partner of Alfred Safford's first brother-in-law Henry Hart Massey.[58] Mary purchased a mortgage Lottie's brother Walter Sammons owed on property he purchased from the Lake Butler Villa Company in 1885.[59] Several years later, Walter married teacher Miss Pond, paid off his mortgage, and moved with her to Blue Island, Illinois.[60] While there, Elizabeth Pond Sammons wrote Mary's short biography for Fidelia's son Merrick Whitcomb's journal *To-Day*. Elizabeth included a description of Mary's working habits:

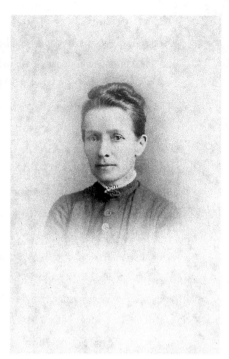

"How did she accomplish so much? She was an absolutely industrious woman, never losing a moment of her waking hours. She invariably conversed with callers and kept her fingers busy with needlework or knitting, not fancy work, but homely, ordinary articles of apparel, and always kept some bit of such work in a convenient place in parlor or office, to pick up when visitors 'dropped in.' Professional callers were made an exception of, and to them she gave her undivided attention. She spent but little time in the so-called social duties, though she entertained frequently and delightfully. Games she was not fond of, but was always willing to take part, so that others might enjoy them.'

'She made few formal calls, though she often ran in, very unceremoniously, all about among her friends, and if obliged to travel by public conveyance, she went well stocked with reading, writing and needlework, or something to study."[61]

Dr. Mary Jane Safford, late 1880s. Courtesy Coppola family.

Mary Safford spent at least part of the miserably hot summer 1888 in Tarpon Springs as Lucie reported the town's July 4th celebration's barbecue with, "Dr. Safford at the helm."[62] The new Library Association provided the food, and Orange Belt Railroad's excursion trains from St. Petersburg and elsewhere brought numerous hungry guests who ran for cover when a sudden downpour commenced concurrently with food service. That storm did not dampen participants' spirits, but an October hurricane's making landfall just north of town may have been concerning. Mary and her family possibly missed the storm, since, reputedly, Miss Pond, Margarita and Gladys returned from an unnamed location in November; undoubtedly, Mary was nearby.[63]

In January 1889, Miss Sage, who accompanied Dr. Safford to Tarpon in 1883, returned in company of, "Mrs. Coman, one of New York's celebrated artists."[64] Acclaimed landscape painter Charlotte Buell Coman sought health in Florida.[65] Miss Sage was having a large home built to accommodate her kindergarten.[66] Avid kindergarten proponent Mary Safford obviously encouraged this enterprise by selling Miss Sage two prime Tarpon Springs' lots for $1 in 1884.[67] In March 1889, Mary hosted George D. Atkins and his father.[68] George was Boston agent for the Nonotuck Silk Company founded by kindergarten proponent Samuel Hill.[69] What if any connection existed between the Atkins' visit, Mary Safford's lectures on kindergartens of Boston, her selling Miss Sage land for $1, and the woman's erecting Tarpon Springs' kindergarten is unknown, but speculation is enticing. Taught by beloved, "Auntie Sage," with her white sausage curls, Tarpon Springs' kindergarten lasted well into the 20th century.[70]

News of Dr. Safford's 1889 activities was otherwise sparse except for a suggestion she visited Illinois relatives.[71] In 1889-90 she was Florida's sole representative to the National Conference of Charities and Correction, a prison reform and watchdog organization that involved her friend Dr. Barrows.[72][73] Reputedly, Mary summered in North Carolina where current Floridians still seek cooler summers. Dr. Barrows recounted Mary's experience there:

"… she was riding through the mountains of North Carolina, among very poor and ignorant people, an old woman happened to see a large gingham apron of Dr. Safford's, and expressed a desire for one like it. 'You shall have one,' was the promise. Some weeks later, when next in the neighborhood, the doctor carried to the old woman the coveted apron. The surprise of the woman was unbounded. 'I didn't suppose there was any one so good this side o' heaven,' was her comment; and the goodness to her was not so much in the generosity as in the fact that Mary Safford had kept her word."[74]

Mary returned to Florida soon after Ex-President Cleveland's sister Rose Elizabeth arrived in December and likely attended A. P. K. and Soledad's afternoon reception for her.[75] The next week, A. P. K., Rose Cleveland and others journeyed to Paola, Florida's Pine Crest Inn.[76] Later, with special friend Mrs. Evangeline Marrs Simpson and Lucie Vannevar, Rose traveled the Orange Belt Railroad back to Tarpon Springs for several days' visit, but Lucie did not report Rose and Evangeline's spending time with Mary Safford.[77][78]

Mary received a special gift that winter:

"Mr. Wm. Cannon has a beautiful little fleet of row boats on the bayou for the use of visitors or others desiring to rent boats. Mr. Cannon has also presented to Dr. Safford, who has been a good friend to him, a fine clinker built boat…"[79]

If she was healthy enough to use the boat, Mary may well have exercised in Spring Bayou, but many people were unhealthy, as a global influenza pandemic's originating in Russia spread rapidly to North America, killing roughly a million worldwide in 1890.[80][81] As Tarpon Springs' winter tourists arrived via crowded conveyances, the town may have experienced a considerable number of cases. Dr. Safford could recognize influenza and its complications but could offer little beyond supportive measures. In February, Aunt Lydia Safford Wilson died at age 98, but with the influenza epidemic and Mary's own failing health, her travel to Vermont is doubtful. Mary did practice medicine that winter as advertised in the, "Professional Cards," section of a local newspaper.[82] A month later, she represented Tarpon Springs at Tampa's national WCTU convention.[83] Well-recognized southern organizer Mrs. Sallie E. Chapin gave a rousing speech interrupted by thunderous applause at Tampa's opera house.[84] Hers was a tough act to follow, but:

"Our Dr. Safford followed Mrs. Chapin and made a speech characteristic of herself. Perhaps no other woman could have followed Mrs. Chapin without being completely overturned. That little woman came to the front and held our attention by her sweet voice and eloquent words. It was like the purling brook following the mountain torrent."[85]

A report of that winter's Universalist Church's, "A Gypsy Camp," fundraiser showed Mary Safford's humor at work:

"…against one side hung the celebrated bed quilt sold by shares, containing (so Dr. Safford assured us) a piece of George Washington's night shirt (I doubt if he ever had one) a fragment of Martha Washington's wedding-dress, part of George the third's shirt worn at the battle of Pompeii, a scrap from the handkerchief used to staunch the blood of Napoleon Boneparte (sic) when wounded at the battle of Waterloo, and many other pieces of equally reminiscent value."[86]

Leandro Safford was proclaimed the handsomest of the gypsies although he was dressed as a girl.

The window to Tarpon Springs' daily activities and Mary Safford's town life closed with Lucie Vannevar's move to Sanford, FL, in spring 1890.[87] Others partly filled the void, as Merrick Whitcomb wrote of Tarpon Springs' events to his Harvard alumni magazine:

"We have recently incorporated the University of Florida located here. The medical courses will be given this winter. We are also trying to establish here, upon the Gulf of Mexico, a Biological Station, similar to the one in Naples, Italy. Mr. Disston, Mr. Chas. E. Sajous, F. A. Davis of Philadelphia, and Professor W. P. Wilson of the University of Pennsylvania are among those interested."[88]

Notes of the fledgling University of Florida at Tarpon Springs Board of Trustees' meeting held May 29, 1890, named A. P. K. Safford President, Merrick Whitcomb Vice President, W. W. K. Decker Secretary and Leandro Safford Treasurer.[89] The group read and approved the Articles of Incorporation, but the Florida State Archives' Corporations Listing shows no record of the University of Florida at Tarpon Springs. The university was to include schools of medicine, law, theology, arts, veterinary services, and dentistry and to have an associated sanitarium.[90] The board moved to appoint a committee to submit by-laws and voted Dr. Charles E. Sajous Provost of, "all the separate Faculties of the Institution of the University of Florida." Subsequently, the Secretary was to inform Dr. Sajous of his appointment, but, by then, he lived in Paris.[91] His absence did not deter his name's use in advertising the new University of Florida at Tarpon Springs and in promoting town land sales.[92] In an ad, the, "American Riviera Company," named Tarpon Springs as site for its, "great Sanitary Colony," with easily accessible medical talent. As a former educator, Mary might have enjoyed helping build a new university, but Dr. Sajous and the other American Riviera Company principals' being male allopathic physicians made her faculty membership chances nil. Her dream of a Tarpon Springs sanitarium withered, as did her health. So, too, the University of Florida at Tarpon Springs and the American Riviera Company's Sanitary Colony's vigor disappeared, as neither passed the paperwork stage.

Mary's days were numbered, but she continued treating patients and did limited traveling. She likely attended Leandro and Helen K. Polk's Tarpon wedding in December 1890.[93] In August 1891, their daughter Mary Safford was born, and possibly, Dr. Mary attended.[94] This was the closest she came to grandmotherhood.

Tarpon Truth editor George Truax wrote of Mary Safford in early December 1891:

"It was only a few weeks ago, while up in North Carolina, that she sent in a communication—we believe the last letter she ever wrote for publication in any journal, in which she expressed great hope that, in the Keeley Cure—a permanent relief from the bondages of intemperance had been found. It was no more than natural, for it reflected her main object in life: To relieve the afflicted, to comfort the distressed, to care for the dying."[95]

Dr. Leslie E. Keeley of Dwight, Illinois, promoted his double chloride of gold cure for alcoholism and drug addiction.[96] Although Drs. Safford and Keeley differed on alcoholism's genetic basis, she was open minded enough to acknowledge his success in treating inebriates.

Mary sought health in North Carolina, and on October 20th, "Miss Mary J. Safford, Tarpon Springs, FL," arrived at Asheville's Battery Park Hotel.[97] The place attracted the era's health seekers and specifically northerners with tuberculosis and southerners with malaria.[98] The newspaper failed reporting Mary's length of stay or participation in hotel activities, but she returned to Tarpon Springs by mid-November. Reportedly, she immediately took to bed with little hope of recovery from an unspecified illness that led to her gradually fading from what has variably been attributed to frailty, chronic overwork, or a, "slow form of typho-malarial fever."[99][100] At 5:55 PM, on Tuesday, December 8, 1891, almost 60-year old Mary Jane Safford died at home, as A. P. K. lay deathly ill in a nearby room.[101]

Two days later, all Tarpon Springs businesses closed for her funeral. Reverend Webster conducted the Universalist

Church service, and other pastors participated. The congregation sang, "Nearer My God to Thee," prior to Rev. Webster's startling mourners by stating:

"Dr. Safford was not a Christian, not in the narrow sense of church membership, for a noble soul of her depth and breadth is too great for the narrow limits of denominationalism."[102]

Of course, the minister provided her life's synopsis, and, before closing the coffin, gave mourners opportunity to view Mary's remains in a gesture that would have made her shudder, confirming the old saying about funerals' being for the living and not the deceased:

"Then it was that the character of 'Our Noble Physician' was revealed to many in that audience, when one poor mother after another passed around and tenderly kissed those pale lips, then lifted her tender infant to glance at her, to whom both were debtors—and tears answered to tears in that vast assemblage."[103]

Mrs. Meres and Professor Smeltz decorated with flowers:

"A lavish and magnificent floral display was made at her home, the church, and at the grave, which was lined with palmetto leaves and roses. A carpet of palmetto leaves was also spread for a wide space around the lot, which is shaded by stately Florida pines; blacks and whites uniting in this work of love."[104]

Her abolitionist parents would have been proud. Obituaries abounded in newspapers and journals across the country. Memorial tributes appeared, and the Boston Homoeopathic Medical Society appointed a committee to draw up resolutions on Mary's death. Her old friend Isabel (Bella) Chapin Barrows' articulate memorial tribute included the following:

"Of late years, Mary Safford has had many a battle with death, her brave, cheerful spirit and her determination to live for her children winning the day time after time. But alas! the last enemy has conquered, and the faithful friend, the skilful surgeon, the unwearied mother, sleeps her last sleep beneath the Southern pines. Dead, but not forgotten. The thousands of lives that she has touched will treasure the memory of her simple goodness, her genuine kindness, her noble sympathy with every effort to uplift humanity, to make the crooked straight and the rough places smooth. The music of her voice in laughter and in speech echoes down the years; again the girlish figure of long ago comes back; and only gratitude for the tender grace of a quarter of a century's friendship can reconcile me to the thought that that voice is forever hushed; that the dear form is forever at rest."[105]

But what of A. P. K.? One of Mary's obituaries noted:

"Gov. Safford who is lying sick in the same house in which his sister died, was reported improving by a late telegram, but his friends are very anxious to the effect the death of his sister will have upon him in the low condition of his health."[106]

A year earlier, when in ill health, A. P. K. wrote his old friend Sam Hughes in Tucson:

" …When I thought that I had but a few hours to live my affections seemed to turn with renewed force and vigor to the old friends in Arizona and the land I love so well."[107]

Whether he saw Arizona again is unknown, but, a week after Mary's death, *The Chicago Daily Tribune* reported A. P. K.'s death of, "nervous prostration," that provided Tarpon Springs' opportunity to repeat the prior week's events.[108][109] In his single page last will and testament, he summed his view of the afterlife:

"This life is only the beginning of another you will miss me but I shall be with you and meet and welcome you on the other shore but you have your work to do here do it bravely do not mourn for me for I shall not be dead I shall only bid you good evening in order to be able to say good morning to you when we meet on the other shore."[110]

If Mary greeted A. P. K. on that other shore, one can rely on her being sensibly dressed and armed with a healthful meal devoid of peppers and limes.

14 WHERE THERE'S A WILL THERE'S AN EPILOGUE AND A FEW LOOSE ENDS

Being a practical and responsible person, Mary Safford planned for the future, and on June 20, 1884, signed her long, complicated last will in Boston.[1] Perhaps her combination of virtual motherhood and failing health inspired her writing bequests she felt useful to specific beneficiaries. Review of them provides a better view of her interests and intimate friends -- a somewhat different group than those with whom she associated publicly.

Mary was particularly generous to Elizabeth Ingalls Sage to whom she proposed leaving the income of several thousand dollars in bonds and a pick of books from her library.[2] If Margarita's and Gladys' deaths preceded Mary's, Elizabeth was to receive thousands more dollars.[3] Miss Sage was later known as Tarpon Springs' beloved kindergarten teacher, and perhaps Mary's generosity was directed specifically to support the kindergarten. Elizabeth died in 1922 and lies near the Saffords in Cycadia Cemetery.[4]

In 1884, Mary's friend Lizzie Sweetser Beal's son George Safford Beal was only an 8-year old boy, but Mary willed him five hundred dollars.[5] That bequest more than covered his tuition for Brown University where he was graduated as a civil engineer in 1901.[6] She also listed Lizzie as book recipient and to potentially receive $500.[7]

To her cousin Sabrina Wood Millar, the only blood relative aside from Margarita mentioned in the will, Mary left two hundred dollars.[8]

Not often does one leave one's banker and lawyer a bequest, but Mary left one hundred dollars each to her banker Edward Church and lawyer Edward A. Hunting while naming both men as back-up executors.[9] The latter man went far above and beyond being merely Mary's lawyer, as Anna Safford wrote to Civil War nurse Mary Ann Bickerdyke in 1897:

"Margarita will be 18 in October--now with a great friend of dear Mary's in Boston who is her Guardian, and he and his family could not do more for her if their own child. They write me she is doing good work in School, growing to be a very helpful generous girl…"[10]

As A. P. K. was Margarita's father, he and Soledad were the logical guardians for Margarita and even Gladys after Mary died. 31-year old widowed Soledad

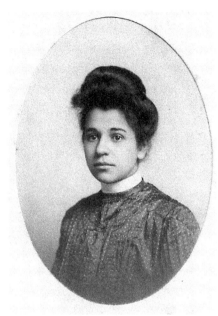

Margarita Safford, about 23 years, A. P. K. Safford's daughter, near her 1903 Smith College graduation. Courtesy Coppola family.

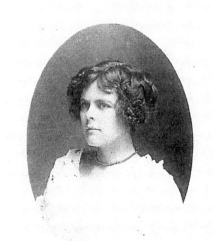

Gladys Safford Sammons Hill, around age 30, after 1912. Courtesy Tarpon Springs Area Historical Society -2013.001.0187.

and 23-year old Leandro with his own wife and baby daughter were the girls' initial guardians.[11] In April 1893, Hunting became Margarita's guardian and brought her to Massachusetts to live with his family and attend the Burnham School aka Miss Capen's School for Girls and Smith College that granted her degree in 1903.[12][13][14] She continued living with the Huntings, attended Radcliffe for post-graduate study, taught school, worked in the WEIU children's bookshop and then lived for many years with her classmate and friend Florence Dunton.[15][16][17] Margarita never married, and A.P.K. Safford's bloodline ended with her 1963 death.[18]

Anna Safford's letter to Mary Ann Bickerdyke continued with a hint about Gladys' caregiver:

"...The other girl is with the lady who cared for and taught the children when and for sometime before..."[19]

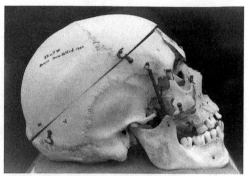

"Skull V. Donor Miss Safford 1903." The skull's origin is unknown but likely came from Margarita's Aunt Mary Safford. Detachable calvarium (skull top), books and springs consistent with a teaching specimen allow further interior study. Photo courtesy of Smith College.

Just six weeks after Mary's death, teacher Elizabeth Pond married Walter W. Sammons in Tarpon Springs' Universalist Church and immediately moved to Blue Island, IL. Possibly, Gladys joined them, as, in 1900, she was listed as a 17-year old student at Waterman Hall girls' boarding school in Sycamore, IL, about 75 miles west of Blue Island.[20] In 1903, Gladys married Walter's younger brother Richard Sammons in Blue Island and moved to Tarpon Springs where they buried their stillborn child in 1907.[21][22] Richard became Tarpon's mayor, but the marriage ended prior to 1912 when she married plumber Robert Cham Hill who died of tuberculosis in 1921.[23][24][25] In 1937, hapless Gladys died of rectal cancer complications at New Orleans' Charity Hospital and supposedly lies in that city's St. Mary's Cemetery.[26][27]

Mary left two hundred dollars to the WEIU and her library of medical books, charts, bones and skeletons to BUSM.[28] Although WEIU received its bequest, BUSM did not. [29][30] Curiously, concurrent with Margarita's college graduation, Smith College's Zoology Department received a gift:

"...from Miss Meta Safford '03, of two human skulls, the one transected, and the other disarticulated, a fine preparation of a human temporal bone, showing the auditory ossicles, entire skeleton of an infant and a case of histological preparations."[31]

Very likely, Margarita acquired these from her Aunt Mary's estate. Although most of the items would be usual for a gynecologic surgeon's collection, the human temporal bone preparation would not. Perhaps Mary acquired this from ex-husband Gorham Blake's first cousin the famous otolaryngologist Clarence J. Blake, MD. Smith College owns a photo of one of the skulls.[32]

To those listed as closest friends, Elizabeth Sage, Bella C. Barrows, "Abbie," Sage Richardson, Alice Chase, Lizzie Beal and Georgianna Davis, Mary offered a selection of books from her library. [33] Nothing is known of Alice and little of Lizzie, but Georgianna worked at WEIU and the Moral Education Association.[34]

Surprisingly, Elizabeth Sage's sister Abby Sage Richardson was among the, "close friends." [35][36] Shakespearian scholar Abby (spelled Abbie in the will) married lawyer Daniel McFarland in the 1850s, but he was reputedly an unsupportive drunkard and physically abusive to her and their sons.[37][38] Having to support herself and her children, she first gave literary readings and taught school but, in 1866, joined Edwin Booth's theater company. [39] Mary Safford attended medical school in New York then and may have met Abby at a reading or, possibly, met her in Chicago in

1871 when both women arrived near the time of the fire.[40] The McFarlands moved to a New York boarding house in January 1867 just before journalist and Civil War correspondent Albert Deane Richardson's relocation to the same house.[41] As he wrote an 1868 biography of U. S. Grant with numerous references to Cairo, IL, and lived there during Grant's Mississippi Valley campaign, Mary may have known Albert in Cairo. Widower Richardson befriended Abby, and Daniel's jealous rages led to her obtaining a legal divorce in Indiana in October 1869.[42] She returned to New York to marry Richardson, but McFarland shot him point blank in the abdomen in the *New York Tribune* lobby on November 25, 1869.[43] Richardson clung to life just long enough to marry Abby at the Astor House but died December 2, 1869.[44][45] McFarland's 7-week murder trial ended with his acquittal by reason of insanity, custody of his and Abby's sons, and no incarceration.[46] Mary was studying in Europe by then but was likely indignant at the trial's outcome that became a cause célèbre for that day's feminists.

Mary requested her friends Georgianna Davis, Mrs. M. B. Bruce and Effie Squires Tilden to join A. P. K. in reviewing her journals to decide publication vs. destruction.[47] A Universalist minister named, "Mrs. E. M. Bruce," was Mary's fellow Moral Education Association member and involved in editing and publishing.[48][49] "Effie Squires Tilden," may have been Effie Squier Tilden. An Effie J. Squier wrote an article on black abolitionist and woman's rights leader Sojourner Truth.[50] Later, Effie married James Tilden.[51] After unsuccessfully searching high and low for years on the possibility that Mary Safford's journals somehow evaded destruction, this author now assumes the journals did not survive. If they do surface, their contents will certainly help fill this book's gaps and rectify suppositions.

To Margarita and Gladys, Mary left the bulk of her money and personal effects.[52] Margarita was to receive albums, books of engravings, sketches, family heirlooms and Mary's microscope while Gladys, who was a toddler at the time Mary wrote the will, was to get Mary's china pin, gold watch and chains. In 1884, Mary could not have predicted Gladys' marrying twice and Margarita's remaining single, without use for her great-great grandmother's wedding gown.

Alfred Safford bequeathed Mary a, "cabinet of curiosities, coins, etc.," and she left it to Cairo's Safford Memorial Library.[53] The library now owns several display cabinets with unusual items including minute people carved from pecan shells, tiny furniture, a small, carved ivory palace, peacock feather fans, and other little treasures. Cairo Librarian Monica Smith says no one knows for sure now who owned these.

Mary requested her body be cremated with its ashes scattered over her brother Alfred's grave in Blue Island and, if cremation was impossible, that she be buried in the most simple and inexpensive manner:

"I want an unstained uncovered board coffin, and if burial is necessary I wish to be conveyed to my place of burial by some other conveyance than a hearse; and if buried I desire the body buried either in the old family burying ground in Cambridge Vermont or in Blue Island Illinois, near the grave of my brother."

"I desire not to be publicly or privately exhibited after death. Nor do I wish to have any church services performed over me and only the presence and expression of those who knew and loved me. If I am buried I desire to have my place of burial marked, if at all by a granite block unhewed, except where the inscription of name is made."[54]

As seen in the prior chapter, almost none of Mary's funerary requests occurred. However, three-foot, gray, granite cubes, both with deeply engraved, erroneous birth years, mark Mary's and A. P. K.'s adjacent graves at Tarpon Springs' Cycadia Cemetery.[55]

But what of the loose ends…

Mary did not name Leandro in her will although (or perhaps because) she knew him well. Even A. P. K.'s 1886 will mentioned him as an afterthought, in line for a monetary bequest only if some was left after Mary, Margarita, and Gladys received theirs.[56] Perhaps Leandro was a known profligate? He was co-executor for A. P. K., but, by 1899, the probate judge removed Leandro for dereliction of executorial duties.[57] He died in Philadelphia around 1940. [58]

31-year old Soledad became A. P. K.'s sole executrix. She remained active in the Tarpon Springs' Women's Town Improvement Society she founded in 1892 and at St. Ignatius Catholic Church, reputedly, named for her brother Ignacio Bonillas.[59][60] He had been A. P. K.'s Tucson helper, was graduated from Massachusetts Institute of Technology, became the Mexican Ambassador to the United States during WWI, and unsuccessfully ran for Mexico's presidency in 1920.[61][62] In 1896, Soledad married William Warwick Parken, an English musician who died in 1903.[63][64] She was known in town as, "Auntie Parken," until she married cigar maker Salvador Martin, and she remained childless.[65] In 1975, the Safford house was placed on the U.S. Department of Interior's National Register of Historic Places, and, in 1994, Tarpon Springs acquired and restored the house to its 1893 appearance, opening it as the Safford House Museum.[66] Soledad died in 1931 and lies in Cycadia Cemetery near her first two husbands.[67]

The Tarpon Springs Hotel that Mary and Fidelia ran as a health resort burned in 1898 and was not rebuilt.[68] By the early 1900s, the town's sponge industry prospered so well the place acquired the title, "Sponge Capital of the World."[69] Greek sponge divers, with their expertise, food, and religion, transformed the former snowbirds' playground until hampered by sponge blight in the late 1930s. Most of the original settlers' and snowbirds' families wandered away although a few descendents still celebrate the town's unique early heritage. Today, at a population of nearly 25,000, Tarpon Springs supports a vibrant tourist industry and an active cultural program with a variety of art, music, museums, and theater available to people of all races and religions. Safford Avenue runs on either side of the Pinellas Trail, a, "rails to trails," project that follows the Orange Belt Railroad's long abandoned route. Pedestrians and bikers' traveling it follow Mary Safford's exercise advice unknowingly.

In 1978, almost a hundred years after Dr. Safford practiced in Florida, Cuban Dr. Lucia Pinon was the first woman physician on the Tarpon Springs General Hospital's staff.[70] This book's author was the fourth in 1981. Now, the modern, 168-bed facility has over 300 allopathic physicians, with many being women in a variety of specialties.[71] About half of the obstetrician/gynecologists are women. No homeopaths are on staff.

Although Mary's dream of a health colony never materialized, she indicated among her will's bequests a desire to help the sick and underprivileged.[72] In 1877, she wrote about bequests:

"It would seem as if the satisfaction that must be derived from planning and executing one's own bequests would stimulate each one who hopes in the end to endow charities to do it while living, and reap the reward of well-doing; and more especially so, since it so frequently is the case that one's wishes, as to the disposal of one's property, are disregarded after death, and the money that was designed for benevolent purposes is squandered in law, through the wranglings and dissensions of relatives."[73]

Had she truly wanted to help little old ladies, invalids, and the poor, Mary should have taken her own advice. Maybe she did. Her will was admitted to probate and record in Boston in January 1892, and Edward A. Hunting was appointed her executor as she requested.[74] Property disputes extended proceedings, and, by 1912, Pinellas County commenced existence following legal separation from Hillsborough County. In November 1925, nearly 34 years after she died, her will was admitted to probate in Pinellas County, as estate settlement remained incomplete.[75] In the interim, lawsuits flew over misappropriated estate funds, and just as Mary predicted, legal fees mounted in litigious tangles.[76] Her family remembered her but not for the reasons she hoped.

Many others should remember Dr. Mary Jane Safford in a more favorable light. By the mid-twentieth century, kindergarten classes became standard in public schools nationwide. Mary's dress reform advocacy helped kill the once ubiquitous, nearly mandatory corset and promote women's heath. Coeducation at universities and graduate schools of all kinds is the rule rather than the exception. Women may vote in all public elections.

Today, Boston University School of Medicine is a top-ranked U.S. school with over 2000 full- and part-time faculty. The school's unique program that works with historically black colleges and universities, those with large Hispanic populations, and the Indian Health Service, to promote increasing the number of MDs among minorities, would impress Mary Safford. For years, BUSM had a Mary Jane Safford Academy of Advisors, an advising, mentoring and career development program assisting students through contact with experienced faculty members as role models. Some had degrees from institutions that refused admitting women in Mary's day. She would be pleased that BUSM remains coeducational and now has over 50% female students and would be amused to learn that Harvard Medical School has an even higher proportion of women students.

Mary's help for the needy materialized. The Women's Educational and Industrial Union continued aiding Boston's poor and started the nation's first public school hot lunch program, the nation's first credit union, and Massachusetts' first transitional housing for battered or homeless women and children.[77] In 2006, the WEIU merged with non-profit service agency Crittenton to form the Crittenton Women's Union, a resource for low-income Boston area women and their families' seeking economic independence. Tarpon Springs' Universalist Church of the Good Shepherd is now called the Unitarian Universalist Church and is a few blocks from the original church founded by Mary, Fidelia Whitcomb, A. P. K. and others.[78] The UU Church helps support the interfaith Shepherd Center that, as northern Pinellas County's largest and most comprehensive community service organization, feeds, clothes, and provides emergency services and educational opportunities for the needy of all ages, races, and religions.

Mary may have been small in physical stature, but her legacy is enormous.

ENDNOTES

APKS = *Anson Peasley Keeler (A. P. K.) Safford*

MJS = *Mary Jane Safford*

MJSB = *Mary Jane Safford-Blake, when MJS used her married name*

FP = *Flora Payne*

LV = *Lucie Buckner Vannevar*

TG = *Tampa Guardian*

TJ = *Tampa Journal*

TWJ = *Tampa Weekly Journal*

TSAHS = *Tarpon Springs Area Historical Society*

NARA = *National Archives and Records Administration*

GPO = *Government Printing Office*

Chapter 1 • IN THE BEGINNING

1   NARA, Passport Applications 1795-1905, New York City, July 3, 1862. Traveling with an image-conscious party, MJS avoided appellation as, "spinster," by lying about her age.

2   Triebold and Monks, *Crete Remembered*, First School (article 54), 2:11.

3   Robinson, *Genealogical History*, 53.

4   Safford ephemera, Cairo Public Library.

5   Wallbridge, *Descendants*, 311-12, 317.

6   Early Marriage Records Cards, Vermont Archives, book 2, 5.

7   Safford, E., *Saffords in America*, Q.

8   Hyde Park, VT, Town Records, vol. 3-4, multiple pages note Joseph Warren Safford was Justice of the Peace.

9   Bazilchuk and Strimbeck, *Longstreet Highroad Guide*, 13.

10   Edmunds, *The Potawatomis*, 217, 247-48.

11   Straus, *Indians of the Chicago Area*, 65.

12   Hyde Park, VT, Town Records, vol. 4, 177.

13   APKS, *Sketch of the Life*, 1.

14   1840 U.S. Census, Thorn Creek Precinct, Will County, IL.

15   Woodruff and Hill, *History of Will County*, 281.

16   Andrews, Hinsdale and Holman, *Hinsdale Genealogy*, 264-65.

17   Triebold and Monks, *Crete Remembered*, 1:7.

18   Baker, M., "Wood's Corners, Papers Read," 10.

19   Triebold and Monks, *Crete Remembered*, 1:7.

20   Woodruff and Hill, *History of Will County*, 263.

21   South Suburban Genealogical and Historical Society records, Will County marriage license issued 2 Apr 1839 to Anna Safford and George Gridley. Also, 1978 and 1993 Crete Cemetery readings found the grave of Anna S. Gridley, wife of George C. Gridley. 1843 death at 27 years suggests her 1816 birth. Gridley was Crete's blacksmith.

22   Triebold and Monks, *Crete Remembered*, 1:46.

23   "Crete's Early History," *Momence-Press Reporter*, 1922, 3.

24   APKS, *Sketch of the Life*, 1.

25   Belden, *Will County*, 8.

26   Bateman and Selby, *Historical Encyclopedia*, 589.

27   Matile, "Was Dr. Conrad Will Really Worth His Salt?" *Ledger-Sentinel*, 22 Jun 2006.

28   Carpenter, "Illinois Constitutional," *Journal of the Illinois State Historical Society*, 1913, 337.

29 Davis, *Frontier Illinois*, 444.

30 APKS, *Sketch of the Life*, 1-3.

31 Sammons, "Mary J. Safford, MD," *To-Day*, Jun 1896, 261.

32 Ibid.

33 APKS, *Sketch of the Life*, 2.

34 Ibid., 1. APKS desired education, but, "my first duty was to care for my parents, regardless of my own personal interests."

35 U. S. Bureau of Education, "History of Public School Education in Arizona," 33. Chapter 3 covers Governor Safford's Administration and development of Arizona's public schools.

36 Jenness, "Dr. Mary J. Safford," *Cottage Hearth*, May 1876, 113. Jenness was a good friend of Katharine Sherwood Bonner McDowell with pen name Sherwood Bonner. In early to mid-1870s Katherine was secretary to Mary Safford's Bostonian acquaintance Dr. Diocletian Lewis (Dio Lewis). Through him both McDowell and Jenness had direct access to Mary Safford.

37 Hyde Park, VT, Town Records, vol. 8 (1846), 357-58, and (1847), 511.

38 Crete Cemetery, lot 40.

39 Death and Administration Notices, Joliet, Will County, IL, 1849-1854, extracted from the *Joliet Signal*, Illinois State Historical Library. Entry read, "Safford, Mrs. Dyantha; formerly of Lamoille Co., Vt., 4/15/1849 in Crete..."

40 *Souvenir of Settlement*, 257. A nationwide cholera epidemic in 1848-1849 affected Will County.

41 APKS, *Sketch of the Life*, 3.

Chapter 2 • ANTEBELLUM LIFE

1 Woodruff and Hill, *History of Will County*, 566.

2 APKS, *Sketch of the Life*, 4.

3 1850 U.S. Census, Crete, Will County, IL.

4 APKS, *Sketch of the Life*, 26-27.

5 Bakersfield North, "8th Annual Catalog," 8.

6 Woodruff and Hill, *History of Will County*, 895.

7 APKS, *Sketch of the Life*, 14.

8 Bakersfield North, "8th Annual Catalog," 4.

9 Ibid., 5-9.

10 Aldrich, *History of Franklin and Grand Isle*, 227-28.

11 Bakersfield North, "8th Annual Catalog," 6, 9.

12 Jenness, "Dr. Mary J. Safford," *Cottage Hearth*, May 1876, 113.

13 Perrin, *History of Alexander*, 2:568.

14 James, *Notable American Women*, 220.

15 Sterling, *Sterling Genealogy*, 509-10.

16 Woodruff and Hill, *History of Will County*, 318, 363. In 1845 then Illinois State Senator Matteson nominated brother-in-law William as an Illinois State's attorney

17 Stevens, *Past and Present of Will County*, 222.

18 Smith, *History of Southern Illinois*, 248.

19 Ferril, "Roswell Eaton Goodell," *Sketches of Colorado in Four Volumes*, 269.

20 Sterling, *Sterling Genealogy*, 702.

21 Knox, *A History of Banking*, 724.

22 Ibid., 712. The bank first opened in 1813.

23 Allen, *Legends & Lore*, 154.

24 "State Banks of Issue," *The Bankers' Magazine*, 1898, 662-63. Bank closed again in 1842.

25 Knox, *A History of Banking*, 714.

26   Musgrave, *Handbook of Old Gallatin*, 58. Although Matteson allegedly bought the building for $15,000 in 1853, Gallatin County property record extracts show A. B. Safford purchased the bank and two lots for $11,500 in 1854.

27   Waggoner, "Shawneetown Bank Project," 11-12. Soon after Alfred Safford purchased the bank he sold it to Matteson's State Bank of Illinois for the same amount.

28   Knox, *A History of Banking*, 712-14.

29   Homans, "Banks of the United States," *The Bankers Magazine and Statistical Register*, May 1857, 995.

30   Safford, A. B., marriage announcement, *Joliet Signal*, last published 25 Apr 1854.

31   Jenness, "Dr. Mary J. Safford," *Cottage Hearth*, May 1876, 113.

32   NARA, Passport Applications 1795-1905, her physical description included height of 4' 4", high forehead, black eyes, ordinary size nose, medium mouth, round chin, dark brown hair, oval face, and sallow complexion.

33   Guthrie, *A Plea*, 4-5.

34   Reynolds, *Pioneer History of Illinois*, 368.

35   Jenness, "Dr. Mary J. Safford," *Cottage Hearth*, May 1876, 113.

36   Williams, W., *Appleton's Southern and Western*, 14.

37   Ackerman, *Historical Sketch*, 86.

38   Kittridge, *Ingersoll*, 39.

39   Ecelbarger, *Black Jack*, 47.

40   Logan, *Reminiscences*, 38-39.

41   Wakefield, *Letters*, 18-19.

42   Author's 2007 and 2012 visits to Shawneetown. Marker is on vacant lot at Cunningham home site across the street from the now derelict and greatly deteriorated Shawneetown bank building.

43   Logan, *Reminiscences*, 29.

44   Logan, *Thirty Years in Washington*, 648.

45   Maher, "Shawneetown Believes," *Illinois Catholic Historical Review*, 1929, 384.

46   Lansden, *A History of the City of Cairo*, 237.

47   Dickens, *American Notes*, 64.

48   Trollope, *North America: 1863*, 285-88.

49   Kionka, *Key Command*, 21.

50   Hawes, *Illinois State Gazetteer*, 25-27.

51   Lansden, *A History of the City of Cairo*, 209.

52   Harrell, *Cairo City Directory*, unnumbered page.

53   Lansden, *A History of the City of Cairo*, 231.

54   Newspaper clipping of unknown source among Safford ephemera in Cairo Public Library and referring to General Grant said, "The General's first headquarters were in the bank building near the rooms occupied by Mr. Safford's family."

55   Shearer, *Home Front Heroes*, 730.

56   Illinois State University archivist's search of student 1857-67 records found no MJS entries.

57   FP, To Nathan, Rome 28 Mar 1864, 218. In typewritten transcriptions of now unavailable lengthy handwritten letters Flora Payne (later Whitney) wrote home from her European trip with MJS. Flora noted MJS' friendship with McChesney.

58   "Second Annual Catalogue of the University of Chicago," 6. "J. H. McChesney, A. M., Professor of Chemistry, Geology, Mineralogy and Agriculture."

59   APKS, *Sketch of the Life*, 20. A. P. K. had a San Francisco excavating business and served in various elected positions including State Representative for Placer County, CA, per, *A Memorial and Biographical History of Northern California*, Illustrated, 183.

60   1860 U. S. Census, Crete, Will County, IL

Chapter 3 • WAR ARRIVES

1   McPherson, *The Political History*, 113.

2   Lansden, *A History of the City of Cairo*, 130.

3   Ibid.

4   "Camp Defiance," *Harper's Weekly*, 1 Jun 1861, 350.

5   Logan, *Reminiscences*, 103-5.

6   "Camp Defiance," *Chicago Tribune* quoted in *Harper's Weekly*, 1 Jun 1861, 350.

7   Logan, *Reminiscences*, 109.

8   Fischer, "Cairo's Civil War Angel," *Journal of the Illinois State Historical Society*, Autumn 1961, 229-30.

9   Greenbie, *Lincoln's Daughters*, 68-69.

10   Hoge, *The Boys in Blue*, 134.

11   Baker, N., *Cyclone in Calico*, 51-52.

12   Fischer, "Cairo's Civil War Angel," 233.

13   Jenness, "Dr. Mary J. Safford," *Cottage Hearth*, May 1876, 114.

14   Baker, N., *Cyclone in Calico*, 5-6.

15   Ibid., 8, 10, 11, 13.

16   Fischer, "Cairo's Civil War Angel," 231.

17   Young, *Women and the Crisis*, 93.

18   Baker, N., *Cyclone in Calico*, 52.

19   Logan, *Reminiscences*, 109.

20   Livermore, *My Story*, 206.

21   Richardson, A., *The Secret Service*, 147-48.

22   Livermore, *My Story*, 136, 159.

23   Greenbie, *Lincoln's Daughters*, 76-82

24   Bellows, "Notes," *Documents of the U. S. Sanitary Commission*, 4-8.

25   Greenbie, *Lincoln's Daughters*, 84.

26   Kionka, *Key Command*, 62.

27   Jolly, *Nuns*, 131.

28   Joseph Brewster Safford's headstone, Crete, IL, cemetery. Death 20 Aug 1861.

29   Lansden, "General Grant," *Journal of the Illinois State Historical Society*, Oct 1915, 421.

30   Grant, *Personal Memoirs*, 135-36.

31   Farina, *Ulysses S. Grant*, 50.

32   Grant, *U. Papers: April-October 1861*, 289-90.

33   Grant, U., *Personal Memoirs*, 138-39. Detailed Belmont battle description is on 137-44.

34   Tucker, *The Civil War Naval*, 59.

35   Logan, *Reminiscences*, 115-16.

36   Grant, U., *Personal Memoirs*, 140.

37   Lloyd, *Battle History*, 54.

38   Eckley, *Lincoln's Forgotten*, 101.

39   Logan, *Reminiscences*, 116-17.

40   Baker, N., *Cyclone in Calico*, 62.

41   Logan, *Reminiscences*, 117.

42 Brockett and Vaughan, *Woman's Work*, 358

43 Livermore, *My Story*, 215.

44 Fischer, "Cairo's Civil War Angel," 238.

45 Kerner, "Diary of Edward W. Crippin," *Transactions of the Illinois State Historical Society for the Year 1909*, 232.

46 Baker, N., *Cyclone in Calico*, 69.

47 Young, *Women and the Crisis*, 93.

48 Grant, J., *Personal Memoirs of Julia*, 93.

49 Grant, U. *Papers: January 1–September 30, 1867*, 28-29.

50 Brockett and Vaughan, *Woman's Work*, 358

51 Logan, *Reminiscences*, 120.

52 *Album of Genealogy and Biography*, Cook County, 502. Entry for H. H. Massey notes Julia's death 31 Jan 1862.

53 Obituary, "Julia Safford," *Cairo City Weekly Gazette*, 6 Feb 1862.

54 Grant, U., *Personal Memoirs*, 147.

55 Kerner, "Diary of Edward W. Crippin," 235.

56 Eddy, *The Patriotism*, 258-59.

57 Trollope, *North America*, 291.

58 Schroeder-Lein, *The Encyclopedia*, 145.

59 Baker, N., *Cyclone in Calico*, 71.

60 Tucker, *The Civil War Naval*, 385.

61 Gibson and Gibson, *Dictionary of Transport*, 146. The "City of Memphis" was 1900 tons, a side-wheel steamer that served at battles of Forts Henry and Donelson and Shiloh in 1862.

62 Young, *Women and the Crisis*, 149.

63 Morris, *Lighting Out*, 23.

64 Grant, U., *Personal Memoirs*, 149.

65 Ambrose, *History of the Seventh*, 25.

66 Heidler and Coles, *Encyclopedia*, 735-36.

67 Ibid.

68 Tucker, *The Civil War Naval*, 385.

69 Grant, U., *Personal Memoirs*, 150-59.

70 Henshaw, *Our Branch*, 53.

71 Young, *Women and the Crisis*, 149, 151.

72 Heidler and Coles, *Encyclopedia*, 730.

73 Livermore, "After the Battle of Fort Donelson," *The Ladies Repository*, May 1868, 371-81.

74 Kerner, "Diary of Edward W. Crippin," 235-36.

75 Logan, *Reminiscences*, 122.

76 Newberry, *Spring Campaign*, 30-31.

77 Ibid., 278.

78 Greenbie, *Lincoln's Daughters*, 117-18.

79 Baker, N., *Cyclone in Calico*, 89.

80 Fischer, "Cairo's Civil War Angel," 238-39.

81 Alger, *The War of Rebellion*, 281.

82 Woodward, *Recollections*, 51.

83 Ibid.

84   Grant, U., *Papers: January 8-March 31, 1862*, 418-19. 24 Mar 1862 from Savanna, TN, to Julia.

85   Grant, U., *Papers: April 1-August 31, 1862*, 8. 3 Apr 1862 from Savanna, TN, to Julia.

86   Grant, J., *Personal Memoirs of Julia*, 99.

87   Lloyd, *Battle History*, 82-88.

88   Ibid.

89   Newberry, *Spring Campaign*, 35.

90   Young, *Women and the Crisis*, 168.

91   Baker, N., *Cyclone in Calico*, 103.

92   Livermore, *My Story*, 214-15.

93   Hoge, *The Boys in Blue*, 67-68.

94   Collyer, "To Pittsburg," *Chicago Tribune*, 18 Apr 1862, 1.

95   Gillett, "Care of the Wounded," *Chicago Tribune*, 24 Apr 1862, 2.

96   Richardson, A., *The Secret Service*, 235-36.

97   Cooper, G., *Lost Love*, 43.

98   Brockett and Vaughan, *Woman's Work*, 359.

99   MJS, "To Frank Moore," explains why MJS could not comply with his request for information recounting her Civil War experiences. He desired to include her in his book *Women of the War: Their Heroism and Self-Sacrifice*.

100 Grant, U., *Papers: April 1-August 31, 1862*, 35, 110, 117-18, 127. Letters all regarded providing funds to Julia through Alfred Safford.

101 Owens, *California Coiners*, 97.

Chapter 4 • ACROSS THE POND

1   NARA, Passport Applications 1795-1905, New York City, 3 Jul 1862.

2   Hickey, "An Illinois First Family," *Journal of the Illinois State Historical Society*, Feb 1976, 104.

3   Ibid., 112.

4   Homans, "Banks of the United States," *The Bankers Magazine and Statistical Register*, May 1857, 995.

5   Haxby, Bellin and Allan, *Standard Catalog*, 325, 364. Cairo Bank issued $1, $2, $3, and $5 notes.

6   Marckhoff, "Currency and Banking," *Journal of the Illinois State Historical Society*, Autumn 1959, 407, 416.

7   Reed, F., personal communication, April 2013.

8   Hickey, "An Illinois First Family," 111-13.

9   Ibid., 104, 113.

10   Curran, N., "General Isaac B. Curran," *Journal of the Illinois Historical Society*, Autumn 1978, 273.

11   Ibid., 275.

12   Ibid., 276.

13   Ibid., 277.

14   Ibid., 277-78.

15   Dennett, *Weird and Wonderful*, 30.

16   Doggett, "Letter from Switzerland," *The Woman's Journal*, 21 Oct 1871, 336. Doggett quoted MJS' letter on Viennese life and thanked her for introduction to feminist Frau von Litrou (aka Littrow).

17   Adams, *E. Pluribus Barnum*, 160.

18   MJS, "To Caroline Crane Marsh," 10 April 1867. MJS' impressions on racial equality.

19   Dugan, *The Great Iron Ship*, 138.

20   "Register of Deaths of Volunteers," Group 94: 108.

21   Hickey, "An Illinois First Family," 112-13.

22   Brockett and Vaughan, *Woman's Work*, 577-79.

23   MJS, "European Correspondence-No. 3," *New Covenant*, 30 Sep 1862, 2. Robers is likely David Roberts, a prominent mid-19th century Scottish painter whose work hangs in the British Museum.

24   FP, To Father, Athens, Greece 31 Oct 1863, 120.

25   MJS, "European Correspondence-No. 3," 2.

26   Ibid.

27   Ibid.

28   Richardson, J., *The Annals*, 285.

29   MJS, "European Correspondence-No. 3," 2.

30   Hickey, "An Illinois First Family," 113.

31   Jenness, "Dr. Mary J. Safford," *Cottage Hearth*, May 1876, 114.

32   Hickey, "An Illinois First Family," 114.

33   Benson, *The Ancestors and Descendants*, 29. Singer marketed his machines in Paris and had four families, some concurrently under different surnames, and had 18 children. He lived in Paris in 1860, but it is unknown if Mary Safford or the Mattesons met him.

34   Hickey, "An Illinois First Family," 113.

35   FP, To brother Oliver, Paris 3 Feb 1863, 5-6.

36   Lopez, *Mon Cher Papa*, 124.

37   Livingston and Rogers, *Franklin and His Press*, 4-5.

38   Ibid., 5.

39   Wack, *The Romance*, 34-35.

40   Johnson and Johnson, *The Social Impact*, 146.

41   Einstein, "Napoleon III and American Diplomacy," 9, 25.

42   FP, To Dear Folks Back Home, London 30 Jan 1863, 2.

43   Adams, T., *Outline of Town*, 103-4.

44   Advertisement, John Munroe and Company, *The Nation*, 4 Nov 1869, 399.

45   Advertisement, John Munroe and Company, *Commercial & Financial Chronicle*, 9 Sep 1865, 352.

46   FP, To Dear Folks Back Home, London 30 Jan 1863, 1-3.

47   White, *The Paynes*, 167.

48   Hoyt, *The Whitneys*, 127.

49   Hirsch, *William C. Whitney*, 35.

50   Ibid.

51   Van Tassel and Vacha, *Beyond Bayonets*, 50.

52   White, *The Paynes*, 167.

53   Obituary of Flora Payne-Whitney, *New York Times*, 6 Feb 1893.

54 Biddle, *Whitney Women*, 97.

55 White, *The Paynes*, 162, 165.

56 Hickey, "An Illinois First Family," 108.

57 White, *The Paynes*, 160.

58 FP, To Dear Folks Back Home, London 30 Jan 1863, 2.

59 FP, To brother Ol, Paris 3 Feb 1863, 5.

60 Ibid, 6.

61 Ibid. Letter implies Flora arrived in Paris 1 Feb 1863.

62 FP, unaddressed, Paris 15 Feb 1863, 12.

63 Ibid.

64 Ibid.

65 College de France website and 3 May 2013 author's email correspondence with archivist Christophe LaBaune. The college admitted women from its inception, but they were not numerous. The school kept no register of students.

66 FP, unaddressed, Paris 15 Feb 1863, 13.

67 Barnard, *Johnson's New Universal*, 178.

68 FP, unaddressed and unsigned, Paris 25 Feb 1863, 17.

69 "United States Ministers and Ambassadors to France," *The World Almanac*, 281.

70 Khan, *Enlightening the World*, 14.

71 FP, To Father, Paris 21 Mar 1863, 24-25.

72 Gray, *Interpreting American Democracy*, 38. Laboulaye lectured on the American Constitution at the College de France and wrote a United States history for a French audience. In 1863 Bigelow wrote of French students' warmly receiving Laboulaye's lectures.

73 Khan, *Enlightening the World*, 10. Bigelow received Laboulaye's permission to distribute copies of his treatise on American-French relations.

74 FP, To Father, Paris 21 Mar 1863, 24-25.

75 Khan, *Enlightening the World*, 11.

76 Doyle, *The Cause of All Nations*, 311.

77 FP, To Mother, Paris 9 Mar 1863, 19.

78 FP, To Father, Paris 21 Mar 1863, 22.

79 Ibid., 23. The 18th to 19th century Greek Temple style Madeleine church contained priceless artworks. Reputedly, church construction cost over $2 million dollars.

80 FP, To Father, Paris 21 Mar 1863, 23.

81 FP, To Mother, Paris 29 Mar 1863, 28.

82 Ibid.

83 Ibid.

84 Ibid., 29.

85 Ibid.

86 Ibid.

87 Chisholm, "Orleanists," *Encyclopedia Britannica*, 281. Orleanist political party appeared after the 1789 French Revolution and promoted a more liberal governmental form with more popular representation within the context of a diminished monarchy.

88   Curran, I., "Diary," 24 Mar 1863, 9. Handwritten diary is partially illegible.

89   FP, To Mother, Paris 29 Mar 1863, 29-30.

90   Ibid.

Chapter 5 • PROCEEDING ON THE GRAND TOUR

1   FP, To Mother, Orleans 9 Apr 1863, 32.

2   Ibid.

3   Ibid., 32-34.

4   Ibid., 35.

5   FP, To Mother, Madrid, Spain 22 Apr 1863, 36.

6   Ibid.

7   Ibid.

8   FP, To Nathan, Geneva 24 Jun 1863, 59.

9   FP, To Mother, Madrid, Spain 22 Apr 1863, 38.

10   *Executive Documents 1863-4*, 33. This notes Koerner's federal appointment.

11   FP, To Mother, Madrid, Spain 22 Apr 1863, 39.

12   FP, To Nathan, Geneva 24 Jun 1863, 59.

13   Koerner, *Memoirs*, 311.

14   Despite Curran, "Diary," 18. Despite Curran's spelling it is clear he meant Cholera morbus, typified by usually self-limited severe gastrointestinal upset and by differing from epidemic cholera.

15   FP, To Father, Sevilla 3 May 1863, 40.

16   FP, To Mother, Orleans 9 Apr 1863, 33.

17   FP, To Father, Sevilla 3 May 1863, 40-41.

18   Ibid., 44.

19   FP, To Nathan, Geneva 24 Jun 1863, 60-61. Flora initially called McChesney, "McChester."

20   Curran, "Diary," 21-22.

21   Ibid., 25.

22   Ibid.

23   Ibid., 29-30.

24   Ibid., 34.

25   Ibid., 35.

26   TALIM, director's blog. Jesse McMath was U.S. Consul from 1862-69. Mark Twain noted McMath in *Innocents Abroad* as holding one of the worst foreign service billets, so desolate and lacking contact with Americans that, "I would seriously recommend to the government of the United States that when a man commits a crime so heinous that the law provides no adequate punishment for it, they make him Consul General to Tangier."

27   Ibid. The 1865 Cap Spartel Lighthouse Convention was a League of Nations forerunner and United Nations precursor.

28   "The Avalon Project." McMath represented the U.S. in the Convention that included numerous European countries on one part and the Sultan of Morocco on the other. Sir John Hay represented Britain. Convention was ratified in 1867 and terminated in 1958.

29   Curran, "Diary," 35.

30   TALIM director Gerald Loftus, via email 20 May 2013.

31   Curran, "Diary," 39.

32   Drummond-Hay, *A Memoir*, 221-22.

33   Ibid., 222.

34   Curran, "Diary," 39.

35   Green, *Moses Montefiore*, 306.

36   Maghraoui, *Revisiting the Colonial*, 30.

37   Dr. Philip Abensur, Pariente's descendant, via email, 20 May 2013.

38   Curran, "Diary," 40.

39   FP, To Mother, "Steamer Guadaira," Mediterranean 6 Jun 1863, 45.

40   Safford, A. B., and Anna Candee, marriage record, 7 Apr 1863.

41   FP, To Mother, "Steamer Guadaira," Mediterranean 6 Jun 1863, 46.

42   Curran, "Diary," 46.

43   FP, To Nathan, Geneva 24 Jun 1863, 59.

44   FP, To Mother, "Steamer Guadaira," Mediterranean 6 Jun 1863, 46. Fearing and Haseltine were both Harvard class of '63 members, the latter being brother of the artist William Haseltine. No Bowden is among the class listing, but a Charles Pickering Bowditch was, according to *Report of the Secretary of the Class of 1863*, 129-30.

45   Ibid., 47.

46   Ibid.

47   Ibid.

48   Ibid., 48.

49   Ibid., 49.

50   Irving, "Legend of the Moor's Legacy," *The Alhambra*, 247-69. Flora imagines inhabiting a fictional room from Van Wart's Uncle Washington Irving's short story.

51   FP, To Nathan, Geneva 24 Jun 1863, 59.

52   FP, To Mother, "Steamer Guadaira," Mediterranean 6 Jun 1863, 49.

53   Ibid., 49-52.

54   FP, To Father, Lyon, France 20 Jun 1863, 54.

55   Ibid.

56   MJSB, "Etiquette and Custom," *The New Age*, May 1876, 239.

57   FP, To Father, Lyon, France 20 Jun 1863, 55-56.

58   Curran, "Diary," 53.

59   Ibid., 59-60.

60   Ibid., 63, 68.

61   Ibid., 69, 72.

62   Musee Calvet website

63   FP, To Mother, Geneva 30 Jun 1863, 62.

64   MJSB, *Science of Health* article in *Evening Post*, 26 Feb 1875, 1.

65   FP, To Father, Lyon, France 20 Jun 1863, 58.

66   FP, To Mother, Geneva 30 Jun 1863, 62.

67   Ibid.

68   FP, To Nathan, Geneva 24 Jun 1863, 60-61.

69   Tselos and Wickey, *A Guide*, 106. Entry #M4 lists McChesney's birth year as 1828.

70   FP, To Mother, Geneva 30 Jun 1863, 63.

71   FP, Letter to Mother, Geneva 13 Jul 1863, 66. Book was Kingslake's *The Invasion of Crimea*.

72   FP, To Mother, Geneva 13 Jul 1863, 67.

73   Jenness, "Dr. Mary J. Safford," *Cottage Hearth*, May 1876, 114.

74   FP, To Mother, Geneva 13 Jul 1863, 67.

75   Ibid., 69-70.

76   FP, To Mother, Interlaken 31 Jul 1863, 71.

77   Ibid., 72.

78   Ibid., 73.

79   Ibid., 75. Cairns are small rock piles left as trail markers by hikers.

80   Ibid.

81   Costa, "On Goiters," *Panminerva Medica*, Apr-Jun 1989, 97-106.

82   FP, To Mother, Interlaken 31 Jul 1863, 75-76.

83   Ibid., 76. CSA is Confederate States of America.

84   Ibid., 77.

85   Ibid., 77-78.

86   Ibid., 78.

87   FP, To Mother, Ragatz 16 Aug 1863, 81, 84.

88   Ibid., 79-80.

89   FP, To Father, Baden Baden and Wiesbaden 30 Aug 1863, 85.

90   Ibid., 87.

91   Ibid.

92   Ibid., 88.

93   "Papers Read at the Fourth Congress," 87. MJSB was one of the Committee of Reform's three members.

94   FP, To Father, Baden Baden and Wiesbaden 30 Aug 1863, 90.

95   FP, To Parents, Constantinople 24 Oct 1863, 99.

96   FP, To Mother, Dresden 3 Sep 1863, 92.

97   Davidson and Stuve, "The Canal Scrip Fraud," *A Complete History of Illinois from 1673 to 1884*, 668-673. The Court ruled against Matteson who was represented by son-in-law Goodell among others. Sale of Matteson's property occurred Apr 1864.

98   FP, To Oliver, Vienna 7 Oct 1863, 96-97.

99   MJS, "Extracts from a Letter," *The Medical Investigator*, Feb 1870, 232-33.

100 FP, To Parents, Constantinople 24 Oct 1863, 103.

101 Ibid., 103-4.

102 Ibid., 105.

103 Comay, *Who's Who in Jewish History*, 88.

104 Stanton et al, *Cultural Sociology*, 198.

105 FP, To Parents, Constantinople 24 Oct 1863, 104-5.

106 Ibid., 107.

Chapter 6 • MIDDLE-EASTERN JOURNEY

1   FP, To Mother, Constantinople 23 Oct 1863, 108.

2   Ibid.

3   Ibid., 109.

4   Ibid., 111.

5   MJSB, "How the Mighty," *The New Age*, 1 Jul 1876, 278.

6   Ibid.

7   MJS, "A Visit to a Harem," *Woman's Advocate*, Jan 1869, 34. "Daughters of Circassia," references Caucasus Mountain women who were considered most desirable harem denizens.

8   FP, To Mother, Constantinople 23 Oct 1863, 116-17.

9   FP, To Father, Athens 31 Oct 1863, 119.

10   Ibid., 123.

11   Ibid., 123-24.

12   Ibid., 124-25.

13   Dubbs, *History of Franklin*, 282-93. This covers Prof. Koeppen's endearing idiosyncrasies.

14   FP, To Father, Athens 31 Oct 1863, 125. King George I married Russian Princess Olga in 1867. A political liaison with Russia trumped Queen Victoria's matchmaking.

15   FP, To Mother, Beyrout and Damascus 28 Nov 1863, 130.

16   FP, To Oliver, Beyrouth (sic) 13 Nov 1863, 128.

17   FP, To Mother, Beyroot and Damascus 28 Nov 1863, 131.

18   FP, To Oliver, Joppa 18 Dec 1863, 163.

19   FP, To Mother, Beyroot and Damascus 28 Nov 1863, 131.

20   MJS "European Correspondence," Beyroot (Syria), *New Covenant*, from reprint in *Humboldt Register*, 11 Jun 1864, 1.

21   Ibid.

22   Ibid.

23   Ibid.

24   Ibid.

25 MJS "European Correspondence." *New Covenant*, Damascus (Syria) 5 Oct 1863. From reprint in *Humboldt Register*, 18 Jun 1864, 1. Date questionable since the events described in this letter followed those of the 28 Nov 1863 letter.

26 Ibid.

27 Ibid.

28 Ibid.

29 Ibid.

30 Commins and Lesch, *Historical Dictionary of Syria*, 199. Reputedly, 5000 Christians were slaughtered.

31 MJS, "European Correspondence." *New Covenant*, Damascus (Syria) 5 Oct 1863. From reprint in *Humboldt Register*, 18 Jun 1864, 1.

32 Ibid. Mary's euphemism, "descendants of Ham," likely implies dark-skinned individuals.

33 Ibid.

34 FP, To Oliver, Joppa 18 Dec 1863, 163.

35 MJS, "European Correspondence." *New Covenant*, Damascus (Syria) 5 Oct 1863. From reprint in *Humboldt Register*, 18 Jun 1864, 1.

36 Ibid.

37 FP, To Mother, Beyroot and Damascus 28 Nov 1863, 135.

38 Ibid., 135-36.

39 Ibid., 136-37.

40 FP, To Oliver, Joppa 18 Dec 1863, 163.

41 FP, To Mother, Beyroot and Damascus 28 Nov 1863, 138.

42 FP, To Oliver, Beyrouth (sic) 13 Nov 1863, 127.

43 Alger, *War of the Rebellion*, vol. 4, 932.

44 FP, To Mother, Beyroot and Damascus 28 Nov 1863, 138.

45 FP, To Mother, Jerusalem 6 Dec 1863, 141. A convent at Ramleh (meaning sand in Arabic) is between Beirut and Jerusalem.

46 Ibid., 142.

47 Ibid.

48 Ibid., 143.

49 Ibid., 145.

50 Ibid., 144.

51 Ibid., 145.

52 Ibid., 146.

53 Ibid.

54 Ibid., 147.

55 Ibid. Dead Sea was 1312' below sea level; extreme salinity made Jericho's inhabitants sick.

56 Ibid., 149.

57 Ibid.

58 Ibid., 150.

59 FP, To Mother, Jerusalem 10 Dec 1863, 151.

60 Ibid., 155.

61 Beeton, *Beeton's Modern*, 217.

62 FP, To Mother, Jerusalem 10 Dec 1863, 155.

63 FP, To Oliver, Joppa 18 Dec 1863, 163.

64 Ibid., 163-64.

65 FP, To Mother, Joppa 18 Dec 1863, 161.

66 FP, To Nathan, Cairo, Egypt 25 Dec 1863, 165.

67 FP, To Parents, Naples, Italy 2 Feb 1864, 172.

68 Ibid.

69 Ibid.

70 Ibid., 174.

71 Ibid. Shepheard's Hotel hosted the Suez Canal's Grand Opening gala in 1869, per website.

72 FP, To Parents, Naples, Italy 2 Feb 1864, 180.

73 Ibid.

74 Ibid., 181.

75 Ibid., 184.

76 Ibid., 185.

77 Ibid., 186.

Chapter 7 • BACK TO EUROPE

1 FP, To Parents, Naples, Italy Feb 1864, 190-91. An overturned lamp began the blaze.

2 Ibid., 195-96.

3 MJS, *Opinions on Cremation*, 37-38. Even 35 years later MJS found Naples' practice shocking.

4 FP, To Mother, Rome 13 Mar 1864, 210, 212.

5 Castellani and Chalmers, *Manual of Tropical Medicine*, 631.

6 U.S. Centers for Disease Control and Prevention website: "If I get malaria." Disease has the potential for reactivation after being asymptomatic for decades if the patient becomes immune compromised. No effective treatment was known when MJS had Roman Fever.

7 Sullivan, "The Roman Fever," *The Medical Times and Gazette*, 12 Jan 1878, 32. A form of Roman fever, "attended with an exaggerated or profoundly nervous prostration resembling or simulating typhoid," may exist. The term, "typho-malarial fever," was in vogue in the mid to late 1800s, but typhoid and malaria are two separate diseases caused by two distinctly unrelated organisms.

8 FP, To Mother, Rome 13 Mar 1864, 213.

9 Hickey, "An Illinois First Family," *Journal of the Illinois State Historical Society*, Autumn 1961, 114.

10 FP, To Mother, Rome 30 Mar 1864, 220. Isaac Curran was to leave for Paris 31 Mar and return to the U.S. rather than proceed to his consular post.

11 FP, To Mother, Rome 13 Mar 1864, 213.

12 FP, To Nathan, Rome 28 Mar 1864, 218.

13 FP, To Mother, Rome 26 Mar 1864, 215.

14 Bacon, *A Life Worth Living*, 162. Emily Bliss' interest in early childhood education may have inspired Mary who later promoted the kindergarten movement.

15   FP, To Nathan, Rome 28 Mar 1864, 218.

16   Ibid.

17   FP, To Father, Florence 5 Jun 1864, 246-48.

18   Ibid., 236.

19   Catalog, "19th Century Paintings and Sculpture," 57-59.

20   Taylor, *The Fine Arts*, 61.

21   Everett, et al, *Powers' Statue of the Greek Slave*, 3-30. As the most famous mid-19th century sculpture, the piece's nudity required a proper sales pitch to prudish Victorian viewers; numerous articles favored the statue's innocent beauty and metaphoric importance.

22   Hall, Alston and McConnell, *Ancient Slavery*, 232.

23   Browning, "The Greek Slave," *The Complete Works of Mrs. E. B. Browning*, 178. Sonnet was written in 1844.

24   FP, To Father, Florence 5 Jun 1864, 240-41.

25   Ibid., 241.

26   Ibid.

27   Powers, *Hiram Powers Papers*. Born in 1835, Nicholas Longworth Powers lived in Hiram's shadow and lacked his father's success.

28   FP, To Father, Florence 5 Jun 1864, 241.

29   Fairman, "Works of Art," 43.

30   FP, To Father, Milan 15 Jun 1864, 250-52.

31   FP, To Father, Lake Como 19 Jun 1864, 257.

32   Ibid., 260.

33   FP, To Father, Munich 26 Jun 1864, 263.

34   FP, To Father, Antwerp 8 Jul 1864, 266.

35   MJS, "European Correspondence No. 53," *New Covenant*, 7 Jan 1865, 1.

36   Ibid.

37   FP, To Father, Munich 27 Jun 1864, 264.

38   MJS, "European Correspondence No. 53," 1.

39   Ibid.

40   FP, To Mother, Oban, Scotland 4 Aug 1864, 267.

41   FP, To Nathan, Rome 28 Mar 1864, 218.

42   Lander, *Lincoln and Darwin*, 72. McChesney was Illinois' Assistant State Geologist in 1858 and vice-president of the Illinois Natural History Society according to, "State Natural History," *Prairie Farmer*, 20.

43   FP, To Mother, Oban, Scotland 4 Aug 1864, 267.

44   Ibid., 269.

45   Ibid., 267. Flora probably meant Fingal's Cave.

46   Ibid.

47   Ibid., 269.

48   MJS, "Physiological Effects of Alcoholic," *Union Signal*, 8 Mar 1883, 5.

49   FP, To Mother, Oban, Scotland 4 Aug 1864, 269.

50   FP, To Mother Wordsworth's Cottage, Grassmere Aug 1864, 270.

51   "Police Search for Portree Fossil Hunters," *Oban Times & West Highland Times*, 22 Nov 2011. Article notes, "reckless fossil hunting."

52   Lander, "Herndon's Auction List," *Journal of the Abraham Lincoln Association*, Summer 2011, 16-49.

53   Ibid.

54   Anne M. Huber, Institute Librarian, Prairie Research Institute email communication 12 Jun 2012.

55   FP, To Mother, Oban, Scotland 4 Aug 1864, 269.

56   FP, To Mother, Wordsworth's Cottage, Grassmere Aug 1864, 270.

57   "Irish News," *The Morning Freeman*, 6 Sep 1864.

58   FP, To Mother Wordsworth's Cottage, Grassmere Aug 1864, 270.

59   Ibid., 271.

60   Quinlan, *Strange Kin*, 82. Conolly attempted blockade-running and knew Jefferson Davis.

61   FP, To Mother Wordsworth's Cottage, Grassmere Aug 1864, 271.

62   FP, To Papa, Stanhope, Durham Court 9 Sep 1864, 274.

63   FP, To Nathan, Warwick 16 Sep 1864, 276.

64   FP, To Mama, London 28 Sep 1864, 278.

65   FP, To Papa, Stanhope, Durham Court 9 Sep 1864, 273.

66   FP, To Nathan, Paris 15 Oct 1864, 283.

67   FP, To Mama, London 28 Sep 1864, 279.

68   FP, To Papa, Paris 16 Oct 1864, 286.

69   Leonard, *Marquis Who's Who*, 940. Later, Professor McChesney worked at the University of Chicago and died 12 Mar 1895. His only child Dora Greenwell McChesney was born in Chicago, 1 Oct 1871, just 8 days before the fire.

70   *Journal of the Executive Proceedings of the Senate*, 12 Apr 1869, 145.

71   *Annual Catalogue of the University of Chicago*, 18. Lists J. H. McChesney, M. A., as Professor of Chemistry, Geology, and Mineralogy.

72   FP, To Nathan, Paris 15 Oct 1864, 283.

73   FP, To Papa, Paris 16 Oct 1864, 286.

74   FP, To Nathan, Paris 15 Oct 1864, 284.

75   FP, To Papa, Paris 16 Oct 1864, 286.

76   FP, To Nathan, Paris 9 Nov 1864, 294.

77   Swanberg, *Whitney Father*, 4, 44.

78   Ibid., 105-6.

79   FP, To Mama, Paris 30 Oct 1864, 291.

80   Digre and Corbett, *Practical Viewing*, 6.

81   Stahnisch, "Graefe," *Dictionary of Medical Biography*, 572.

82   MJSB, "What Ladies Should Wear," *The Health Reformer*, Jul 1874, 204. Dr. Graefe theorized that women's wearing spotted lace veils was a main cause of blindness.

83 MJS, "An Evening at a German Professor's," *The Woman's Advocate*, Jun 1869, 286-91.

84 Ibid., 291.

85 Woolson, *Dress Reform: A Series of Lectures*, 28-29.

86 MJS, "An Evening at a German Professor's," *The Woman's Advocate*, Jun 1869, 291.

87 Jenness, "Dr. Mary J. Safford," *Cottage Hearth*, May 1876, 114.

88 MJSB, "Etiquette and Custom," *The New Age*, 27 May 1876, 239.

89 Jones, *Una and Her Paupers*, 490.

90 MJSB, "Etiquette and Custom," 239.

91 Michelet, *Glimpses from Agnes Mathilde*, 138. Norwegian portraitist and feminist Aasta Hasteen wrote from Boston to Dr. Wergeland in Norway of meeting the day's great reformers.

92 Bjornson, *Land of the Free*, 68.

93 MJS, "Remembrances of Moscow," *The Woman's Advocate*, Feb 1869, 89-93.

94 Ibid., 90.

95 Ibid., 91.

96 *Register of the Members of the Vieusseux*, files 218 and 256.

97 MJS, "To George Perkins Marsh," Florence, Italy 30 Dec 1865.

98 Marsh and Ducci, *George P. Marsh Correspondence*, 15, 194.

99 Jenness, "Dr. Mary J. Safford," 113.

100 Livermore, *My Story*, 215.

101 Sarti, *Italy: A Reference*, 395.

102 Willson, *The University of London*, 1858-1900, 85-86.

103 Hart, "To Mary."

104 Gantz, "Hiram Powers and Joel Tanner Hart."

105 Berry, *Joel Tanner Hart*, 40.

106 Hart, "Portrait of Mary Morgan Hart Weaver." Mary died at 39 in 1845.

107 APKS, Sketch of the Life, 26.

108 NARA, *New York, Passenger Lists, 1820-1957*, arrival 1 Feb 1866, on the *Atlantic* from Aspinwall, Panama.

109 NARA, *Passport Applications 1795-1905*, New York City, 6 May 1866.

110 APKS, *Sketch of the Life*, 26-27.

111 Sammons, "Mary J. Safford, MD," *To-Day*, Jun 1896, 262. MJS was fluent in German, French and Italian.

112 Anonymous, "European Correspondence," *Humboldt Register*, 29 Sep 1866 and 6 Oct 1866. Although the writer is anonymous, APK's Humboldt County domicile and MJS's coincident presence in Florence suggests either of them could have written the letters. Dated Florence, Italy, 6 Jul 1866, the first told of French political intrigue, descriptions of Paris, Marseilles and Florence. The writer visited sculpture studios of Hiram Powers, Mr. Ball of Boston (probably Thomas Ball who just finished a marble statue of Lincoln) and Mr. Hart of Kentucky who worked on a statue with description matching that of, "Woman Triumphant." The second letter, from Milan, told of the political situation regarding the Italian-Austrian war, Italian government, Garibaldi, described Italian hospitals and how both Italian and enemy combatants received equally good care.

113 "Americans in Paris," *Anglo-American Times*, 1 Sep 1866, 12. MJS listed in, "Americans registered in the offices of Messrs. John Munroe and Co," from " 21st to the 28th August." Same publication's 14 Sep edition (2: no.47, 13) lists, "Mr. A. P. H. (sic) Safford," but not MJS.

Chapter 8 • MEDICAL EDUCATION AND EARLY WOMEN'S RIGHTS WORK

1   MJS, "To Caroline Crane Marsh," New York City 10 April 1867.

2   Ibid.

3   Ibid.

4   Ibid.

5   Livermore, *The Story of My Life*, 589.

6   New York Medical College for Women, *Fifth Annual Announcement*, 3.

7   Griffith, *In Her Own Right*, 187.

8   Ullman, *Homeopathic Revolution*, 221-22.

9   Davidson, *Century of Homeopaths*, 10.

10   Grant, T., *Women in Medicine*, 12.

11   Haller, *History of American Homeopathy*, 138.

12   *Fifth Annual Announcement*, 7.

13   Kirschmann, *A Vital Force*, 58-59.

14   Ibid.

15   Ibid., 61.

16   King, *History of Homeopathy*, 125, 129.

17   *Fifth Annual Announcement*, 4.

18   Ibid., 8.

19   *Sixth Annual Announcement*, 7.

20   *Fifth Annual Announcement*, 8.

21   Barrows, Memorial statement on MJS' death, *Tarpon Springs Truth*, 12 Dec 1891.

22   *Seventh Annual Announcement*, 6.

23   Cleave, *Cleave's Biographical*, 289-90. In 1869 Millard resigned to marry New York Mayor Harper's daughter.

24   *Seventh Annual Announcement*, 8,11. *Gray's Anatomy* was first published in 1858 per Richardson, *The Making of Mr. Gray's*, 201.

25   *Seventh Annual Announcement*, 8-9.

26   *Sixth Annual Announcement*, 9.

27   Ullman, *Homeopathic Revolution*, 221.

28   MJS, To Frank Moore, Cairo, IL 28 Dec 1866.

29   Grant, *U. Papers: January 1–September 30*, 1867, 28.

30   King, *History of Homeopathy*, 132. Dr. Lozier gave $6000 for a dispensary and pledged an additional $10,000 for the school later.

31   Kirschmann, *A Vital Force*, 62.

32   Ibid.

33   Cole, *Centennial History of Illinois*, 428.

34   Stanton, et al, *History of Woman*, 564.

35   Ibid., 570.

36   "New--York Medical College for Women," *New York Times*, 24 Mar 1869.

37   Note, *Woman's Advocate*, April 1869, 229.

38   "New--York Medical College for Women," *New York Times*, 24 Mar 1869.

39   "Item," *Cairo Evening Bulletin*, 27 Mar 1869, 3.

40   Stewart, *Reminiscences*, 252.

41   DeLong, *The History of Arizona*, 85.

42   Pickard, *Letters of John Greenleaf*, 194.

43   Kirschmann, *A Vital Force*, 62.

44   MJS, Letter, *Anti-Slavery Standard*, 17 Apr 1869, 3.

45   Hering, *Materia Medica*, 77.

46   Society of Homeopaths website.

47   Hering, *Materia Medica*, 76.

48   Ibid., 79-80.

49   Ibid., 81, 84, 95, 103, 111, 122-23.

50   Lilienthal, *Homeopathic Therapeutics*, 515, 668.

51   "Local News," *Cairo Evening Bulletin*, 7 May 1869, 3.

52   Hunt, "Golden Jubilee," 525.

53   Hart, "Last Rail Laid."

54   "Married," *Cairo Evening Bulletin*, 17 Aug 1869, 3. "At Tucson, Arizona, on Wednesday evening, July 25th, the Hon. A. P. K. Safford and Miss Jennie L Tracey (sic) of San Diego California."

55   "Specimens of Silver," *Cairo Evening Bulletin*, 11 Jun 1869, 3.

56   MJS, "To Mr. and Mrs. Marsh," Vienna, Austria 7 Oct 1869.

57   MJS, "Concerning European," *The Medical Investigator*, May 1872, 218-20.

58   S. L., Correspondence, *The Medical Investigator*, Feb 1870, 232-33. "S. L." was likely Sophia Clemence Lozier who toured Europe in 1867 and possibly made Viennese medical connections. S. L. mentions, "Mrs. Barrows and Miss Safford, both M. D.'s from our college, now in Vienna…"

59   Bonner, *To the Ends*, 1.

60   MJS, "Concerning European," 218-20.

61   Barrows, Memorial statement on MJS' death, *Tarpon Springs Truth*, 12 Dec 1891.

62   Doggett, "Letter from Luxor, Egypt," *Cairo Daily Bulletin*, 7 May 1871, 1. Doggett visited MJS in Vienna October 1870.

63   S. L., Correspondence, 232-33.

64   MJS, "Letter from Austria," *New Covenant*, 27 May 1871, 1.

65   Barrows, "Hospital Life," *The Phrenological Journal and Packard's Monthly*, Mar 1870, 170-71.

66   "Periscope," *The Medical Investigator*, Jan 1870, 190.

67   "Obituary of Carl Rudolph Braun," *Medical Record*, 2 May 1891, 517.

68   "Memorial to Carl Braun," *The American Journal of Obstetrics and Diseases of Women and Children*, Jun 1891, 711.

69   Connolly et al, *Autopsy Pathology*, 5-6.

70   S. L., Correspondence, 233. In cord prolapse the umbilical cord precedes the head on delivery. A hemi-cephalous monster lacks certain brain parts.

71   "Periscope," *The Medical Investigator*, Jan 1870, 190.

72   "Memorial to Carl Braun," *The American Journal of Obstetrics and Diseases of Women and Children*, Jun 1891, 711.

73   Barrows, Memorial statement on Mary Jane Safford's death, *Tarpon Springs Truth*, 12 Dec 1891.

74   MJS, "To Mr. and Mrs. Marsh," Vienna, Austria 7 Oct 1869.

75   Rummel, *Illinois Handbook*, 32. Jay's title was, "Envoy Extraordinary and Minister Plenipotentiary of the United States of America, Vienna."

76   "Periscope," *The Medical Investigator*, Jan 1870, 190. Angina in this sense suggests severe pain of unspecified location, possibly a headache or menstrual cramps.

77   Doggett, "Letter from Switzerland," *The Woman's Journal*, 21 Oct 1871, 336.

78   Nightingale, *Florence Nightingale*, 410.

79   Eigler, *The Feminist*, 29.

80   MJS, "Austrian Correspondence," *New Covenant*, 28 Feb 1871, 1.

81   MJS, "Grillparzer," *Boston Daily Advertiser*, 30 Jan 1872.

82   MJS, "Sights in Vienna," *The Revolution*, 25 Aug 1870, 115-16.

83   Ibid.

84   Anonymous German correspondent, "Letter from Hesse-Darmstadt," *The Woman's Journal*, 5 Aug 1871, 245.

85   Doggett, "Letter from Switzerland," 336.

86   MJS, "To Clara Barton," 6 Mar 1870. At letter's top in writing different than MJS' is, "Miss Mary J Safford Ansd 16 March 1870," implying Miss Barton responded.

87   MJS, "To George Marsh," Vienna 30 Oct 1869.

88   MJS, "Letter from Mary Safford," *The Herald of Health*, Sep 1870, 132-34.

89   Gurney et al, *Phantasms*, 88.

90   Society for Psychical Research website.

91   Gurney et al, *Phantasms*, 88.

92   MJS, "Correspondence," *The Medical Investigator*, May 1870, 378.

93   Semmelweis, *The Etiology*. This is a direct translation of Semmelweis' 1860 puerperal fever monograph.

94   Hellman, *Great Feuds*, 44.

95   Semmelweis, *The Etiology*, 86.

96   Daintith, *Biographical Encyclopedia*, 762.

97   Howard, "European Letter," *Cincinnati Medical Advance*, Dec 1873, 595-96.

98   MJS, "Correspondence," *The Medical Investigator*, May 1870, 379.

99   MJS, "The Skoda Ovation," *New England Medical Gazette*, May and June 1871, 249-50. Dr. I. T. Talbot edited this journal and would play a significant role in Mary Safford's future in Boston.

100 Baas and Handerson, *Outlines of the History*, 1083.

101 MJS, "Concerning European," 219.

102 MJS and Allen, M., *Health and Strength for Girls*.

103 Baas and Handerson, *Outlines of the History*, 954.

104 Ibid., 957.

105 MJS, "Letter from Vienna," *The New England Medical Gazette*, Jan 1871, 36-37.

106 MJS, "The Skoda Ovation," 249-50.

107 "Obituary of Johan Oppolzer," *Medical Times and Register*, 1 Jun 1871, 327. He died 16 Apr 1871, age about 63.

108 MJS, "Letter from Germany," *New Covenant*, 27 May 1871, 1.

109 MJS, "How They Treat," *Herald of Health*, Sep 1871, 129-31.

110 Anonymous German correspondent, "Letter from Hesse-Darmstadt," 245.

111 Clarke and O'Malley, *The Human Brain*, 113-14.

112 U.S. National Library of Medicine, NIH website for Waldeyer-Hartz. Waldeyer was 5 years younger than Mary and donated parts of his body to Berlin's Institute of Anatomy.

113 Geitz, et al, *German Influences*, 242.

114 Obituary of Dr. Otto Spiegelberg, *The Boston Medical and Surgical Journal*, 29 Dec 1881, 623.

115 "Notes of the 61st Regular Meeting," *Journal of the Gynaecological Society of Boston*, Jan 1872, 2-3.

116 Ibid., 3.

117 MJS, "How They Treat," 130.

118 MJS, To James Jackson Putnam, Breslau 16 Apr 1871.

119 "Obituary of James Jackson Putnam," *The Harvard Graduates' Magazine*, 1918-1919, 229.

120 "Notes of the 61st Regular Meeting," *Journal of the Gynaecological Society of Boston*, Jan 1872, 3.

121 "Obituary of C. P. Putnam," *Harvard Alumni Bulletin*, 1913, 487. This mentions Charles Putnam's 1869 Viennese study and marriage to Lucy Washburn.

122 Madsen and Plunz, *The Urban Lifeworld*, 58. Brothers Charles and James Putnam shared a vacation home with Harvard Medical School classmate Dr. Wm James, brother of author Henry Jmes

123 James and James, *William and Henry James*, 530. Ellen Washburn Freund is sister of Dr. Charles Putnam's wife Lucy and is German physician Maximilian Bernard Freund's spouse.

124 Cleave, *Cleave's Biographical*, 466-67.

125 MJS, "Concerning European," 218-20.

126 Doggett, "Letter from Switzerland," 336. Kate's letter quoted Mary.

127 MJS, "Case of Ovariotomy," *Proceedings of the Gynaecological Society of Boston*, Jul 1872, 12-20.

128 Ibid., 12-13. Dr. W. Freund knew Dr. Norris who communicated another of Freund's articles to the society; noted in the Jan 1872 issue of the same journal, 2-3.

129 "Sixty Eighth Regular (Annual) Meeting," *Proceedings of the Gynaecological Society of Boston*, Jul 1872, 11, and Nov & Dec 1872, 336.

130 Safford, Miss, "Indications for Ovariotomy," *Proceedings of the Gynaecological Society of Boston*, Jul 1872, 19-20.

131 MJS, "How They Treat," 131.

132 MJS, "Concerning European," 219.

133 Doggett, "Letter from Switzerland," 336.

134 Doggett, "Letter from Luxor, Egypt," 1.

135   Epler, *Life of Clara Barton*, 167-68.

136   Safford, Frank Alfred, death notice, *Arizona Citizen*, 9 Sep 1871, 3.

137   "Brevities," *Cairo Daily Bulletin*, 17 Oct 1871, 4.

Chapter 9 • REESTABLISHING AMERICAN LIFE

1   News item, *Arizona Citizen*, 30 Dec 1871, 4.

2   Cooper, *Fighting Fire*, 52.

3   Sheahan and Upton, *The Great Conflagration*, 185-91.

4   Duncan, "Medical View," *Homeopathic World*, 1 Dec 1871, 277-79.

5   "Dr. Mary Safford," *Cairo Daily Bulletin*, 19 Dec 1871, 4.

6   "Dr. Mary Safford," *Cairo Daily Bulletin*, 3 Jan 1872, 4.

7   "All Sorts of Items," *Cairo Daily Bulletin*, 3 Jan 1872, 4.

8   "Brevities," *Cairo Daily Bulletin*, 6 Jan 1872, 4.

9   News item, *Ottawa Free Trader*, 2 Mar 1872, 1.

10   MJS, "The Folly of Fashion," *Terre Haute Daily Gazette*, 29 Feb 1872, 3.

11   Willard, *Glimpses*, 216.

12   "Catalogue and Circular Evanston College, 1871-72," 4, and 1872-73 catalogue, 10.

13   "Evanston College for Ladies, Contracts," 11.

14   Willard, *Glimpses*, 216.

15   Cook, B., *Women and War*, 289.

16   Bradford, *Homoeopathic Bibliography*, 541.

17   Duncan, "Medical View," *Homeopathic World*, 1 Dec 1871, 277-79.

18   "List of Permanent Members," Illinois Homoeopathic Medical Association 1875, 142.

19   "Illinois Homoeopathic Medical," *American Observer Medical Monthly*, Sep 1872, 384-85.

20   King, *History of Homoeopathy*, 341.

21   Kirschmann, *A Vital Force*, 164.

22   "Clifford Mitchell, MD," *Biographical Dictionary and Portrait Gallery of Representative Men of Chicago*, 721.

23   "Of Interest to All Women," *The Arrow*, 7.

24   "Report of the Illinois Homoeopathic Medical," 1872 *AIH Transactions*, 275.

25   *Proceedings of the Twenty-Fifth Session*, 185.

26   "Cook County Medical," *U.S. Medical Investigator*, 1872, 365.

27   "Notice," *The Medical Investigator*, Nov 1872, 492.

28   "Chicago Letter July 14," *Cairo Daily Bulletin*, 18 Jul 1872, 2.

29   "Proceedings of the AAAS," 1872, xli.

30   Ibid., xxvi.

31 Ibid., xxxii. Mitchell joined in 1850. As many members used initials only, true number of women members is unknown.

32 Livermore, "After the Battle," *The Ladies Repository*, May 1868, 376.

33 "Oak Park Unity Church Dedication," *New Covenant*, 8 Aug 1872, 3.

34 "Marriage of Dr. Mary J. Safford," *Cairo Daily Bulletin*, 1 Oct 1872, 2.

35 "Illinois Cook County Marriages," film 1030079.

36 Blake, S., *A Genealogical History*, 44, 61-62.

37 Ibid.

38 Ibid., 61.

39 1850 U.S. Census, Newton, Middlesex, MA.

40 Cushing,T., *Historical Sketch*, 91.

41 "Memorial of James Barnard Blake," 5.

42 Blake, C. J., "John Harrison Blake," *Proceedings of the American Academy of Arts & Sciences*, May 1900-01, 565-68.

43 Obituary, "Gorham Blake Buried," *San Francisco Call*, 20 Dec 1897, 9. A supercargo is one who oversees cargo on a merchant ship.

44 Blake, G., "Correspondence," *Journal of Psychical Research*, Jul 1884, 104-5.

45 1850 U.S. Census, Newton, Middlesex, MA.

46 Passenger Listing, "Bark Kepler," from Sumatra, *New York Evening Post*, 11 Dec 1850.

47 Owens, *California Coiners*, 87.

48 Blake, S., *A Genealogic History*, 75.

49 "Murder by the Indians," *Sacramento Daily Union*, 8 July 1852, 2.

50 Kagin, *Private Gold*, 170-71.

51 APKS, *Sketch of the Life*, 20.

52 1860 U.S. Census, Grass Valley, Nevada (county), CA.

53 Owens, *California Coiners*, 96-97. Quote from, "Letter to Louisa," tells of mining conditions and miners. Original letter is in the Francis P. Farquhar Collection, Bancroft Library.

54 "Resident Members," *Proceedings of the California Academy*, vii.

55 Meek and Gabb, *Paleontology*, 1, xiv, x, 19, 28-29, 35. Corbula blakei, Orthoceratites blakei.

56 Blake, G., Letter to sister Mary C. Young, 1 Oct 1890. To his sister Gorham describes long study of William Denton's 1863 work, *The Soul of Things*.

57 Powell, *William Denton*, 28-33.

58 Denton, *The Soul*, numerous pages describe the psychometer.

59 Blake, G., Letter to sister Mary C. Young, 1 Oct 1890.

60 Bankruptcy Notice, *Daily Alta California* 18 Jan 1869, 4.

61 Bankruptcy notice, *Daily Alta California*, 20 Feb 1869, 4.

62 1870 U.S. Census, Boston, Ward 16, Suffolk, MA.

63 1870 U.S. Census, Worcester, Ward 8, Worcester, MA. Census taken 9 Jun 1870.

64 "Memorial of James Barnard Blake," 5-6.

65 Ibid., 8.

66 Ibid., "The Obsequies of James Barnard Blake," 23-25.

67 "Clarence J. Blake vs. Gorham Blake," *Massachusetts Reports 110 Cases Argued and Determined*, 202-3.

68 Essex Institute, 1 Feb 1875 meeting, 28. "Mr. Bell, in conjunction with Dr. Clarence J. Blake, the aurist, or Boston, has conducted a series of experiments, the remarkable result of which were now first exhibited to a public audience." Dr. Blake provided a cadaver eardrum.

69 Warner, *Against the Spirit*, 311. Dr. Blake wrote letters home to Boston on his Vienna experiences of 1866-69.

70 "Clarence J. Blake vs. Gorham Blake," 202-3.

71 Per Earl Taylor, Dorchester Historical Society, Boston. 1874 record listed James Blake as homeowner who was reportedly ill.

72 "The Boston Directory," 1872, under business listings.

73 MJSB, "The Prayer Gauge," *New York World*, 22 Nov 1872, 7.

74 Gunter, *Alice in Jamesland*, 28-29. Author Henry James' sister Alice was a Second Radical Club member concurrently with Mary Safford. Although Henry did not belong, the club discussed his works. James' character Dr. Mary J. Prance in his 1886 novel *The Bostonians* resembles Dr. Mary J. Safford-Blake though Dr. Prance is more likely a composite of the era's, "doctresses."

75 Ibid., 29. The FRA never established its own churches but published religious materials and functioned as the, "voice of radical religion and a force on Unitarianism."

76 Hillerbrand, *The Encyclopedia*, 86.

77 Free Religious Association website, membership roll.

78 MJSB, "The Prayer Gauge," 7.

79 MJSB, "A Visit to Dr. Harriet K. Hunt," *Woman's Journal*, 23 Nov 1872, 376.

80 Campbell, *Disasters*, 131.

81 Conwell, *History*, 53.

82 Ibid., 91.

83 Campbell, *Disasters*, 132.

84 Conwell, *History*, 91, 98.

85 Ibid., 70 and illustration on unnumbered page before 77.

86 Phelps, Letter to the Editor, *New England Medical Gazette*, Jan 1873, 29.

87 Kaufman, *Boston Women*, 39.

88 Davidson, *A Century*, 37-38.

89 "Obituary of Israel Tisdale Talbot," *Transactions of the Fifty-sixth Session*, 839.

90 *Transactions of the World's Congress*, 55.

91 "Personal," *New England Medical Gazette*, Jan 1873, 48.

92 King, *History of Homeopathy*, chapter 5 by John Preston Sutherland, MD, recounts Boston University School of Medicine, 159-213.

93 "American Institute of Homoeopathy Twenty-Sixth Session," *The American Observer*, Jul 1873, 386-87. Note on expulsion of the Massachusetts homeopaths from the allopathic Massachusetts Medical Society.

94 "The Boston University," *New England Medical Gazette*, Feb 1873, 129-33. Massachusetts Supreme Court ruled it lacked jurisdiction over the allopathic society's expulsion of homeopaths and removed an earlier injunction placed against dismissal.

95 Kirschmann, *A Vital Force*, 64.

96 King, *History of Homeopathy*, Sutherland, "Boston University School of Medicine," 181.

97 "Homoeopathic Association," *The American Observer*, Jul 1873, 342-43.

98 King, *History of Homeopathy*, Sutherland, "Boston University School of Medicine," 183.

99 Ibid., 183-85.

100 MJS, "Pruritis," and "Complete Inversion," *The New England Medical Gazette*, May 1873, 222-30.

101 MJS, "Complete Inversion," 228.

102 Zweifel, "Occlusion of the Os Uteri, *New England Medical Gazette*, Oct 1873, 456.

103 MJS, "Sure Test of Death," *Brisbane Australia Courier*, 14 Jun 1873, 7. This referred to an undated item from the *Boston Transcript*.

104 *Transactions of the Twenty-Sixth Session*, 184.

105 "The Consumptive Home," 7.

106 "Acts," *Acts, Resolutions and Memorials*, 1873, 17.

107 Hickey, "An Illinois First Family," *Journal of the Illinois State Historical Society*, Feb 1976, 105.

108 Skrabec, *The 100 Most Significant*, 70-72.

109 "Tilghman's," 14. Lists Gorham Blake as General Agent for the United States.

110 "American Institute of Homeopathy," *The American Observer*, 1873, 385.

111 MJSB, "Inversion of the Uterus," 503-7.

112 Reports in: *New England Medical Gazette*, Jul 1873, 327: *American Observer Medical Monthly*, Jul 1873, 385: *The Medical Union*, Jun 1873, 142.

113 "History of the Association for the Advancement of Woman," *Souvenir Program*, 121-27.

114 *Papers and Letters Presented*, 1873, Stanton's lecture, 39-52: Woolson and Burleigh's lectures, 109-20.

115 Ibid., Temperance, 147-53: Suffrage, 126-32: Women Professors, 60-67: Dr. Jacobi's talk, 168-78.

116 *Papers Read Before the Association*, 1887, 3.

117 "Report of Regular Meeting," *Bulletin of the Essex Institute*, Oct 1873, 164.

118 "The Essex Institute," *Bulletin of the Essex Institute*, Jan 1873, 3. The descendant organization Peabody Essex Museum is one of the oldest continuously operating U.S. museums.

119 "General Calendar," *Boston University Yearbook*, vol. 1, 6.

120 "Homoeopathic Association," *The American Observer*, 1873, 342-43.

121 Kirschmann, *A Vital Force*, 65.

122 MJSB, "Boston News," *The Medical Investigator*, Jan 1874, 249-50.

123 "Special Notices," *The Woman's Journal*, 7 Mar 1874, 80.

124 Notice, *New England Medical Gazette*, Jun 1874, 272.

125 Ballou, "Help for Women," *The Index*, 29 Oct 1874, 9, 525.

Chapter 10 • THE DRESS REFORM CRUSADER

1   MJS, "Ornament and Dress," *Herald of Health*, Jan 1873, 10-13: Mar 1873, 120-23: Jun 1873, 265-68.

2   Ibid., 266.

3   Ibid. Article cited the Massachusetts State Board of Health's 1872 report on green cloth's arsenic content and its detriment to both wearer and dressmaker. Magenta dye was worse.

4   Ibid., 266-67.

5   Ibid., 267.

6   *Papers and Letters Presented*, 109-15.

7   Croly, *The History*, 41.

8   Woolson, *Dress Reform*, xvi. MJSB's lecture is on 1-41.

9   "Dress Reform. A Lecture to Ladies," *Boston Morning Journal*, 26 Feb 1874, 2.

10   Ibid., 1.

11   Woolson, *Dress Reform*, 38.

12   Ibid., 38-41. MJS learned the last caveat from Berlin's Dr. Graefe in 1864.

13   "What Ladies Should Wear," *The Health Reformer*, Jul 1874, 203. Anonymous author recounted MJS' 25 Feb 1874 lecture.

14   "Editor's By-Hours," *The Repository*, 469.

15   "Notes and Comments," *The Index*, 16 Apr 1874, 1.

16   Birch, *The Unsheltered Woman*, 146.

17   McDowell, *A Sherwood Bonner Sampler*, 409-14. As Dio Lewis' secretary and friend of MJS biographer Jenness, Bonner may have known MJS was on the New England Women's Club Dress Reform Committee with Lewis and his wife (lxii, 15).

18   Ibid., 412.

19   "Library Chat," *The Cambridge Tribune*, 22 Nov 1890, 4.

20   "The Dress Reform Lectures," *New England Medical Gazette*, May 1874, 215-16. The author given only as, "B," was undoubtedly MJSB.

21   MJSB, "Article XLV. Lac Defloratum," *North American Journal of Homoepathy*, May 1874, 541-44.

22   Cicchetti, *Dreams*, 177.

23   MJS, "How a Daughter," *Herald of Health*, May 1874, 205-9.

24   Ibid., 207.

25   "Transactions of the Twenty-Seventh," *The North American Journal of Homeopathy*, 141.

26   MJSB, "The Etiology and Infectiousness," *Transactions of the Twenty-Seventh Session*, 379-83.

27   Burroughs, "Women in the Institute," *Transactions of the Forty-Seventh Session*, 76.

28   "The Dress Reformers," *New York Times*, 15 Jun 1874, 8.

29   "The Dress Reform Meeting in Boston," *Frank Leslie's Illustrated Newspaper*, 20 Jun 1874, 229 and cover illustration.

30   "Dress Reform in Boston," *Herald of Health*, Nov 1874, 72, 74, 82.

31   MJSB, "A New Dress for Women," *Science of Health*, 1 Mar 1875, 103-7.

32   Advertisement, "Ladies' Garment Suspenders," *Herald of Health*, Dec 1874, 287.

33   "Local News," *Daily Illini*, Oct 1874, 20. Item dwelled more upon the university women's enthusiastic acceptance of MJSB's words (without reporting their content) and her high praise for the nascent school, favorably comparing it to, the, "Hub," (Boston) and, "all New England."

34   Arnold, *Four Lives*, 83-84.

35   MJSB, "Hopeful Things," *The Woman's Journal*, 28 Nov 1874, 386.

36   *Tenth Report of the Board of Trustees of the Illinois Industrial University*, 7. Lists "Don Carlos Taft, M. A., Professor of Geology and Zoology."

37   Zeller, *The Autobiography of George Zeller*, 13.

38   Russler, "A Museum's Life Story," *Daily Illini*, 13 Feb 1927, 1. Famous sculptor Lorado Taft was Don Carlos Taft's son.

39 "College of Natural Sciences," *The Illio*, 33.

40 "Historical Sketch," *Tenth Report of the Board of Trustees of the Illinois Industrial University*, 15. Lists Taft's achieving full professorship March 1872.

41 "In the matter of the Guardianship of Leandro Taft, a minor." "Orphan," Leandro's named parents were Carlos Taft and Margrisio Maldonado (another male name, no feminine name given), and birthplace was Hermosillo, Sonora, Mexico, March 1868. That birth date correlates with a summer 1867 liaison. It is unknown if Don Carlos Taft was on John Wesley Powell's first western expedition in summer 1867. Although, "Don," could have been a title of courtesy, it is unknown if geologist Don Carlos Taft and Carlos Taft were the same individual.

42 MJSB, "Hopeful Things," *The Woman's Journal*, 28 Nov 1874, 386.

43 "Women's Congress," *Friends' Intelligencer*, 21 Nov 1874, 612.

44 Leach, *True Love*, 259.

45 "The Women's Congress in Chicago," *Daily Graphic*, 21 Oct 1874, 805.

46 *Souvenir Nineteenth Annual Congress*, 127.

47 MJSB, "A Visit to Cornell University," *The Woman's Journal*, 12 Dec 1874, 397.

48 Bishop, *A History of Cornell*, 111.

49 "Dr. Mary Safford Blake's Lecture," *Lowell Daily Citizen and News*, 8 Mar 1878.

50 "Obituary for Dr. Mary J. Safford," *Lasell Leaves*, Feb 1892, 95.

51 Janney (Derby), to Mother Rebecca Smith Janney, 23 May 1875.

52 Kirschmann, *A Vital Force*, 70.

CHAPTER 11 • FURTHER NORTHERN LIFE

1 MJSB, "Prenatal Influence," *Herald of Health*, Jan 1875, 1-9. Yet another iteration of Mary's evening at the German professor's house, "A Delightful Memory," is on 228-29.

2 Ibid., 4.

3 Ibid., 5.

4 Ibid., 6.

5 Ripley, "Some Overlooked Causes," *Transactions of the Forty-Fifth Session*, 640.

6 "Obituary for Dr. Mary J. Safford," *Lasell Leaves*, Feb 1892, 95. It included, "She was radical in her opposition to fashionable follies of social life in dress, diet, etc. To eat mince-pie was, to her a sin..."

7 Winslow, *Lasell*, 56.

8 Carpenter, C., Letter, *Herald of Health*, Jul 1875, 34.

9 Arnold, *Four Lives*, 83-84.

10 Gregory, transcription of MJSB' lecture, "Womb and Menstruation." Louisa Allen's later married name was Gregory.

11 Gregory, transcription of MJSB' lecture, "Beginnings of Life."

12 Gregory, transcription of MJSB' lecture, "Food Lecture."

13 MJSB, "Glastonbury Criticized," *The Woman's Journal*, 25 April 1874, 130.

14 "Obituary for Dr. Mary J. Safford," *New England Medical Gazette*, Jan 1892, 48.

15 Kaufman, *Boston Women*, 39, 55.

16 "The American Froebel Union," *Kindergarten Messenger*, Sep 1877, 152-53, 155.

17 "Virtual Tours," Northampton, MA, website. Florence is near Northampton, site of Smith College that started in September 1875. Perhaps while

visiting Florence MJS investigated that institution, but no record of such a visit exists. MJS' niece Margarita was graduated from Smith in 1903.

18 "About Hill Institute," website.

19 MJSB, "The Ideal Sunday School," *The Index*, 23 Aug 1877, 404-5.

20 Warwick, *Warwick's Keystone*, 331.

21 "School of All Sciences," 105.

22 "Lecture Subjects: Professor Mary S. Blake," 94.

23 Janney (Derby), To Parents, 13 Feb 1876.

24 "Preceptors," 88.

25 Coachman, "Fidelia Jane Merrick Whitcomb," *Sunland Tribune*, 2008-9, 60-64.

26 "Massachusetts Homoeopathic Hospital." *Publications of the Massachusetts Homoeopathic Medical Society*, 195. Boston women held public fairs in May 1872 netting $76,000 to purchase land on E. Concord Street. The hospital opened May 1876.

27 "Massachusetts Homoeopathic Hospital," 196-97.

28 MJSB, "A Supposed Uterine Tumor," *United States Medical Investigator*, 1 Sep 1877, 259-61.

29 "Local Brevities," *Los Angeles Daily Herald*, 23 Jul 1875, 3. "Dr. Mary Safford Blake of Boston is at the St. Charles." Just below is, "Gov. Safford of Arizona is expected to-day, to meet his brother A. B. Safford and wife of Cairo, Ill., Dr. Mary Safford Blake of Boston and J. S. Dennis and wife of Chicago, who stop at the St. Charles."

30 MJSB, "Women in Utah," *The Woman's Journal*, 14 Aug 1875, 258. Bryant's poem, "The Battle-Field," appeared in The *U.S. Democratic Review*, October 1837, 15-16.

31 Breslin, *Brigham Young*, 212.

32 Turner, *Brigham Young*, 376. Young's wife may have been British feminist and poet Hannah Tapfield King, "sealed," to him in 1872 for her, "salvation," as her husband was a not a Mormon.

33 Ware, *Forgotten Heroes*, 125.

34 MJSB, "Women in Utah," *The Woman's Journal*, 14 Aug 1875, 258.

35 Ibid.

36 Ibid.

37 Van Wagoner, "Sarah Pratt," *Dialogue: A Journal of Mormon Thought*, 79.

38 Foster, *Women, Family and Utopia*, 148-50.

39 "Pratt, Sarah Marinda Bates," "The Joseph Smith Papers," The Church Historian's Press online. Sarah Pratt's excommunication date was 4 Oct 1874.

40 "The Utah Theocracy," *The New York Herald*, 18 May 1877, 4. The long article recounts Sarah Pratt's interview, "Orson Pratt's Harem," Sarah's son's report, and Brigham Young's possible connection to the 1857 Mountain Meadow Massacre.

41 MJSB, "Women in Utah," *The Woman's Journal*, 14 Aug 1875, 258.

42 MJSB, "A Glimpse of California," *The Woman's Journal*, 18 Sep 1875, 304.

43 "Local Brevities," *Los Angeles Daily Herald*, 29 Jul 1875, 3.

44 MJSB, "A Glimpse of California," *The Woman's Journal*, 18 Sep 1875, 304.

45 "Lotta's Fountain," website. San Francisco vaudevillian Lotta Crabtree, grateful to the city where her career began, donated the water fountain.

46 MJSB, "A Glimpse of California," *The Woman's Journal*, 18 Sep 1875, 304.

47 *Souvenir Nineteenth Annual Congress*, 128.

48 "Travels in the East," *Sacramento Daily Union*, 22 Mar 1876, 3. Original said to be in Boston Globe, 1 Mar 1876.

49   Ibid.

50   Blake, Mary J. vs. Gorham Blake (divorce). Paperwork lists Mary as the libellant suing Gorham for divorce on his desertion, "the first day of May A. D. 1876…" Also, registered letter receipt for divorce papers signed by Gorham Blake 16 Jul 1879, Loudsville, White County, GA.

51   Lowell, *The Historic Genealogy of the Lowells*, 37.

52   "Passengers Sailed," *New York Times*, 5 Nov 1876, 12.

53   "Moral Education Association," *Boston Post*, 2 Jun 1876, 4.

54   Janney (Derby), to Mother Rebecca Smith Janney, 9 Jun 1875.

55   Blake, G., To Mary C. Young, 1 Oct 1890.

56   Blake, G., "Correspondence," *Journal of Society for Psychical Research*, 1885, 104.

57   Fulton County, GA, Marriage Book E, 797, Gorham Blake married Mrs. Mary A. Gordon 8 May 1885.

58   Blake, M. A., To Mary C. Young, 22 Feb 1898. Letter from Oakland, CA.

59   Ibid.

60   "International Exhibition 1876 Official Catalogue," 90. "195 Blake, Mary J. S., Boston, Mass.—Surgical instrument. Sec. C"

61   Author's conversation with U. S. Patent Office employee Dennis Taylor, 10 Apr 2008. 1870s era patents were filed by invention and not by inventor's name. Searching for MJS' patent would be like seeking a needle in a 500-acre hayfield.

62   "World's Homeopathic Convention," *United States Medical Investigator*, 15 Sep 1876, 290, 292.

63 MJS, To Caroline Severance, East Gloucester, MA 14 Jul 1876.

64   Ibid.

65   Ibid.

66   *Papers Read at the Fourth Congress of Women*, 87-88.

67   "The Boston Anniversaries," *New York Daily Tribune*, 1 Jun 1877, 3. "The Moral Education Association elected Dr. Mary J. Safford Blake, President; Georgianna Davis, Secretary; and Mrs. C. P. Nickles, Treasurer."

68   Kaufman, *Boston Women*, 74.

69   News Item, *The Index*, 14 Mar 1878, 121, and 19 Dec 1878, 609.

70   Kirschmann, *A Vital Force*, 42.

71   Croly, *The History*, 620.

72   *Report of the Women's Education & Industrial Union for the Year Ending May 7, 1879*, 3, 28.

73   Ibid., 25. Report of the Committee on Moral and Spiritual Development.

74   "Gamma Delta," *Boston University Annual Index for 1885-86*, 21.

75   "Field Meeting," *Bulletin of the Essex Institute*, Jul 1877, 99-102.

76   Perrin, *History of Alexander*, 56E.

77   " 'I'll Try.' Mr. Safford's Last Words," undated news clipping from unnamed source, page 11 of a scrapbook possibly assembled by Anna Candee Safford and now in Cairo Public Library. Reputedly, rescued in 2012 from a flooded house near Cairo, IL, the book came to librarian Monica Smith. Within the fragile, black cloth protected cardboard covers was a very old collection of Safford/Candee family items, primarily newspaper clippings, obituaries and letters of condolence on Alfred Safford's death. The scrapbook is called the, "Memorabilia Book," for these citations. It first arrived at the library on the one day the author of this book came to Cairo's library for research in 2013.

78   APKS To Anna Safford, "Memorabilia Book," 26.

79   Alfred Safford's death record, Vermont Vital Records 1760-1954. Death 26 Jul 1877. Listed death cause was, "apoplexy," and he was 54 years 6 months old.

80   "Gone East," newspaper clipping, "Memorabilia Book," unnumbered page.

81 Willcox, Jessie, To Anna Safford, 6 Aug 1877, "Memorabilia Book," 69.

82 *Boston University Yearbook 1877*, 95. Jessie Willcox was Mary's only 1878 preceptee.

83 "First Annual Convention of the Illinois," *Chicago Daily Tribune*, 5 Oct 1877, 7.

84 "City News," *Cairo Daily Bulletin*, 19 Oct 1877, 3.

85 Ballard County, Kentucky, records website. Anna was executrix. She and Mary passed through conveyance about 1000 acres in Ballard County, KY, along the Mississippi River.

86 Wilson, E., "Memorial Library," *Parson's Memorial and Historical Library Magazine*, Jan 1885, 81-83.

87 MJSB, "W.C. and L. L. A.," *Cairo Bulletin*, 13 May 1877, 3. Letter to young ladies of Cairo's, "Juvenile Wide Awakes."

88 "City News," *Cairo Daily Bulletin*, 4 Dec 1877, 3.

89 Obituary of Dr. Mercy Jackson, *New England Medical Gazette*, Jan 1878, 27-28.

90 News Item, *Lowell Daily Citizen and News*, 8 Mar 1878.

91 "Important Events," *Nunda News*, 4 Jul 1953.

92 News Item, *Arizona Citizen*, 2 Aug 1878, 1.

93 Per U.S. Grant National Historic Site Curator Karen Maxwell. Grants' world tour was May 1877 to Oct 1879.

94 News Item, *Daily Alta California*, 9 Oct 1878, 1.

95 Hubbard, *Hubbard's Newspaper*, 2278.

96 Schweikart, *A History of Banking*, 17.

97 "The Mining Wealth of Arizona," *The Weekly Arizona Miner*, 19 Sep 1879, 1.

98 Faulk, *Tombstone Myth*, 66.

99 "Arizona in Philadelphia," *The Arizona Citizen*, 20 Jun 1879, 2.

100 McClintock, *Arizona*, 411. APKS was president of Tombstone Gold and Silver Milling and Mining Company that owned the Tough Nut and other mines. Disston et al purchased the Schieﬄin brothers' interest in the Tough Nut group for $1,000,000 in March 1879.

101 News Item, *The Arizona Citizen*, 14 Dec 1878, 2.

102 Sprague, "New England Women's Club," *The Woman's Journal*, 26 Jun 1880, 206.

103 "Sixth Annual Commencement," 84-89.

104 Lockwood, "Vosburgh Conversation," 4.

105 Given wedding date of 11 Dec 1878, and Margarita's death at age 20 in early 1880, she was either 18 or 19 at marriage. Death 7 Jan 1880, Woodlawn Cemetery Register of Interment #19175, Folio 235, "Margaretta" G. Safford.

106 Safford, Margarita, unsigned letter to APKS, Boston 2 Oct 1879.

107 News Item, *Arizona Citizen*, 18 Oct 1879, 2. "Born in Boston, October 11, 1879, to the wife of Ex Governor A. P. K. Safford, a daughter."

108 Births Registered in the City of Boston For the Year 1879, #10159 Marguerita Safford, Beacon Street, Boston; APKS is listed as father and banker, born in Hyde Park, VT.

109 APKS, Handwritten biography of Margarita Grijalva Safford.

110 R. M. H., Letter, *Weekly Arizona Star*, 29 Jan 1880, 1.

111 Obituary of Marguerite G. Safford, *New York Times*, 9 Jan 1880. "SAFFORD—In this city, on the 7th inst., of consumption, Marguerite G., wife of ex-Gov. Safford, of Arizona."

112 R. M. H., letter, *Weekly Arizona Star*, 29 Jan 1880, 1.

113 APKS, handwritten biography of Margarita Grijalva Safford.

114 1880 U.S. Census, Boston, Suffolk, MA. Census dated 5 Jun 1880, lists 12-year old, "son," "And." and 8/12ths year old daughter, "M." Listed, "at school," Leandro's birthplace was Mexico as was his mother's. Space for a father's birthplace is blank.

115 Napheys, *Physical Life*, 215, 220-21.

116 Wilson, L., To Niece Mary, Burlington, VT 15 Dec 1880.

117 Obituary of Lydia Safford Wilson, *Cambridge Transcript*, 13 Feb 1890. She died at 98.

118 "Local Matters," *Arizona Citizen*, 1 Jul 1876, 3. Leandro received fourth place in First Class of Ollendorff (a language program). The same column noted Ignacio Bonillas' first place in Algebra and U.S. History. The following week's newspaper (6: no. 40, 3) reported Soledad Bonillas' recitations.

119 Attendees, "Programme of the Thirty-First," 89.

120 "Proceedings of the American Association for the Advancement of Science," 1882, A. G. Bell's, "Electrical Experiments to Determine the Bullet's Location in the Late President Garfield's Body," 151: "A Proposed Method of Producing Artificial Respiration by Means of a Vacuum Jacket," 224: Sir William Osler's tuberculosis paper, 528. He also presented one of the first descriptions of blood platelets.

121 Ibid., 496.

122 Sheridan, *Los Tucsonenses*, 100.

123 Acuna, *Corridors*, 89.

124 *Register of Former Students*, Massachusetts Institute of Technology, 56.

125 Lockwood, *Early Arizona*, 4.

126 Ibid.

127 Obituary of Soledad Safford Martin, *Arizona Historical Review*, Jul 1931, 80.

128 Obituary of Soledad Safford Martin, *Arizona Citizen*, 26 Mar 1931. Soledad was born 25 May 1860 in Magdalena, Sonora, Mexico.

129 Boston City Tax Records, *Real Estate for 1880*, 360-61.

130 "Courses of Instruction," *Boston University Yearbook*, 1880, 124.

131 "Lecture of Dr. Mary Safford-Blake," *Boston Medical and Surgical Journal*, 12 Feb 1880, 163.

132 MJS, "Artificial Alimentation," *The New England Medical Gazette*, Apr 1880, 109-10. This featured ways to feed patients unable or unwilling to take food orally. MJS described feeding tubes and food types to instill nourishment via skin or rectum. She preferred the latter route for infusing broth or milk. Article never became a classic, as the rectal mucosa's ability to absorb nutrients is questionable.

133 Sammons, "Mary J. Safford," *To-Day*, Jun 1894, 262.

134 "Report on the Women's Congress," *Annual Report of the Association for the Advancement of Women*, 1881, 5.

135 "The Woman's Congress," *Unitarian Review*, Nov 1880, 498-99.

136 MJS, To Dr. Mary Holywell Everett, from Boston, 11 Mar 1881.

137 "The Institute of Heredity," *Boston Post*, 18 May 1881, 3. It is unknown if Mary was a member or a guest speaker.

138 Untitled news item, *The Index*, 28 Jul 1881. MJS began investigating consanguineous marriage outcomes by soliciting voluntary responses to 8 questions concerning genealogic and medical history of such families and their resultant offspring. She promised confidentiality should results be published, but report of study is unknown.

139 "American Institute of Homeopathy 34th Annual Meeting," *Hahnemannian Monthly*, Aug 1881, 511-12.

140 "The Committee on Medical Legislation," *The Homoeopathic World*, 1 Oct 1881, 476-77.

141 McMullin and Walker, *Biographical Directory*, 31.

142 "Congratulations," *Arizona Weekly Star*, 15 Sep 1881.

143 MJS to APKS, Boston, 18 Nov 1881.

144 *Massachusetts Death Index, 1901-1980*, 16. APKS' daughter and MJS' niece Margarita (Margaret) Safford died in Lynnfield, Massachusetts, in 1963.

Chapter 12 • FLORIDA DREAMS AND SCHEMES

1   Gambier, *Florida*, 3.

2   News Item, *The Weekly Arizona Miner*, 8 Jul 1881, 2.

3   "Special Notice," *Real Estate Record and Builder's Guide*, 10 Dec 1881, 1145.

4   APKS, To Sam Hughes, 31 Dec 1888.

5   Shaw, *The Story of a Pioneer*, 142.

6   MJS, "Last Will," 25th paragraph. For the will's purposes, MJS desired Gladys be treated as legally adopted although she was not.

7   Safford, A. E., To Mary Ann Bickerdyke, undated. Context puts this in 1897, as letter states Margarita will be in 18 in October.

8   1900 U.S. Census, Sycamore Township, Dekalb, IL. Waterman Hall School. Gladys' listing gives Massachusetts' birth in December 1882.

9   MJS, "Lacerated Cervix," *New England Medical Gazette*, Oct 1881, 301-3.

10 Trehy, Deborah, M. D., email communication 4 Feb 2015.

11 MJS, "Physiological Effects of Alcoholic Beverages," *The Union Signal*, 8 Mar 1883, 5.

12 MJS, To Caroline Severance, Tarpon Springs, 14 Mar 1885.

13 Mountain, *Tarpon Springs*, 7.

14 Cushing, "Preliminary Report," *Proceedings of the American Philosophical Society*, 6 Nov 1896, 352-54. Reputedly, the mound held over six hundred burials of archaic people.

15 Stoughton, *Tarpon Springs*, 5, 6.

16 Pent, *History of Tarpon Springs*, 3, 7, 8.

17 Straub, *History of Pinellas County*, 162-63.

18 Schnur, "Springing into Action," *Punta Pinal*, Fall 2006, 10.

19 "Art," *Florida: A Guide to the Southern-Most State*, 158.

20 Schnur, "Springing into Action," *Punta Pinal*, Fall 2006, 11.

21 Stoughton, *Tarpon Springs*, 10.

22 Straub, *History of Pinellas County*, 163.

23 Obituary of Elizabeth Ingalls Sage, *Tarpon Springs Leader*, 28 Feb 1922, 6.

24 MJS, "Personal and News Items," *New England Medical Gazette*, Apr 1883, 128.

25 School Document No. 22-1883, *Annual Report of the School Committee*, 1883, 36, 215.

26 MJS, "Nervous Prostration," *The Union Signal*, 17 May 1883, 5.

27 News Item, *Nunda News*, 14 Apr 1883, 3.

28 MJSB, "Reminiscences of German Hospitals," *The New England Medical Gazette*, May 1874, 216-17.

29 Richardson, "Hygeia."

30 MJS, "Personal and News Items," *New England Medical Gazette*, Apr 1883, 128.

31 News Item, *Union Signal*, 10 May 1883, 9.

32   Abstracts of Title, #24416 of Guaranty Title and Trust Company, Clearwater, FL, Sheet #1, Lines 9-13—owners: Fidelia's husband Walter B. Whitcomb, daughter Eva Olney and son-in-law E. C. Olney, son Merrick, brother-in-law Samuel P. Whitcomb and his wife Juliet. Line 8: May 2, 1883, 40.05 acres.

33   Van Bibber, "Peninsular and Sub-Peninsular Air," *Journal of the American Medical Association*, 16 May 1885, 536-42.

34   Brown, *Gulfport*, 36-37.

35   Author's interview of Lily McCrady Styles' granddaughter Betty Styles Hammock in Seminole, FL, 17 Feb 2006; Mrs. Hammock died in 2008. Her father Louis was about 4 on his 1883 Florida arrival with the Saffords.

36   "Tarpon Springs, Florida: The Gem of the Gulf Coast." This promotional booklet was possibly written by APKS.

37   News Item, *Union Signal*, 25 Oct 1883, 11-12. Massachusetts temperance activity report.

38   "Reading for Health," The Christian Union, 7 Feb 1884, 136. This was a review of *Chautauqua Annual* essays.

39   Safford and Allen, *Health and Strength for Girls*.

40   Ibid., 48.

41   MJS, "Protest Against Pepper," *Woman Suffrage Cookbook*, 122-23.

42   Safford and Allen, *Health and Strength for Girls*, 49-50.

43   "Literature Reviews," *Musical Herald*, May 1884, 135.

44   *Report of the Women's Education & Industrial Union for the Year Ending May 1, 1884*, 6.

45   MJSB, "Annie Conway Damer," *The Woman's Journal*, 24 Apr 1875, 130.

46   "Report of the Social Affairs Committee for the Year Ending May, 1892,"*Report of the Women's Educational and Industrial Union for the Year Ending May, 1892*, 29.

47   MJS, "Last Will," paragraph 11.

48   Whiting, "Lilian Whiting's Pen," *The Inter-Ocean*, 25 June 1881, 9.

49   *Report of the Women's Education & Industrial Union for the Year Ending May 1, 1884*, 28.

50   Obituary for Dr. Arvilla Britton Haynes, *The New England Medical Gazette*, Feb 1884, 64.

51   *Publications of the Massachusetts Homoeopathic Medical Society 1884*, 196-98.

52   Ibid., 11.

53   *Report of the Women's Education & Industrial Union for the Year Ending May 1, 1884*, 26.

54   MJS "An Extraordinary Case of Constipation," *New England Medical Gazette*, Feb 1884, 48-50.

55   "Passenger Lists," *Daily Alta California*, 12 Jul 1884, 4. Saffords' listed home was Tucson.

56   "Real Estate Transactions, *Daily Alta California*, 23 Jul 1884, 7.

57   Report extracted from the Mining Index, *Gulf Coast Herald*, 26 Jul 1884, 3.

58   "An Act No. 13," *Acts, Resolutions and Memorials of the Eighteenth*, 44-46.

59   Hillsborough County Deed No. 59, *Old Hillsborough County Deed Book P, 19*. Pinellas County Clerk of the Circuit Court Office, Clearwater, FL.

60   "Plat of the Subdivision," 480. Survey of 25 Apr 1884, recorded 26 Apr 1884. L-shaped land divided into 40 equal lots.

61   Whitcomb, F., "Our Florida Letter," *Nunda News*, 12 Jan, 19 Jan, 16 Feb 1884. Letters read like, "Florida the Sunshine State," advertisements.

62   MJS, "Letter to the Herald," *Gulf Coast Herald*, 13 Oct 1884, 3. Top of same page had C. D. Webster's, "Meteorological Phenomena," report of prior week's temperatures.

63   Conway, *Atmospheric Science at NASA*, 167.

64   "Tarpon Topics," *Gulf Coast Herald*, 1 Nov 1884, 3.

65   Buckner, "Fraud Exposed Governor A. P. K. Safford a Liar," *Gulf Coast Herald*, 13 Dec 1884, 3. After being exonerated of murder charges Lucie wrote scathing articles in the newspaper's last issue. Paper contained its own obituary.

66   Buckner, "Tarpon Topics," *Gulf Coast Herald*, 27 Sep and 15 Nov 1884, 3.

67   Kilgo, *Tarpon Springs*, 23.

68   Notice, *Nunda News*, 1 Nov 1884, 1.

69   Author has found no earlier trained women physicians' practicing in Florida. References name Mary J. Safford, MD, as first physician while ignoring unfamiliar Dr. Whitcomb.

70   Hand, *Centennial History*, 258.

71   "Book-Store for Sale," *Publishers Weekly*, 5 Mar 1887, 352. "Book-Store for Sale-Owing to ill health, I am compelled to give up a large and profitable trade—Bradford Co. S. P. Whitcomb."

72   LV, "Our Tarpon Letter," *Tampa Journal*, 3 Jun 1887, 1. Widowed Lucie Buckner remarried and became Mrs. George Vannevar by 1886. After she put her own paper *Gulf Coast Herald* out of its misery in 1884 she wrote under the name, "Lucie Vannevar," for several Tampa Bay area newspapers.

73   "History of Early Amateur Journalism," website. Truax published the *Diminutive News* from 1883-86.

74   *History of the Counties of McKean, Elk, Cameron and Potter, Pennsylvania*, 173, 408.

75   Mountain, *Tarpon Springs*, 10.

76   Stoughton, *Tarpon Springs*, 18.

77   Mountain, *Tarpon Springs*, 7-8.

78   "A Bradford Reunion," *The Bradford (Pa.) Era*, 27 Mar 1888, 1.

79   LV, "Tarpon Springs FLA, October, '86," *Tampa Guardian*, 17 Nov 1886, 2. Lucie's columns noted Seymour Thornton and C. B. Thornton families.

80   Abstract #38109, Tarpon Springs Abstracts of Title. Seymour Thornton bought his land from the Lake Butler Villa Company Dec 1885.

81   "New Loose-Skinned Orange—The Thornton," *Yearbook of the United States Department of Agriculture*, 336.

82   *Harvard College Class of 1879 Secretary's Report*, 5, 91. Although Merrick was not in the class of 1879 his name is among those listed as, "Non-Graduate Members."

83   Stoughton, *Tarpon Springs*, 29.

84   Buckner, "Tarpon Topics," *Gulf Coast Herald*, 1 Nov 1884, 3. "W. H." was Heman Whelpy Massey. Buckner transposed his initials.

85   Webb, "Tarpon Springs," *Webb's Historical Industrial and Biographical Florida*, 59.

86   "45. Mary A. Bigelow House," notes from the Tarpon Springs Cultural Center's, "Historic Tarpon Springs Self Guided Tour," 1989. Emily E. Massey was the original owner.

87 MJS, To Caroline Severance, Tarpon Springs 14 Mar 1885.

88 Ibid.

89 "Woman's Work," *Boston Daily Courier*, 21 Jun 1885. Among attendees were MJS' reform associates Mary Livermore, Kate Gannett Wells, and Abby Morton Diaz.

90 "Transactions of Societies," "Society for Promoting the Welfare of the Insane," *The Medico-legal Journal*, 439. Society's founder Henry R. Stiles, MD, was a homeopath MJS surely knew from AIH.

91 "Editorial Notes," *The Index*, 5 Nov 1885, 221. The Parker Memorial Science Class was the Free Religious Association's adult Sunday school lecture series.

92 Croly, *The History of the Woman's Club*, 43.

93 "A Crematory for Boston," *Chicago Daily Tribune*, 27 Nov 1885, 5.

94 *Transactions of the New England Cremation Society 1893*, 9-10. MJS was dead before the society's successful rebirth in 1892.

95 *Opinions on Cremation*, 37-38. MJS described numerous ghastly methods for disposing human remains and touted cremation as the most efficient and healthful.

96 MJS, "Last Will," 19th paragraph.

97 Advertisement, *Florida Medical and Surgical Journal*, Nov 1885, 45.

98 "Tarpon Springs," and, "Physicians," *Florida State Gazetteer and Business Directory*, 434, 631. Only Drs. Safford & Whitcomb's names are listed and labeled homeopaths. Tarpon had no allopaths.

99 Webb, "Tarpon Springs," *Webb's Historical*, 59.

100 Pent, *History of Tarpon Springs*, 26.

101 Hardy, *Oranges and Alligators*, 195-96. Ms. Hardy told young Englishmen to expect little return for hard work in Florida.

102 Stoughton, *Tarpon Springs*, 30.

103 Pent, *History of Tarpon Springs*, 59.

104 MJS, "The Effects of Stimulants," *Papers Read Before the Association for the Advancement of Women 14th Women's Congress*, 121-32.

105 Ibid., 121.

106 Ibid., 122.

107 Ibid., 124-25.

108 Ibid., 129.

109 "Current Topics," *The Index*, 4 Nov 1886, 217.

110 Advertisement for BUSM, *New England Medical Gazette*, Dec 1886, 645.

111 "Faculty, School of Medicine," *Boston University Year Book for 1887-1888*, 132, 135. MJS was Professor of Diseases of Women and on BUSM Women's Dispensary Staff.

112 Sammons, "Mary J. Safford," *To-Day*, Jun 1894, 262.

113 "Standing Committee Members," *Publications of the Massachusetts Homoeopathic Medical Society*, 84.

114 Member listing, *Transactions of the Forty-First Session of the AIH*, 744.

115 Burroughs, "Women in the Institute," *Transactions of the Forty-Seventh Session of the American Institute of Homoeopathy*, 76.

116 Boston City Assessor's Record # 2100-004, 308 Columbus Avenue, Boston.

117 Obituary for Dr. Mary J. Safford, *Report of the WEIU for the Year Ending May 1892*, 29.

Chapter 13 • THE SNOWBIRD TAKES WING

1   LV, "Tarpon News," *Tampa Guardian*, 24 Nov 1886, 2. Under her own byline Lucie Vannevar (LV) wrote Tarpon Springs' gossip columns for the *Tampa Guardian* (TG) then *Tampa Journal* (TJ) and *Tampa Weekly Journal* (TWJ) until spring 1890.

2   1880 U.S. Census, Wrentham, Norfolk, MA. School teacher Lizzie B. Pond was 22 years old.

3   LV, "Our Tarpon Letter," TJ, 29 Dec 1886, 2.

4   LV, "Our Tarpon Letter," TJ, 13 Jan 1887, 2.

5   Cooper, H. J., "A Visit to Tarpon," TG, 24 Nov 1886, 2.

6   "Florida State Statistics," *The Universalist Register*, 14. Church of the Good Shepherd began in winter 1886.

7   Thomas, *Centenary Voices*, xix, 1.

8   Mountain, *Tarpon Springs*, 25.

9   Kilgo, *Tarpon Springs*, 60.

10 Stoughton, *Tarpon Springs*, 39.

11 Rooks and Mountain, *Tarpon Springs, Florida*, 71. Reference gives Tarpon Springs' African-American perspective.

12 Denominational Column, *Manford's New Monthly Magazine*, Dec 1885, 710.

13 LV, "Correspondence—Our Tarpon Letter," TJ, 31 Mar 1887, 1.

14 LV, "Our Tarpon Letter," TJ, 2 Feb 1887, 2.

15 LV, "Our Tarpon Letter," TJ, 9 Feb 1887, 2.

16 Abstract #29703 prepared for John H. Cheyney by Guarantee Title & Trust Company, Clearwater, FL. Page 7 notice lists Tarpon Springs' 46, "duly qualified electors," who desired the town's incorporation.

17 Mountain, *Tarpon Springs*, 17.

18 LV, "Lucie Vannevar's Letter," TWJ, 16 Feb 1888, 8. Train tracks ran north and south down the middle of today's Safford Avenue, and the depot is now home of the Tarpon Springs Area Historical Society's Depot Museum.

19 LV, "Our Tarpon Letter," TJ, 26 May 1887, 1.

20 LV, "Our Tarpon Letter," TJ, 2 Jun 1887, 1.

21 LV, "Our Tarpon Letter," TJ, 26 May 1887, 1.

22 *Register of Former Students*, MIT, 432. Leandro Safford, class of '87 II, 1883-86.

23 Pent, *History of Tarpon Springs*, 21.

24 Advertisement, *The Tarpon*, 5 Jan 1887, 4.

25 Advertisement, *The Tarpon*, 18 Aug 1887, 6.

26 LV, "Our Tarpon Letter," TJ, 2 Jun 1887, 1.

27 LV, "Our Tarpon Letter," TJ, 28 Jul 1887, 8.

28 Sammons, "Mary J. Safford," *To-Day*, June 1894, 263.

29 LV, "Our Tarpon Letter," TJ, 16 Jun 1887, 1.

30 Wall, "The Yellow Fever," 60-75.

31 LV, "Our Tarpon Letter," TJ, 16 Jun 1887, 1.

32 Wall, "The Yellow Fever," 61.

33 News Item, *Tampa Tribune*, 11 Aug 1887, online.

34 LV, "Tampa As Seen by Tarpon Eyes," TWJ, 15 Sep 1887, 5.

35 News Item, *Tampa Tribune*, 11 Aug 1887, online. Letter from V. Martinez Ybor & Co. tells of financial hardship cigar manufacturers would face if Cuban cigar workers left because Hillsborough County went, "dry."

36 News item, TJ, 5 Oct 1887, online. Referendum results report.

37 Weatherford, *Real Women*, 92.

38 "Donors," TWJ, 27 Oct 1887.

39 Weatherford, *Real Women*, 95, 109.

40 Weatherford, *They Dared to Dream*, 149, 158-59.

41 LV, "Our Tarpon Letter," TWJ, 6 Oct 1887, 8.

42 News item, "Personals," *The Tarpon*, 18 Aug 1887, 4.

43 LV, "Our Tarpon Letter," TJ, 12 Jan 1888, 8.

44 News item, "Personals," *The Tarpon*, 17 Nov 1887, 4.

45 LV, "Sensation at Tarpon," TWJ, 9 Feb 1888, 8.

46 *Report of the International Council of Women*, 10-11.

47 Obituary of Fidelia Merrick Whitcomb, *The Nunda News*, 7 Apr 1888, 3.

48 Cycadia Cemetery census. Listing is: Whitcomb, T. (sic) J. M. (Mrs.) d. 4/1/88. Grave is currently unmarked.

49 Wilson and Fiske, *Appleton's Cyclopaedia*, 48.

50 LV, "Lucie Vannevar's Letter," TWJ, 29 Jun 1888, 5. Professor Johonnot was a prolific author whose works included *Ten Great Events in History*. He ran a series of teachers' institutes and was involved with NY's teacher certification.

51 Scott, *The Story of a Bird Lover*, 253.

52 Obituary of W. E. D. Scott, *The Auk*, Oct 1910, 486-88.

53 Advertisement, *The Tarpon*, 5 Jan 1887, 1.

54 Cassino, *The Naturalists' Universal Directory*, 138. Listing in the U.S. & Canadian section was, "3606 Safford, Mary J., M.D., Tarpon Springs, Fla. Phaen.Bot., Ferns, Diurnal Lepid.*"

55 LV, "Lucie Vannevar's Letter," TWJ, 22 Mar 1888, 8.

56 Sammons, "Mary J. Safford," 264.

57 LV, "Lucie Vannevar's Letter," TWJ, 23 Jun 1888, 8.

58 Volp, *The First Hundred*, 214.

59 Abstract #27308. Walter paid his mortgage in full 11 Feb 1893.

60 Illinois Deaths and Stillbirths Index 1916-1947. Death of Elizabeth B. Sammons 3 Oct 1924, Blue Island, IL. Husband was Walter W.

61 Sammons, "Mary J. Safford," 264.

62 LV, "The Fourth at Tarpon," TWJ, 13 Jul 1888, 1.

63 LV, "Lucie Vannevar's Letter," TWJ, 22 Nov 1888, 3.

64 LV, "Lucie Vannevar's Letter," TWJ, 24 Jan 1889, 8.

65 Benson, "Five Women Artists of New York," *The Year's Art as Recorded in the Quarterly Illustrator*, 42-45.

66 LV, "Lucie Vannevar's Letter," TJ, 9 May 1889, 6.

67 Indenture, *Old Hillsborough County Deeds*, N, 763-64. Mary sold lots 27 and 28 in her subdivision for $1 to Elizabeth Sage on 2 Jun 1884.

68 LV, "Lucie Vannevar's Letter," TJ, 7 May 1889, 8.

69 King, M., *Harvard Register*, 251.

70 Stoughton, *Tarpon Springs*, 14.

71 Safford ephemera at Cairo Public Library includes an untitled news clipping of unspecified origin referencing the *Cairo Telegram's* account of Dr. Safford's late 1891 death and noting she, "was a relative of Mrs. C. E. Allen of Malone, and visited here about two years ago."

72 Smith and Sanborn, "State Legislation for the Insane," *Proceedings of the National Conference of Charities and Correction at the Sixteenth Annual Session*, 78.

73 "Report from the Committee on Commitment," *Proceedings of the National Conference of Charities and Correction at the Seventeenth Annual Session*, 251. Mary's friend Bella Chapin Barrows, MD, edited the proceedings.

74 Barrows, "In Memoriam Mary J. Safford, M.D."

75 LV, "Three Days with Rose Cleveland," TJ, *West Coast Department*, 26 Dec 1889, unnumbered page.

76 LV, "West Coast Department," TJ, *West Coast Department*, 19 Dec 1889 unnumbered page.

77 D'Emilio and Freedman, *Intimate Matters*, 192. 41-year old spinster Rose Cleveland met much younger Evangeline Simpson in Naples, FL, in winter 1889, and the two began a lengthy lesbian relationship.

78 LV, "Mrs. Vannevar's Party," TJ, *West Coast Department*, 20 Feb 1890, 3.

79 LV, "Three Days with Rose Cleveland," TJ, *West Coast Department*, 26 Dec 1889, unnumbered page. A clinker-built boat could be either a rowboat or sailboat.

80 Ryan, *Pandemic Influenza*, 16.

81 Shally-Jensen, *Encyclopedia of Contemporary*, 1510.

82 "Professional Cards," newspaper clipping, 8 Mar 1890, no further identification.

83 LV, "Lucie Vannevar's Letter—Her Impression," TJ, 6 Mar 1890, 8.

84 Harbert, "Mothers to the Rescue," *The New Era*, Sep 1885, 282.

85 LV, "Lucie Vannevar's Letter—Her Impression," TJ, 6 Mar 1890, 8.

86 LV, "A Gypsy Camp," TJ, 20 Mar 1890, 5.

87 "Clear Water Notes," TJ, 29 May 1890, 2.

88 Whitcomb, M., *Harvard College Secretary's Report*, No. IV, 79-80.

89 MSS 253, *Dr. Charles Sajous Papers*, 29 May 1890.

90 "Florida University," *The New York Medical Times*, Dec 1890, 277.

91 "Dr. Sajous Knighted," *The Medical Fortnightly*, 1 Oct 1892, 176.

92 Sajous, "Reasons Why Far-sighted Investors are Purchasing Lots in Tarpon Springs," *Annual of the Universal Medical Sciences*, 19. American Riviera Company's report on the "great Sanitary Colony." On pages D-18-19 of the same journal are testimonials for Tarpon Springs, Asheville, NC, and Colorado Springs as tuberculosis treatment centers.

93 Disston, Mary Safford, Daughters of the American Revolution Descendants Record #282693 gives Leandro and Helen Polk Safford's marriage date of 16 Dec 1890.

94 Disston, Mary Safford, death certificate lists father Leandro T. Safford and mother Helen. Commonwealth of Pennsylvania, Department of Health and Vital Statistics, Local Reg. # 25633, # 119204-62. *New York, New York, Marriage Index 1866-1937* shows in New York, NY, 3 Jul 1909, Mary married Hamilton R. Disston, a cousin of Hamilton S. Disston.

95 Truax, "A Tribute," *The Truth*, 12 Dec 1891.

96 Blocker et al, *Alcoholism and Temperance*, 346-48.

97 "The Hotels, Who are at Them," *Ashville Daily Citizen*, 20 Oct 1891, 3.

98 Martin, *Tourism in the Mountain South*, 30-31.

99 "Death of Dr. Mary J. Safford, the Eminent Female Physician," Sharlot Hall Museum, "Obituary Book," 396. The column attributes her death to a slow form of typho-malarial fever, seemingly a contradiction in terms, as typhoid's cause is bacterial and malaria's a protozoan. However, some late 19th century physicians recognized, "Typho-malaria." Co-infection of the two organisms could occur, especially in someone with decreased immune function and history of travel to endemic regions. Mary traveled to the West Indies, northern Africa, Europe and the Mideast prior to 1872—long before her death. The possibility such diseases could lie dormant and reappear due to an aging and suppressed immune system is a remote possibility. Supposedly, she had malaria (then called Roman Fever) in Rome in 1864. Personnel at the Malaria Branch of the U. S. Centers for Disease Control disclosed a 19th century tendency to overdiagnose malaria, and recovery without treatment was rare. If she truly had malaria and somehow recovered without treatment she could have developed a chronic infection with later re-emergence.

100 Cheong Mun Keong, and Sulaiman, "Typhoid and Malaria Co-Infection," *Malaysian Journal Medical Sciences*, Jan 2006, 74-75.

101 Obituary for Dr. Mary J. Safford, "Died in Florida," newspaper clipping from unknown source but with context suggesting a Cairo, IL, paper.

102 Hafner, "Died: In Tarpon Springs," *The Tarpon Springs Truth*, 12 Dec 1891.

103 Ibid.

104 Obituary of Dr. Mary J. Safford, *New England Medical Gazette*, Jan 1892, 48.

105 Barrows, "In Memoriam Mary J. Safford, M.D."

106 Obituary for Dr. Mary J. Safford, "Died in Florida."

107 "Gov. Safford" letter to Sam Hughes, *Arizona Daily Citizen*, 16 Dec 1890, 1.

108 "A.P. K. Safford Dies in Florida," *The Chicago Daily Tribune*, 16 Dec 1891, 2.

109 Although several newspapers reported APKS' death date of 14 Dec 1891, his official death date was 15 Dec 1891, as shown in Citrus County, FL, Will Book Index, 15.

110 "Last Will and Testament Safford, Anson P. K.," 15 Nov 1886, Codicil 1 Nov 1889, proven 22 Dec 1891, Filed 13 Jun 1893, Hernando County, FL, Book A, 157, Book 1, 40-48. Noted in Citrus County Will Book Index, 15.

Chapter 14 • WHERE THERE'S A WILL THERE'S AN EPILOGUE

1   MJS, "Last Will," signed and witnessed in Boston 20 Jun 1884.

2   Ibid., paragraph 1

3   Ibid., paragraph 24, section 4.

4   Sage, Elizabeth I., Death certificate. Cycadia Cemetery Section I, lot 35, grave 5.

5   MJS, "Last Will," paragraph 23.

6   Leonard, *Who's Who in Engineering*, 121. Entry for George Safford Beal. Brown University tuition in was $105/year according to a 1900-01 catalog.

7   MJS, "Last Will," paragraphs 10 and 24, section 9.

8   Ibid., paragraph 4.

8   Ibid., paragraphs 5, 6.

10   Safford, A. E., To Mary Ann Bickerdyke, 1897 (per context).

11   *Hillsborough County, Florida, Guardianship Records*, vol. A, 1886-1895, roll 27, 257. On 9 Jan 1892 Judge C. E. Harrison appointed Soledad and Leandro guardians for both girls.

12   Ibid., 329-32. On 18 Apr 1893 Soledad, Leandro and Edward A. Hunting applied for Hunting's guardianship of Margarita on the grounds that Mary Safford wished her a northern education. Judge C. E. Harrison granted this on 21 Apr 1893.

13   Hunting family listing, *Blue Book of Newton 1910*, 86. Similar entries were in 1899-1903 and 1911-12 books.

14   "Class News." *The Smith Alumnae Quarterly*. Margarita was called Meta.

15   2007 email correspondence with Jane S. Knowles, Radcliffe Archivist, Schlesinger Library, Cambridge, MA. "Marguerite" Safford was a candidate for A. M. degree in History and attended Radcliffe 1903-04 and 1904-05 but withdrew before finishing. She returned in 1920-21 and took Greek.

16   File of news items and correspondence regarding Margarita Safford, presumably from Smith College alumni office, in Safford House Museum docents' book, Tarpon Springs, Florida. Margarita's friend Florence Dunton was called, "Donc." "Meta and Donc" were friends at Capen and lived together since 1923 in Boston and Melrose, MA. Donc died in 1959, and Meta in 1963. Donc's nephews Dr. Frank Dunton and Mr. Charles Dunton knew Margarita as Aunt Meta in Boston and inherited her belongings.

17   1910 U. S. Census: Newton Ward 3, Middlesex, MA. 30-year old "Margherita" Safford lived with 76-year old Edward A. Hunting and 46-year old Anna Hunting with two servants. Miss Safford's occupation was, "teacher...private school."

18   Safford, Margarita, death. *Massachusetts Vital Records Index to Deaths (1916-1970)*. She died in Lynnfield, MA, 27 Jul 1963, at age 83.

19   Safford, A. E., To Mary Ann Bickerdyke, 1897.

20   1900 U.S. Census, Sycamore Township, Dekalb, IL. Waterman Hall School, 297/19A.

21   "Illinois, Cook County Marriages, 1871-1920." Richard Sammons, age 30, married Gladys Safford, age 20.

22   "Sammons, infant of Dick, d. 6/5/07," USGenWeb Archives Cycadia Cemetery listing, Tarpon Springs. Cycadia Cemetery census lists the infant in Block J, Lot 37, space 5, as child of Gladys and Richard Sammons.

23   Tarpon Springs' Safford House Museum docents' book contains a series of short newspaper clippings and town directory fragments of unknown date and provenance that document Gladys' marriage to plumber Cham Hill.

24   "Former Mayor and Banker," *Tarpon Springs Evening Leader*, 27 Nov 1915, 1.

25   Hill, Robert Cham, death, *North Carolina Death Certificates 1909-1976*, 144. He died in Asheville of pulmonary and meningeal tuberculosis on 5 Apr 1921. Home listed was Tarpon Springs, FL.

26 Hill, Gladys Safford, death. *Louisiana Vital Records Indices*, New Orleans death Indices 1937-1948; vol.: 210; 244.

27 "Mrs. Gladys Hill Dies in New Orleans," unnamed, undated Tarpon Springs newspaper in Docents' book of Safford House Museum; reputedly, Gladys was buried at New Orleans' St. Mary's Cemetery.

28 MJS, "Last Will," paragraphs 7 and 8.

29 *Report of the Women's Education & Industrial Union for the Year Ending May 1894*, 12.

30 2008 emails with Dr. Julie H. Sandell, Professor and Vice Chairman Department of Anatomy and Neurobiology, Boston University School of Medicine. She found no record of BUSM's receiving any of these bequeathed items. Emily L. Beattie, BUSM's Head of Technical Services & Archives in 2008 also found nothing.

31 "Faculty Notes," *Smith College Monthly*, Oct 1903-Jun 1904, 602.

32 2007 emails with Biology Professor Virginia Hayssen, Smith College. Her search for the skull resulted in finding a photograph of it tucked away in a colleague's desk drawer but not the actual skull.

33 MJS, "Last Will," paragraph 10.

34 *Report of the Women's Education & Industrial Union for the Year Ending May 3, 1881*. Georgianna Davis was Chairman of the Visiting the Sick Committee then and in 1882.

35 *The National Cyclopaedia*, "Richardson, Abby Sage," 553. She lived in Manchester, NH, and her grandmother was named Elizabeth Ingalls Sage.

36 1850 U.S. Census, Manchester, NH. Abby Sage was 13 and her sister Elizabeth Ingalls Sage was 10 with father William and mother Abegail Sage. The unusual spelling of Elizabeth's mother's name is also on Elizabeth's 20 Feb 1922 FL death certificate that gives birth date as 6 Jan 1840. She was about 43 on first FL arrival with MJS.

37 "Mrs. McFarland's Statement," *The Richardson-McFarland Tragedy*, 103-4.

38 Cooper, G., *Lost Love*, 210. At the 1870 MacFarland-Richardson trial "Lizzie Sage," testified to Abby's husband's drunkenness.

39 *The National Cyclopaedia*, "Richardson, Abby Sage," 553.

40 Cooper, G., *Lost Love*, 240. Abby arrived in Chicago two weeks before the 1871 fire and reported it for the *New York Tribune*.

41 "Mrs. McFarland's Statement," *The Richardson-McFarland Tragedy*, 104.

42 Ibid., 108.

43 "The Trial," *The Richardson-McFarland Tragedy*, 56.

44 "Opinions of the Press on the Main Question," *The Richardson-McFarland Tragedy*, 46. Wedding officiants were Henry Ward Beecher, Henry M. Field, and O. B. Frothingham.

45 "The Appearance of the Body," *The Richardson-McFarland Tragedy*, 30.

46 Harper, *The Life and Work of Susan B. Anthony*, 351-52.

47 MJS, "Last Will," paragraph 18.

48 "Moral Education Association," *Boston Post*, 2 Jun 1876, 4.

49 Advertisement for *The Myrtle*, 137. Mrs. Bruce was editor of this Universalist children's publication.

50 Squier, "Sojourner Truth," *The Christian at Work*, 28 Sep 1882, 12.

51 "Marriages solemnized in 1884," 34. Marriage was on 24 Apr 1884.

52 MJS, "Last Will," paragraphs 11-13, 15-17.

53 Ibid., paragraph 14.

54 Ibid., paragraph 21-22.

55 Cycadia Cemetery, Tarpon Springs, FL, Section J, Lot 37, Mary and A. P. K. are in spaces 4 and 3 respectively.

56 APKS, "Last Will," 157, 40-48.

57   "In Re Estate of A. P. K. Safford, deceased," 50. Judge C. E Harrison, on 28 Mar 1899 removed Leandro as executor.

58   Disston, Hamilton R., to Mr. A. Hanna at Rollins College, 16 Jun 1947, from Philadelphia. Leandro Safford's son-in-law was a cousin of the original Hamilton S. Disston and noted Leandro's death 7 years earlier.

59   Kilgo, *Tarpon Springs*, 60.

60   Stoughton, *Tarpon Springs*, 34.

61   Sheridan, *Los Tucsonenses*, 100.

62   Coerver et al, *Mexico*, 133.

63   Marriage license of William Warwick Parken and Soledad B. Safford, Issued by Hillsborough County's Judge C. E. Harrison, 11 May 1896.

64   William Warwick Parken's grave adjoins those of Mary and A. P. K. Safford in Cycadia Cemetery, Section J, Lot 37, space 1.

65   Stoughton, *Tarpon Springs*, 34-35.

66   City of Tarpon Springs, website: ci.tarpon-springs.fl.us, Safford House Museum narrative.

67   Cycadia Cemetery, Tarpon Springs, Section J, Lot 37, space 7 is Soledad Bonillas Safford Parken Martin's grave.

68   "A $20,000 Fire," *The Tampa Morning Tribune*, 2 Dec 1898, 3. Fire's cause was unknown but the $20,000 hotel was insured for only $8000.

69   Mountain, *Tarpon Springs*, 8.

70   2015 communication with retired Dr. Lucia Pinon, Clearwater, FL. She trained in Cuba and the U.S. before her 1960 return to Cuba, later escaped and returned to the U.S.

71   Statistics provided by Medical Staff Coordinator Marcella Pertsas, Florida Hospital-North Pinellas, Tarpon Springs, FL.

72   MJS, "Last Will," paragraphs 17, 23-24.

73   MJS, "The Ideal Sunday-School," *The Index*, 23 Aug 1877, 404-5.

74   Will and Probate documents of MJS, Arizona State Historical Society Archives, *Safford Papers*, MS 0704. Tucson, Arizona. Probate #88867, 11 Jan 1892. Recorded in *Suffolk County Probate of Will Book*, 654: 329.

75   "In Re Estate of Mary J. Safford."

76   Swift, "Edward A. Hunting," 157-60. Case of 23 Jan 1903-16 Mar 1903. Mentions Soledad and Leandro's 1893 resignation of Margarita's guardianship and dispute over Margarita and Gladys' inheritance.

77   Davidson, *A Century of Homeopaths*, 12.

78   Unitarian Universalist Church of Tarpon Springs, "History," and, "Shepherd Center," online: uutarpon.org.

BIBLIOGRAPHY

PRIMARY SOURCES

Dr. Philip Abensur, Paris, France

Abraham Lincoln Presidential Library and Museum, Buckmaster-Curran Family Papers, and photos, Springfield, Illinois

Alexander County Records, Cairo, IL

American Antiquarian Society, Worcester, MA

American Association for the Advancement of Science, Washington. DC

Andover-Harvard Theological Seminary Library, microfilms, Newton, MA

Arizona Historical Foundation, Tempe, AZ

Arizona Historical Society Research Collections, Tucson

Arizona State Archives and Public Records, Phoenix

Auburn Avenue Research Library, Atlanta

Ballard County, Kentucky, property records, Wickliffe, KY

Bancroft Library, California Manuscripts and Francis P. Farquhar Collection, University of California, Berkeley

Blue Island Historical Society, Blue Island, IL

Boston Athenaeum, Boston City Archives, and Boston Public Library, Boston

Boston University School of Medicine Archives, Boston

Bradford Landmark Society Archives, Bradford, PA

Cairo Custom House Museum, Cairo, IL

Cairo Public Library, Safford Family Items and Ephemera, Cairo, IL

California Digital Newspaper Collection

Chapel Hill-Chauncy Hall School Archives, Boston

Church of Jesus Christ of the Latter Day Saints, Family Search collections

College de France Archives, Paris, France

Commonwealth of Pennsylvania, Department of Health and Vital Statistics

Cook County, IL, Department of Public Health Records

Cornell University, Carl A. Kroch Library, Division of Rare and Manuscript Collections, Flora Payne Whitney Letters #3852, Ithaca, NY

Cycadia Cemetery records and census, Tarpon Springs, FL

Dorchester Historical Society, Dorchester, MA

Mr. Charles Dunton and Dr. Frank Dunton, recipients of Margarita Safford's belongings

Emory Women Writers Resource Project Collection, Women's Advocacy Collection

Florida State Library and State Archives, Tallahassee

Gabinetto Scientifico Letterario G. P. Vieusseux Archives, Florence, Italy

John M. Germany Public Library, Old Florida Newspapers Microfilms, Tampa, FL

J. Paul Getty Museum, Open Content Program

U. S. Grant National Historic Site, St. Louis

Greentree Foundation, Manhasset, NY

Harvard Medical Library in the Francis A. Countway Library of Medicine, Boston

Harvard University, Widener Library Collection Development Department, Open Collections Program at Harvard University, Women Working 1800-1930

Fred Holabird, Holabird Americana, Reno, NV

Hillsborough County Clerk of the Circuit Court records, Hillsborough County Guardianship Records, Tampa, FL

Hoosier State Chronicles, Indiana's Digital Historic Newspaper Program

Huntington Library, Caroline M. Seymour Severance Collection, San Marino, CA

Hyde Park Town and Village Records, Hyde Park, VT

Illinois Deaths and Stillbirths Index 1916-1947

Illinois Digital Newspaper Collections

Illinois State Historical Library and Illinois State Historical Society, Springfield

Illinois State University Archives, Bloomington

Kansas State Historical Society and Archives, Topeka

Kentucky State Digital Library

Knox College Archives, Galesburg, IL

Lasell College, Brennan Library, Winslow Archives, Auburndale, MA

Library of Congress, Clara Barton Papers, Washington, DC

Library of Congress, Chronicling America Historic American Newspapers, Washington, DC

Library of Congress, Prints and Photographs Division, Washington, DC

Library of Congress, Rare Books and Manuscripts Collection, Washington, DC

Louisiana State Archives, Vital Records Indices, Baton Rouge

Massachusetts State Historical Society Library and Archives, Boston

NARA, Census, Passport Applications, 1795-1905, Adjutant General's Office Records, 1780s-1917, and Passenger Lists 1820-1957,   Washington, DC

Nevada Historical Society Library, Reno

Newberry Library, Everett Family Papers, Chicago

New England Historic Genealogical Society, Registry of Vital Records and Statistics, Boston

New York Academy of Medicine, Annual Announcements of the New York Medical College for Women, New York

New York Historical Society, American Historical Manuscripts Collection, New York

North Carolina State Archives, Division of Archives and Records, Raleigh

Northwestern University Archives, Evanston, IL

Nunda Historical Society, Nunda, NY

Ohio Historical Society, Janney Papers, Columbus

Peabody Essex Museum (successor to the Essex Institute), Salem, MA

Pinellas County Clerk of the Circuit Court records, Old Hillsborough County Land Records books, Clearwater, FL

Pinellas County Historical Society, Largo, FL

Prairie Research Institute, Illinois State Geological Survey, Champaign

Fred Reed, Editor and Publisher of Paper Money

Dr. Patricia L. Ricci, Associate Professor of History and Art and Director Fine Arts Division and Performing Arts, Elizabethtown College, Elizabethtown, PA

Rollins College Archives, Winter Park, FL

Safford House Museum, Tarpon Springs, FL

San Joaquin County Historical Society, Lodi, CA

Schlesinger Library, Cambridge, MA

Sharlot Hall Museum Library, Prescott, Arizona

Shawneetown Public Library, Shawneetown, IL

Shiloh National Military Park, Savannah, TN

Smith College Archives, Northampton, MA

Smithsonian Institution, Archives of American Art, Hiram Powers Papers, Washington, DC

South Suburban Genealogical and Historical Society Library, Hazel Crest, IL

Suffolk County Clerk's Office, Boston

Tampa Bay History Center Archives, Tampa, FL

Tangier American Legation Institute for Moroccan Studies, Tangier, Morocco

Tarpon Springs Area Historical Society Archives, Depot Museum, Tarpon Springs, FL

Tarpon Springs Public Library, Tarpon Springs, Florida

Dennis Taylor, U. S. Patent Office, Washington, DC

Deborah Trehy, MD, gynecologist, Tampa, FL

Triebold Family, Crete, IL

Unitarian Universalist Church of Tarpon Springs, FL

University of Delaware Library, Special Collections, Dr. Charles A. Sajous Papers, Newark

University of Illinois Archives, Louisa A. Gregory Notebooks, Urbana

University of Michigan, William L. Clements Library, Mary Young Papers, Ann Arbor

University of Mississippi, J. D. Williams Library, Archives & Special Collections, Dr. Anne Gowdy/Sherwood Bonner Collection, University, MS

University of Nevada Library, Las Vegas

University of South Florida Library, Special Collections, Tampa

University of Vermont Library, Special Collections, George Perkins Marsh Collection, Burlington

U.S. Department of State, Policy Studies Division, Washington, DC

Vermont History Center, Barre

Vermont State Archives, Early Marriage Records Cards, Deaths Microfilms, Middlesex

Frances E. Willard Memorial Library and Archives, Evanston, IL

Woodlawn Cemetery Records, Bronx, New York City

Yale Law School, Lillian Goldman Law Library, The Avalon Project: Cape Spartel Lighthouse—May 31, 1865, New Haven

SECONDARY SOURCES

APKS = *Anson Peasley Keeler (A. P. K.) Safford*
MJS = *Mary Jane Safford*
MJSB = *Mary Jane Safford-Blake, when MJS used her married name*
FP = *Flora Payne*
LV = *Lucie Buckner Vannevar*
TG = *Tampa Guardian*
TJ = *Tampa Journal*
TWJ = *Tampa Weekly Journal*
TSAHS = *Tarpon Springs Area Historical Society*
NARA = *National Archives and Records Administration*
GPO = *Government Printing Office*

"A $20,000 Fire." Tampa Morning Tribune. 4: no. 282. Tampa: Tribune Publishing Co., 2 Dec 1898.
"A Bradford Reunion." The Bradford Era. Bradford, PA, 27 Mar 1888. Bradford Landmark Society Archives.
A Memorial and Biographical History of Northern California, Illustrated. Chicago: Lewis Publishing Co, 1891.
"About Hill Institute," @ www.hillinstitute.com/about_us.cfm
Abstract # 24416-Whitcomb family land. Abstracts of Title for lands in and around Tarpon Springs. Tarpon Springs, FL: TSAHS Archives.
Abstract # 27308-Walter W. Sammons land. Abstracts of Title for lands in and around Tarpon Springs. Tarpon Springs, FL: TSAHS Archives.
Abstract #29703-Tarpon Springs' Town Incorporation. Tarpon Springs, FL: TSAHS Archives.
Abstract # 38109-Thornton family land. Abstracts of Title for lands in and around Tarpon Springs. Tarpon Springs, FL: TSAHS Archives.
Ackerman, William K. Historical Sketch of the Illinois Central Railroad. Chicago: Fergus Printing Co, 1890.
"A Crematory for Boston… New England Cremation Society to Begin Operations." Chicago Daily Tribune. Chicago: Tribune Co, 27 Nov 1885.
"Acts." Acts, Resolutions and Memorials Adopted by the Seventh Legislative Assembly of the Territory of Arizona. Tucson: Office of the Arizona Citizen, 1873.
Acuna, Rodolfo, F. Corridors of Migration: The Odyssey of Mexican Laborers, 1600-1933. Tucson: University of Arizona Press, 2007.
Adams, Bluford. E. Pluribus Barnum: The Great Showman and the Making of U. S. Popular Culture. Minneapolis: University of Minnesota Press, 1997.
Adams, Thomas. Outline of Town and City Planning. New York: Russell Sage Foundation, 1935.
Adams, William Henry Davenport. The Queen of the Adriatic, Or, Venice Past and Present. Boston: Lothrop and Co, 1869.
Advertisement for Bank of Tarpon Springs. The Tarpon. 1: no. 6. Tarpon Springs: Truax, 5 Jan 1887.
Advertisement for Boston University School of Medicine. New England Medical Gazette. 21: no. 12. Boston: Otis Clapp & Son, Dec 1886.
Advertisement for John Munroe and Company. The Commercial & Financial Chronicle. New York: William B. Dana and Co, 9 Sept 1865.
Advertisement for John Munroe and Company. The Nation. New York, The Nation, 4 Nov 1869.
Advertisement for, "Ladies' Garment Suspenders." Herald of Health. 24: no. 6. New York: Wood & Holbrook, Dec 1874.
Advertisement for Leandro Safford's Muck Business. The Tarpon. 1: no. 38. Tarpon Springs: Truax, 27 May 1887.
Advertisement for Safford, Morris and Candee Insurance. Cairo Bulletin. Cairo, IL: Oberly, 15 Nov 1872.
Advertisement for The Myrtle. The Universalist Register: Containing the Statistics of the Church. 58. Boston: Universalist Publishing House, 1898.
Advertisement for Tarpon Springs Hotel. Florida Medical and Surgical Journal. Jacksonville, FL: Times-Union, Nov 1885.
Advertisement for W. E. D. Scott. The Tarpon. 1: no. 6. Tarpon Springs: Truax, 5 Jan 1887.
Album of Genealogy and Biography Cook County, Illinois. 4th edition. Chicago, Calumet Book & Engraving Co, 1896.
Aldrich, Lewis Cass, ed. History of Franklin and Grand Isle Counties, Vermont. Syracuse, NY: Mason & Co, 1891.
Alger, Russell A. The War of Rebellion, a Compilation of the Official Records of the Union and Confederate Armies. series 2. 3. Washington, DC: GPO, 1898.
Alger, Russell A. The War of Rebellion, a Compilation of the Official Records of the Union and Confederate Armies. series 2. 4. Washington, DC: GPO, 1899.
"All Sorts of Items." Cairo Daily Bulletin. Cairo, IL, Oberly, 3 Jan 1872.
Allen, John W. Legends & Lore of Southern Illinois. Carbondale, IL: Southern Illinois University Press, 1963.
Alvord, Clarence Walworth. "The Era of the Civil War 1848-1870." The Centennial History of Illinois. 3. Chicago: A. C. McClurg and Co, 1922.
Ambrose, D. Leib. History of the Seventh Regiment Illinois Volunteer Infantry. Springfield, IL: Illinois Journal Co, 1868.
"American Institute of Homoeopathy Twenty-Sixth Session," The American Observer. 10. Detroit: Lodge's Pharmacy, Jul 1873.
"American Institute of Homoeopathy 34th Annual Meeting." Hahnemannian Monthly. 16. Philadelphia: Hahnemannian Club of Philadelphia, Aug 1881.
"Americans in Paris." Anglo-American Times. 2: no. 45. London, G. W. Bacon & Co, 1 Sep 1866.
"Americans in Paris." Anglo-American Times. 2: no. 47. London, G. W. Bacon & Co, 14 Sep 1866.
"An Act No. 13." Acts, Resolutions and Memorials of the Eighteenth Legislative Assembly of the Territory of Arizona. Phoenix: Herald Book and Job Print, 1895.
Andrews, Cornelius, Hinsdale, Charles and Holman, Alfred L. Hinsdale Genealogy. Lombard, IL: A. Hinsdale Andrews, 1906.
Annual Catalogue of the University of Chicago. Chicago: University of Chicago, 1869.
Annual Report of the School Committee of the City of Boston 1874. Boston: Rockwell & Churchill, 1874.
Annual Report of the School Committee of the City of Boston 1883. School Document no. 22. Boston: Rockwell & Churchill, 1884.
Annual Report of the St. Louis Mercantile Library Association. St. Louis, MO: St. Louis Mercantile Library Association, 1851.
Anonymous German Author. "Letter from Hesse-Darmstadt." Darmstadt, 9 Jul 1871. The Woman's Journal. Boston, 5 Aug 1871.
"A.P. K. Safford Dies in Florida." Chicago Daily Tribune. 50: no. 349. Chicago, Tribune Co, 16 Dec 1891.

"Arizona in Philadelphia." The Arizona Citizen. 9: no. 36. Florence, AZ Territory, Wasson, 20 Jun 1879.

Arnold, Lois Barber. Four Lives in Science. New York: Schocken Books, 1984.

"Art." Florida: A Guide to the Southern-Most State. State of Florida: Writers' Program of the Works Progress Administration, 1939.

Attendees. "Programme of the Thirty-First Meeting of the American Association for the Advancement of Science, Commencing Wednesday, August 23, and Closing Wednesday, August 30, 1882, in Montreal Canada." Montreal: Local AAAS Committee, 1882.

Baas, Johan Hermann and Handerson, Henry Ebenezer. Outlines of the History of Medicine and the Medical Profession. New York: J. H. Vail & Co, 1889.

Bacon Leonard Woolsey. A Life Worth Living: Memorials of Emily Bliss Gould, of Rome. New York: Anson D. F. Randolph & Co, 1879.

Baker, Minnie Hewes. "Wood's Corners, Papers Read at the Local History Day Meeting of the Crete Woman's Club, January 19, 1922." Momence Press-Reporter, Momence, IL, 1922.

Baker, Nina Brown. Cyclone in Calico, The Story of Mary Ann Bickerdyke. Boston: Little, Brown and Co, 1952.

Bakersfield North Academy. "8th Annual Catalog of the Officers & Students of Bakersfield North Academy for the Year Ending November 1852." Bakersfield, VT, 1852. Vermont History Center, Barre, VT.www.kykinfolk.com/ballard/DeedAIndex.html

Bakst, Henry Jacob. The Story of the Massachusetts Memorial Hospital. Boston: Massachusetts Memorial Hospital, 1955.

Ballard County, Kentucky, property record deed book A at: www.kykinfolk.com/ballard/DeedAIndex.html

Ballou, Alice Dutton. "Help for Women." The Index. 5: no. 253. Boston: Index Association, 29 Oct 1874.

Bankruptcy Notice. Daily Alta California. 21: no. 6865. San Francisco: MacCrellish, 18 Jan 1869.

Bankruptcy Notice. Daily Alta California. 21: no. 6912. San Francisco: MacCrellish, 20 Feb 1869.

Barnard, Frederick A. P., ed. Johnson's New Universal Cyclopaedia: A Scientific and Popular Treasury of Useful Knowledge. New York: Alvin Johnson and Son, 1880.

Barnum, Phineas Taylor. Struggles and Triumphs: Or, Forty Years' Recollections of P. T. Barnum. Buffalo, NY: The Courier Co, 1883.

Barrows, Bella. "Hospital Life in the Old World. May Woman Practice Medicine?" The Phrenological Journal and Packard's Monthly. 1: no. 3. New York: Samuel R. Wells, Mar 1870.

Barrows, Isabella Chapin, MD, as "BCB." "In Memoriam Mary J. Safford, M. D." "Memorial Statement." Tarpon Springs Truth. Tarpon Springs, FL: George Truax, 12 Dec 1891. Undated paper, Safford Family ephemera, Cairo, IL, Public Library.

Bartlett, David W., Vandewater, David and Bartlett, Golden. Paris: with Pen and Pencil: Its People and Literature, Its Life and Business. New York: C. M. Saxton, 1858.

Bateman, Newton and Selby, Paul. ed. Historical Encyclopedia of Illinois. Chicago: Munsell Publishing Co, 1906.

Bazilchuk, Nancy, and Strimbeck, Rick. Longstreet Highroad Guide to the Vermont Mountains. Marietta, GA: Longstreet Press, 1999.

Beeton, Samuel Orchart. Beeton's Modern European Celebrities, A Biography of Continental Men and Women of Note. London: Ward, Lock and Tyler, 1874.

Belden, David A. Will County. Charleston: Arcadia Publishing, 2009.

Bellows, H. W. "Notes of a Preliminary Sanitary Survey of Forces of the United States in the Ohio and Mississippi Valleys, Near Midsummer, 1861." Documents of the U. S. Sanitary Commission. 1: 26. New York: U. S. Sanitary Commission, 1866.

Benson, Frances M. "Five Women Artists of New York." The Year's Art as Recorded in the Quarterly Illustrator. 1: no. 1. New York: Harry C. Jones, 1893.

Benson, Ned Harold. The Ancestors and Descendants of John Lewis Benson and His Sisters and Brother. Bloomington, IN: Anchor House, 2011.

Berry, Carrie Williams. Joel Tanner Hart. Kentucky Digital Library, undated (?1914).

Bickford-Smith, Roandeu Albert Henry. Greece Under King George. London: Richard Bentley and Son, 1893.

Biddle, Flora Miller. Whitney Women and the Museum They Made: A Family Memoir. New York: Arcade Publishing, 1999.

Biographical Dictionary and Portrait Gallery of Representative Men of Chicago. Chicago: American Biographical Publishing Co, 1892.

"Biographical Notice of Henry Ingersoll Bowditch, M.D." Proceedings of the American Academy of Arts and Sciences. 20. Boston: University Press, 1893.

Birch, Eugenie Ladner. The Unsheltered Woman: Women and Housing. New Brunswick, NJ: Transaction Publishers, 2012.

Bishop, Morris. A History of Cornell. Ithaca: Cornell University Press, 1962.

Bjornson, Bjornstjerne. Land of the Free-Bjornstjerne Bjornson's America Letters, 1880-1881. Northfield, MN: Norwegian-American Historical Association, 1978.

Blake, Clarence J. "John Harrison Blake." Proceedings of the American Academy of Arts & Sciences. 36. Boston: Published by the Academy, May 1900-1901.

Blake, Gorham. "Correspondence." Journal of Psychical Research. 1. Westminster, England: Society of Psychical Research Rooms, Jul 1884.

Blake, Gorham. Letter to Mary C. Young 1 Oct 1890. Mary C. Young Papers. University of Michigan, William L. Clements Library.

Blake, Mary Ann Gordon. Letter to Mary C. Young 22 Feb 1898. Mary C. Young Papers. University of Michigan, William L. Clements Library.

Blake, Mary J. vs. Gorham Blake (divorce). Commonwealth of Massachusetts Supreme Judicial County, Suffolk County September Term 1879. Case #2852.

Blake, Samuel. A Genealogical History of William Blake, of Dorchester, and His Descendants. Boston: Ebenezer Clapp, Jr., 1857.

Blocker, Jack S., Fahey, David M., and Tyrell, Ian R. Alcoholism and Temperance in Modern History: An International Encyclopedia. 1. Santa Barbara: ABC-CLIO, 2003.

Blue Book of Newton 1910. Boston, Boston Suburban Book Co, 1910 and subsequent years.

Bonner, Thomas Neville. To the Ends of the Earth. Cambridge, MA: Harvard University Press, 1992.

"Book-Store for Sale." Publishers Weekly. 31: no. 788. New York: Bowker Co, 5 Mar 1887.

Bormio, Italy website: www.bormio3.com/stelvio-pass/.

Boston City Assessing Records. Collection #2100-004, 308 Columbus Avenue, Boston, 1891. Courtesy of Boston City Archives.

Boston City Tax Records, Real Estate for 1880, Ward 11, Block 10, Line 7. Assessors' Plan No. 3, Back Bay District, Section 4.Courtesy of Boston City Archives.

Boston University Yearbook. 4-7. Boston: Houghton, 1877-1880.

Bradford, Thomas Lindsley. Homoeopathic Bibliography of the United States. Philadelphia, Boericke & Tafel, 1892.

Breslin, Ed. *Brigham Young: A Concise Biography of the Mormon Moses*. Washington, DC: Regnery History, 2013.

"Brevities." *Cairo Daily Bulletin*. Cairo, IL: Oberly, 6 Jan 1872.

Brockett, Linus P. *The Cross and the Crescent: Or, Russia, Turkey, and the Countries Adjacent in 1876-7*. Philadelphia: Hubbard Brothers, 1877.

Brockett, Linus P. and Vaughan, Mrs. Mary C. *Woman's Work in the Civil War: A Record of Heroism, Patriotism and Patience*.
    Philadelphia: Zeigler, McCurdy & Co, 1867.

Brown, Lynne S. *Gulfport: A Definitive History. 1*. Charleston: The History Press, 2004.

Browning, Elizabeth Barrett. "The Greek Slave." *The Complete Works of Mrs. E. B. Browning*. New York: The Riverdale Press, 1903.

Bruce, Robert V. *Bell: Alexander Graham Bell and the Conquest of Solitude*. Ithaca: Cornell University Press, 1973.

Bryant, William Cullen. "The Battle-Field." *The U.S. Democratic Review. 1: no 1*. Washington, DC: Langtree & O'Sullivan, Oct 1837.

Buckner, Lucie. "Fraud Exposed Governor A. P. K. Safford a Liar and the Lake Butler Villa Company a Humbug." *Gulf Coast Herald. 1: no. 23*.
    Tarpon Springs: Camp & Buckner, 13 Dec 1884.

Bunting, Josiah. *Ulysses S. Grant: The American Presidents Series: The 18th President, 1869-1877*. New York: Henry Holt and Co, 2004.

Burroughs, Amelia, M.D. "Women in the Institute and in the Medical Profession." *Transactions of the Forty-Seventh Session
    of the American Institute of Homoeopathy*. Philadelphia: Sherman & Co, 1894.

"Camp Defiance, Cairo, Ill., May 10, 1861." *Chicago Tribune of that date, quoted in Harper's Weekly. 5. no. 231*. New York: Harper's Magazine Co, 1 Jun 1861.

Campbell, Ballard C. *Disasters, Accidents, and Crises in American History*. New York: Facts on File, Inc, 2008.

Cannon, Cornelia James. *The History of the Women's Educational and Industrial Union 1877-1927*. Boston: WEIU, 1927.

Carpenter, Carrie. Letter. *Herald of Health. 26: no. 1*. New York: Wood & Holbrook, Jul 1875.

Carpenter, Richard W. "The Illinois Constitutional Convention of 1818. With Introduction and Notes." *Journal of the Illinois State Historical Society. 6 no. 3*.
    Springfield, IL: Illinois State Historical Society, 1913.

Cassino, Samuel E. *The Naturalists' Universal Directory*. Boston: S. E. Cassino, 1888.

Castellani, Aldo, M. D. and Chalmers, Albert J. *Manual of Tropical Medicine*. New York: William Wood & Co, 1910.

"Catalogue and Circular of the Evanston College for Ladies, 1871-72." Chicago, Sewell, 1871.

Cheong Mun Keong, Brian, and Sulaiman, Wahinuddin. "Typhoid and Malaria Co-Infection—An Interesting Finding in the Investigation of a Tropical Fever."
Malaysian Journal Medical Sciences. 13: no. 1. Kelantan, Malaysia: Universiti Sains, January 2006.

"Chicago Letter July 14, 1872, Miss Dr. Mary J. Safford." *Cairo Daily Bulletin*. Cairo, IL: Oberly, 18 Jul 1872.

Chisholm, Hugh, ed. "Orleanists." *Encyclopedia Britannica. 11th Ed*. Cambridge, England: The Encyclopaedia Britannica Company, 1911.

Cicchetti, Jane. *Dreams, Symbols, and Homeopathy: Archetypal Dimensions of Healing*. Berkeley: North Atlantic Books, 2003.

"City News." *Cairo Daily Bulletin. 9: no. 248*. Cairo, IL: Oberly, 19 Oct 1877.

"City News." *Cairo Daily Bulletin. 9: no. 276*. Cairo, IL: Oberly, 4 Dec 1877.

"Clarence J. Blake vs. Gorham Blake." *Massachusetts Reports 110 Cases Argued and Determined in the Supreme Judicial Court of Massachusetts
    March 1872-November 1872*. Cambridge: Houghton, Mifflin & Co, 1874.

Clarke, Edwin and O'Malley, Charles Donald. *The Human Brain and Spinal Cord: A Historical Study Illustrated with Writings from
    Antiquity to the Twentieth Century*. San Francisco: Norman Publishing, 1996.

"Class News." *The Smith Alumnae Quarterly. 7: no. 2*. Northampton, MA: Smith College Alumnae Association, Feb 1916.

"Clear Water Notes." *TJ. 4: no. 23*. Tampa: Cooper, 29 May 1890.

Cleave, Egbert. *Cleave's Biographical Cyclopaedia of Homeopathic Physicians and Surgeons*. Philadelphia: Galaxy Publishing, 1873.

Cline, Bruce. *More History, Mystery, and Hauntings of Southern Illinois*. Rockford, IL: Black Oak Media, 2012.

Coachman, Elizabeth, MD. "Fidelia Jane Merrick Whitcomb: A Nearly Forgotten Florida Medical Pioneer." *Sunland Tribune. 33*.
    Tampa: Tampa Historical Society, 2008-9.

Coerver, Don M., Pasztor, Suzanne B., and Buffington, Robert M. *Mexico An Encyclopedia of Contemporary Culture and History*.
    Santa Barbara, CA: ABC-CLIO, 2004.

Cole, Arthur Charles. *Centennial History of Illinois. 3* Chicago: A. C. McClurg & Co, 1919 and 1922.

College de France @ www.college-de-france.fr/site/en-institution/index.htm#\p=/site/en-about-college/index.htm

"College of Natural Sciences," *The Illio. 2*. Champaign, IL: Junior Class of the University of Illinois, 1895.

Collyer, Robert. "To Pittsburg Landing and Back. An Interesting Letter from Rev Robert Collyer." *Chicago Tribune*. Chicago: Tribune Co, 18 Apr 1862.

Comay, Joan. *Who's Who in Jewish History: After the Period of the Old Testament*. London: Routledge, 2002.

Commins, David and Lesch, David. *Historical Dictionary of Syria. 3rd ed*. Lanham, MD: Scarecrow Press, 2014.

"Congratulations." *Arizona Weekly Star*. Tucson: Hughes & Fay 15 Sep 1881.

Connolly, Andrew J., Finkbeiner, Walter E., Ursell, Philip C., and Davis, Richard L. *Autopsy Pathology*. Philadelphia, Elsevier, 2015.

Conway, Erik M. *Atmospheric Science at NASA: A History*. Baltimore: Johns Hopkins University Press, 2008.

Conwell, Col. Russell H. *History of the Great Fire in Boston November 9 and 10, 1872*. Boston: B. B. Russell, 1873.

Cook, Bernard A. *Women and War: A Historical Encyclopedia from Antiquity to the Present*. Santa Barbara, CA: ABC-CLIO, 2006.

"Cook County Medical Society." *The United States Medical Investigator. 9: no.8*. Chicago: C. S. Halsey, August 1872.

Cooper, George. *Lost Love: A True Story of Passion, Murder, and Justice in Old World New York*. New York: Pantheon Books, 1994.

Cooper, H. J. "A Visit to Tarpon." *Tampa Guardian. 12: no. 32*. Tampa: Magbee, 24 Nov 1886.

Cooper, Michael L. *Fighting Fire!: Ten of the Deadliest Fires in American History and How We Fought Them*. New York: Henry Holt and Co, 2014.

"Correspondence." *Bulletin of the Essex Institute. 5-7*. Salem, MA: Salem Press, 1874-1876.

Costa, A. "On Goiters and the Stupidity Which in Some Countries Accompanies Them, Endeavours of Vincenzo Malacarne, from Saluzzo." Panminerva Medica. 31: no. 2. Rome, Italy: Italian Medical Association, Apr-Jun, 1989.

"Courses of Instruction Diseases of Women: Professor Mary J. Safford-Blake." Boston University Yearbook. 7. Boston: Houghton, 1880.

"Crete's Early History, Papers Read at the Local History Day Meeting of the Crete Woman's Club, January 19, 1922." Momence Press-Reporter. Momence, IL: McNichols, 1922.

Croly, Jane Cunningham. The History of the Woman's Club Movement in America. New York: H. G. Allen, 1898.

Curran, Isaac Bush. "Isaac B. Curran Diary." Buckmaster-Curran Family Papers, Box 4, Folder 1, Springfield, IL: Abraham Lincoln Presidential Library, diary covers 24 Mar 1863 to June 1863.

Curran, Nathaniel. "General Isaac B. Curran: Gregarious Jeweler." Journal of the Illinois Historical Society. 69: no.4. Springfield, IL: Illinois State Historical Society, Autumn 1978.

"Current Topics." The Index. 7: no. 19. Boston: Index Association, 4 Nov 1886.

Cushing, Frank Hamilton. "Preliminary Report on the Exploration of Ancient Key-dweller Remains on the Gulf Coast of Florida." Proceedings of the American Philosophical Society Held at Philadelphia for Promoting Useful Knowledge. 35. Philadelphia: The American Philosophical Society, 6 Nov 1896.

Cushing, Thomas. Historical Sketch of Chauncy-Hall School with Catalogue of Teachers and Pupils 1828-1894. Boston: W. B. Clarke, 1894.

Cycadia Cemetery census. Tarpon Springs, FL. Canvassed by private individuals. Online @ files.usgwarchives.net, 1995.

Daintith, John. Biographical Encyclopedia of Scientists. Boca Raton, FL: CRC Press, 1994.

Dana, Bruce E. The Apostleship. Springville, UT: CFI, 2006.

Davidson, Alexander and Stuve, Bernard. "The Canal Scrip Fraud." A Complete History of Illinois from 1673 to 1884. Springfield, IL: H. W. Rokker, 1884.

Davidson, Jonathan. A Century of Homeopaths: Their Influence on Medicine and Health. New York: Springer, 2014.

Davis, James Edward. Frontier Illinois. Bloomington, IN: Indiana University Press, 1998.

"Death of Dr. Mary J. Safford, the Eminent Female Physician." Newspaper clipping of unknown source in, "Obituary Book." Prescott, AZ: Sharlot Hall Museum.

Dellenbaugh, Frederick S. A Canyon Voyage: The Narrative of the Second Powell Expedition. 1908. Tucson: University of Arizona Press, 1996.

DeLong, Sidney R. The History of Arizona. San Francisco: Whitaker & Ray Co, 1905.

DelPlato, Joan. Multiple Wives, Multiple Pleasures: Representing the Harem, 1800-1875. Cranbury, NJ: Associated University Presses, 2002.

D'Emilio, John and Freedman, Estelle B. Intimate Matters: A History of Sexuality in America. Chicago: University of Chicago Press, 1997.

De Saulcy, F. Les Derniers Jours de Jerusalem. Paris: Librairie de L. Hachette et C., 1866.

Dennett, Andrea Stulman. Weird and Wonderful: The Dime Museum in America. New York: New York University Press, 1997.

Denominational Column. Manford's New Monthly Magazine. 29: no. 12. Chicago: Mrs. H. B. Manford, Dec 1885.

Denton, William. Our Planet, Its Past and Future; or, Lectures on Geology. 2nd ed. Boston: William Denton, 1869.

Denton, William. The Soul of Things. Boston: Wade, Wise and Co, 1863.

Department of Public Health, Registry of Vital Records and Statistics, Massachusetts Vital Records Index to Deaths (1916-1970), vol. 35 77. Index 132/133: Margarita Safford's death. Boston: New England Historic Genealogical Society.

Dickens, Charles. American Notes for General Circulation. New York: Harper Brothers, 1842.

Digre, Kathleen B. and Corbett, James John. Practical Viewing of the Optic Disc. Burlington, MA: Elsevier Science, 2003.

Disston, Hamilton R. To Mr. A. J. Hanna 16 Jun 1947, from Philadelphia. Safford House Museum Docent Book, Tarpon Springs. Original reportedly in Rollins College Library Archives, Winter Park, FL.

Doggett, Kate. "Letter." 16 Feb 1871, Luxor, Egypt. Cairo Daily Bulletin. Cairo, IL: Oberly, 7 May 1871.

Doggett, Kate. "Letter from Switzerland." The Woman's Journal. 42. Boston: 21 Oct 1871.

"Donors to the Tampa Relief Fund." Tampa Weekly Journal. 1: no. 45. Tampa: Cooper 27 Oct 1887.

Doyle, Don. The Cause of All Nations: An International History of the American Civil War. New York: Basic Books, 2015.

"Dr. Mary Safford." Cairo Daily Bulletin. Cairo, IL: Oberly, 19 Dec 1871.

"Dr. Mary Safford." Letter to the Editor. Cairo Daily Bulletin. Cairo, IL: Oberly, 3 Jan 1872.

"Dr. Mary Safford-Blake's Lecture." Lowell Daily Citizen and News. 6778. Lowell, MA: Brown & Morey, 8 Mar 1878.

"Dr. Sajous Knighted," The Medical Fortnightly. 2: no. 7. St. Louis: Bransford Lewis, MD, 1 Oct 1892.

"Dress Reform. A Lecture to Ladies. Corsets, Bustles, Long Skirts and False Hair Condemned." Boston Morning Journal. Boston: Sleeper & Rogers, 26 Feb 1874.

"Dress Reform in Boston." Herald of Health. 24: no. 5. New York: Wood & Holbrook, Nov 1874.

Drummond-Hay, Sir John Hay and Drummond-Hay, Alice Emily. A Memoir of Sir John Drummond-Hay. London: John Murray, 1896.

Dubbs, Joseph Henry. History of Franklin and Marshall College. Lancaster, PA: Franklin and Marshall College Alumni Association, 1893.

Dugan, James. The Great Iron Ship. New York: Harper & Brothers, 1953.

Duncan, Dr. T. C. "Medical View of the Chicago Fire." Homeopathic World. 6. London: Jarrold & Son, 1 Dec 1871.

Eagle, Mary Kavanaugh Oldham, ed. The Congress of Women Held in the Woman's Building, World's Columbian Exposition. 2, Chicago: W. B. Conkey, 1894.

Ecelbarger, Gary. Black Jack Logan: An Extraordinary Life in Peace and War. Guilford, CT: Lyons Press, 2015.

Eckley, Robert. Lincoln's Forgotten Friend, Leonard Swett. Carbondale, IL: Southern Illinois University Press, 2012.

Eddy, T. M. The Patriotism of Illinois. Chicago: Clarke & Co, 1866.

"Editorial Notes." The Index. 6: no. 19. Boston: Index Association, 5 Nov 1885.

"Editor's By-Hours." The Repository. 51. Boston: Universalist Publishing House, 1874.

Edmunds, R. David. The Potawatomis: Keepers of the Fire. Norman, OK: University of Oklahoma Press, 1978.

Eighth Census of the U.S., 1860, Crete, Will County, IL. NARA

Eighth Census of the U.S., 1860, Grass Valley, Nevada, CA. NARA

Eigler, Friederike and Kord, Susanne, ed. *The Feminist Encyclopedia of German Literature*. Westport, CT: Greenwood Press, 1997.

Einstein, Lewis. "Napoleon III and American Diplomacy at the Outbreak of the Civil War." Address in French before the Societe d'Histoire Diplomatique, 9 Jun 1905.

Epler, Percy H. *The Life of Clara Barton*. New York: MacMillan, 1930.

Essex Institute. *Bulletin of the Essex Institute*. 5: no.10, Salem, MA: Essex Institute, Oct 1873.

Essex Institute. *Bulletin of the Essex Institute*. 7: no.2, Salem, MA: Salem Press, Feb 1875.

"European Correspondence." *Humboldt Register*. 4: no. 23 and 24. Unionville, NV: William J. Forbes, 29 Sep and 6 Oct 1866.

Evanston College for Ladies, contracts. Evanston: Northwestern University Archives/Records of the Evanston College for Ladies, 1872.

Everett, Edward, Dewey, Rev. Orville, Tuckerman, H. T., Cushman, Clara, Kirkland, Clara Matilda, Migliarini, A. M., and Calvert,
    G. H. *Powers' Statue of the Greek Slave*. Boston: Eastburn's Press, 1848.

Executive Documents Printed by Order of the House of Representatives During the First Session of the Thirty-Eighth Congress 1863-1864.
    Document no. 6. 9 Dec 1862. Washington, DC: GPO, 1864.

"Faculty Notes." *Smith College Monthly*. 11. Northampton, MA: Senior Class, Smith College, October 1903-June 1904.

"Faculty, School of Medicine." *Boston University Year Book for Year 1887-1888*. 14. Boston: University Offices, 1887.

Fairman, Charles E. "Works of Art in the United States Capitol Building Including Biographies of the Artists." *United States Government
    Congressional Serial Set 63rd Congress, 1st Session Senate Document No. 169*. Washington, DC: GPO, 1913.

Farina, William. *Ulysses S. Grant, 1861-1864: His Rise from Obscurity to Military Greatness*. Jefferson, NC: McFarland & Co, 2007.

Farrar, Jeremy, Hotez, Peter, Junghanss, Thoma, Kang, Gagandeep, Lalloo, David, and White, Nicholas. *Manson's Tropical Diseases*. 23rd ed.
    Philadelphia: Elsevier/Saunders, 2013.

Faulk, Odie, B. *Tombstone Myth and Reality*. New York: Oxford University Press, 1972.

Ferguson, Gillum. *Illinois in the War of 1812*. Springfield, IL: University of Illinois Press, 2012.

Ferguson, William R. *Technician's Guide for Postmortem Examinations*. Xlibris, 2010.

Ferril, Will C. ed. "Roswell Eaton Goodell." *Sketches of Colorado in Four Volumes*. I. Denver: Western Press Bureau Company, 1911.

"Field Meeting at Boxford, Tuesday, June 26, 1877." *Bulletin of the Essex Institute*. 9: no. 7. Salem, MA: Essex Institute, Jul 1877.

"First Annual Convention of the Illinois Association." *Chicago Daily Tribune*. Chicago: Tribune Co, 5 Oct 1877.

Fischer, Leroy. "Cairo's Civil War Angel, Mary Jane Safford." *Journal of the Illinois State Historical Society*. 54: no. 3, Springfield, IL: State of Illinois, Autumn 1961.

"Florida State Statistics." *Universalist Register: Giving Statistics of the Universalist Church, and Other Denominational Information, Etc. for 1887*.
    Boston: Universalist Publishing House, 1887.

"Florida University." *The New York Medical Times*. 18: no. 12. New York: E. B. Coby, Dec 1890.

"Former Mayor and Banker Is Back in City." *Tarpon Springs Evening Leader*. Tarpon Springs: Tarpon Springs Publishing Co, 27 Nov 1915.

Foster, Lawrence. *Women, Family, and Utopia: Communal Experiments of the Shakers, the Oneida Community, and the Mormons*.
    Syracuse, NY: Syracuse University Press, 1991.

Fowkes, Henry L. *Historical Encyclopedia of Illinois*. 1. Chicago: Munsell Publishing, 1918.

Frazar, Caroline M. "The Moral Education Society of Boston." *Report of the International Council of Women*.
    Washington, DC: National Woman Suffrage Association, 30 Mar 1877.

Free Religious Association membership list: www.emersonhouston.org/classMaterial/history/UU/historyTowwwi.pdf

Gabb, William More. *Paleontology*. 2. Sacramento: Legislature of California, 1869.

Gambier, Capt. James William. *Florida: Its Resources and Natural Advantages for the Emigrant, the Capitalist, the Manufacturer*.
    London: Florida Land and Mortgage Company (Limited), 1883.

"Gamma Delta Ladies Literary Society." *Boston University Annual Index for 1885-86*. Boston: Boston University Students, 1886.

Gantz, Theodore A. "Hiram Powers and Joel Tanner Hart: Two Sculptors, A Voyage from Cincinnati Ohio to Florence Italy and the Friendship That Developed."
    Paper presented 11 Oct 2008 at, "Proceedings of the City and the Book V International Conference on the Americans in Florence's English Cemetery III."
    Florence, Italy, Lyceum Club and the English Cemetery.

Geitz, Henry, Heideking, Jurgen and Herbst, Jurgen. *German Influences on Education in the United States to 1917*. Cambridge,
    England: Press Syndicate of the University of Cambridge, 1995.

Gibson, Charles Dana and Gibson, E. Kay. *Dictionary of Transport & Combatant Vessels Steam and Sail Employed by the Union Army 1861-1868*.
    Camden, ME: Ensign Press, 2001.

Gill, H. Z. "Letter from Philadelphia, Visiting Europe for the Purpose of Observation and Study of Medicine." *The Cincinnati Lancet and Observer*. 29.
    Cincinnati: E. B Stevens, MD, 1868.

Gillett, Dr. H. C. "Care of the Wounded." *Chicago Tribune*. Chicago: Tribune Co, 24 Apr 1862.

Godwin, Joscelyn, Chanel Christian and Deveney, John P. *The Hermetic Brotherhood of Luxor*. York Beach, ME: Samuel Weiser, 1995,

Gordon, Sarah H. "Mary Jane Safford." *American National Biography*. New York: Oxford University Press, 1999.

Gowdy, Dr. Anne Razy. *A Sherwood Bonner Sampler*. Knoxville: University of Tennessee Press, 2000.

Grant, Julia Dent. *The Personal Memoirs of Julia Dent Grant (Mrs. Ulysses S. Grant)*. Carbondale, IL: Southern Illinois University Press, 1975.

Grant, Ted. *Women in Medicine: A Celebration of Their Work*. Richmond Hill, Ontario: Firefly Books 2004.

Grant, Ulysses S. *Personal Memoirs of U. S. Grant*. 1885. Cambridge, MA: Da Capo, 2001.

Gray, Walter D. *Interpreting American Democracy in France: The Career of Edouard Laboulaye, 1811-1883*. Cranbury, NJ: Associated University Presses, 1994.

Green, Abigail. *Moses Montefiore: Jewish Liberator, Imperial Hero*. Cambridge, MA: Harvard University Press, 2010.

Greenbie, Marjorie Barstow. *Lincoln's Daughters of Mercy*. New York: G. P. Putnam and Sons, 1944.

Greenwood, John T. and Berry, F. Clifton. *Medics at War: Military Medicine from Colonial Times to the 21st Century.*
    Annapolis, MD: Association of the United States Army, Naval Institute Press, 2005.
Gregory, Louisa A. "Dr. Blake's Lecture to the Gannett School: Womb & Menstruation." "Sex," notebook. *Louisa A Gregory Notebooks 1873-1879.*
Champaign, IL: Courtesy University of Illinois Archives (214), May 1875.
Gregory, Louisa A. "Food Lecture of Dr. Blake May '75." "Sex," notebook. *Louisa A Gregory Notebooks 1873-1879.*
    Champaign, IL: Courtesy University of Illinois Archives (214), May 1875.
Gregory, Louisa A. "Gannett Institute May 25 Beginnings of Life." "Sex," notebook. *Louisa A Gregory Notebooks 1873-1879*
    Champaign, IL: Courtesy University of Illinois Archives (214), May 1875.
Gregory, Louisa A. "Generation." "Sex," notebook. *Louisa A Gregory Notebooks 1873-1879.* Champaign, IL: Courtesy University of Illinois Archives (214), May 1875.
Griffith, Elisabeth. *In Her Own Right: The Life of Elizabeth Cady Stanton.* Oxford, England: Oxford University Press, 1984.
Gunter, Susan E. *Alice in Jamesland: The Story of Alice Howe Gibbens James.* Lincoln, NE: University of Nebraska Press, 2009.
Gurney, Edmund, Myers, Frederic and Podmore, Frank. *Phantasms of the Living. 2.* London: Rooms of the Society of Psychical Research, 1886.
Guthrie, Thomas. *A Plea for Ragged Schools, or Prevention Better than Cure: Supplement to A Plea for Ragged Schools.* Glasgow, Scotland: William Collins, 1847.
Hafner, Albert. "Died: In Tarpon Springs, Florida, Tuesday, Dec. 8th, Dr. Mary J. Safford." *The Tarpon Springs Truth.* Tarpon Springs: George Truax, 12 Dec 1891.
Hall, Edith, Alston, Richard, and McConnell, Justine. *Ancient Slavery and Abolition: From Hobbes to Hollywood.* Oxford: Oxford University Press, 2011.
Haller, John. *The History of American Homeopathy: The Academic Years, 1820-1935.* Binghamton, NY: Haworth Press, 2005.
Hand, Henry Wells. *Centennial History of the Town of Nunda.* Rochester, NY: Rochester Herald Press, 1908.
Harbert, Elizabeth Boynton. "Mothers to the Rescue." *The New Era. 1: no. 9.* Chicago: Elizabeth Boynton Harbert, Sep 1885.
Harbert, Elizabeth Boynton. "The Woman's Congress, Guests of the New England Woman's Club." *The Daily Inter-Ocean. 7: no. 181.* Chicago: Inter Ocean, 20 Oct 1880.
Hardy, Iza Duffus. *Oranges and Alligators. 2 ed.* London: Ward and Downey, 1887.
Harper, Ida Husted. *The Life and Work of Susan B. Anthony. 1.* Indianapolis: Hollenbeck Press, 1898.
Harrell, Moses B. "The Inundation of Cairo in 1858." *Cairo City Directory of 1864.* Cairo, IL: Harrell, 1864.
Hart, Alfred A. "Last Rail Laid at Promontory Point, May 10th, 1869." albumen silver print. Courtesy J. Paul Getty Museum Open Content Program.
Hart, Joel Tanner. "Portrait of Mary Morgan Hart Weaver." *Kentucky Historical Society Object Catalog: 1939.997, circa 1830.*
Hart, Joel Tanner. "To Mary." Florence, Italy, 9 Jul 1866. Unpublished handwritten poem. Safford ephemera at Cairo Public Library.
Harvard College Class of 1879 Secretary's Report. No. III. Commencement, 1885. Buffalo: Bigelow Brothers, 1885.
Hawes, G. W. *Illinois State Gazetteer and Business Directory for 1858-1859.* Chicago: George W. Hawes, 1858.
Haxby, James, Bellin, Barbara Ann and Allan, Walter D. *Standard Catalog of United States Obsolete Bank Notes 1782-1966. 1.* Iola, WI: Krause Publications, 1988.
Heidler, David S., Heidler, Jeanne T. and Coles, David J., ed. *Encyclopedia of the American Civil War.* New York: W. W. Norton & Company, 2000.
Hellman, Hal. *Great Feuds in Medicine: Ten of the Liveliest Disputes Ever.* Hoboken, NJ: John Wiley & Sons, 2001.
Henshaw, Sarah Edwards. *Our Branch and Its Tributaries: Being a History of the Work of the Northwestern Sanitary Commission.* Chicago: Alfred L. Sewell, 1868.
Hering, Constantine. *Materia Medica.* New York: Boericke & Tafel, 1877.
Hickey, James T. "An Illinois First Family: The Reminiscences of Clara Matteson Doolittle." *Journal of the Illinois State Historical Society. 69: no. 2.*
    Springfield, IL: Illinois State Historical Society, Feb 1976.
Hill, Gladys Safford, death. *Louisiana Vital Records Indices.* New Orleans death Indices 1937-1948.
    Baton Rouge, LA: Secretary of State, Division of Archives, Records Management, and History.
Hill, Robert Cham, death. *North Carolina Death Certificates 1909-1976.* NC State Board of Health, Bureau of Vital Statistics.
Hillerbrand, Hans Joachim. *The Encyclopedia of Protestantism.* New York: Routledge, 2004.
Hillsborough County Deed No. 59. Old Hillsborough County Deeds. Book P. Clearwater, FL: Pinellas County Clerk of the Circuit Court Office.
Hillsborough County, Florida Directory-Census 1890, Hillsborough County Marriage Records. Tampa Bay History Center L3154.
Hillsborough County, Florida, Guardianship Records. vol. A 1886-1895. Circuit Court, Thirteenth Judicial Circuit, Hillsborough County. Office of the Clerk, Tampa, FL.
Hirsch, Mark D. *William C. Whitney Modern Warwick.* New York: Dodd, Mead Co, 1948.
"History of Early Amateur Journalism in Pennsylvania." website of the American Private Press Association online reference
    @ www.thefossils.org/horvat/aj/states/Pennsylvania.html.
"History of the Association for the Advancement of Woman." *Souvenir Nineteenth Annual Congress of the Association for the Advancement of Woman.*
    Washington, DC: Todd Brothers, 1877.
History of the Counties of McKean, Elk, Cameron and Potter, Pennsylvania. Chicago: J. H. Beers, 1890.
"History of the University of California Berkeley." www.berkeley.edu.
Hoge, Jane Currie. *The Boys in Blue.* New York: E. B. Treat & Co, 1867.
Homans, Edward, ed. "Banks of the United States." *The Bankers Magazine and Statistical Register. 11,* New York: J. Smith Homans, Jr., May 1857.
"Homoeopathic Association of Boston University Organized." *The American Observer. 10.* Detroit: Lodge's Homoeopathic Pharmacy, 1873.
Howard, Elmira Y., M. D. "European Letter." Allgemeines Krankenhaus, Vienna 24 Nov 1873. *Cincinnati Medical Advance. 1: no. 10.*
    Cincinnati, OH: T. P. Wilson, MD, Dec 1873.
Hoyt, Edwin Palmer. *The Whitneys: An Informal Portrait, 1635-1975.* New York: Weybright and Talley, 1976.
Hubbard, Harlan Page. *Hubbard's Newspaper and Bank Directory of the World. 2.* New Haven: Hubbard, 1882.
Hughes, Nathaniel Cheairs. *The Battle of Belmont.* Chapel Hill, NC: University of North Carolina Press, 1991.
Hugo, Victor. *Les Miserables.* New York: Dodd, Mead and Co, 1862.
Hunt, Harriot. *Glances and Glimpses; or Fifty Years Social, Including Twenty Years Professional Life.* Boston: John P. Jewett, 1856.
Hunt, Rockwell D. "Golden Jubilee of the Pacific Railroad." *Overland Monthly and Out West Magazine. 72: no. 6.* San Francisco: Overland Monthly Co, June 1919.

Hurricanes Affecting Tarpon Springs, FL, City Database @ hurricanecity.com.

"Illinois Homoeopathic Medical Association." *American Observer Medical Monthly.* 9. Detroit, MI: Dr. E. A. Lodge, Sep 1872.

"Important Events of Horse and Buggy Days, 75 Years Ago." *Nunda News.* Nunda, NY: Sanders, 4 Jul 1953.

Indenture. Old Hillsborough County Deeds. Book N. 2 Jun 1884. Clearwater, FL: Pinellas County Clerk of the Circuit Court Office.

"In Re Estate of A. P. K. Safford, deceased." Order Pro. Min. 0, filed 12 Jun 1900. Abstracts drawer, TSAHS Archives, Tarpon Springs, FL.

"In Re Estate of Mary J. Safford." Order Admitting to Probate and Record of Certified Copy of Foreign Will.
        Pinellas County Florida Foreign Wills Book. 9: 386, 10 Nov 1925, Case #2243.

"Institute of Heredity." *Boston Post.* Boston: Beals & Greene, 18 May 1881.

"International Exhibition 1876 Official Catalogue, Part III, Machinery Hall, Annexes, and Special Building, Department V-Machinery."
        Cambridge, MA: Centennial Catalogue Co, 1876.

"In the matter of the Guardianship of Leandro Taft, a minor." Record #109. Probate Court Pima County, Arizona Territory, 24 Mar 1875,
        Guardianship of, "Orphan," Leandro Taft to A. P. K. Safford, Arizona State Archives, Phoenix, AZ.

"Irish News." *The Morning Freeman.* 14: no. 93. Saint John, New Brunswick, 6 Sep 1864.

Irving, Washington. "Legend of the Moor's Legacy." *The Alhambra.* 1849. New York: G. P. Putnam, 1863.

James, Edward T. *Notable American Women 1607-1950, Vol. III P-Z.* Cambridge, MA: Belknap Press of Harvard University Press, 1971.

James, William and James, Henry. *William and Henry James: Selected Letters.* Charlottesville, VA: University of Virginia Press, 1997.

Janney (Derby), Frances. *Letter to Mother Rebecca Smith Janney.* Columbus, OH: Ohio Historical Society Archives, Janney Family papers, 23 May 1875.

Janney (Derby), Frances. *Letter to Mother Rebecca Smith Janney.* Columbus, OH: Ohio Historical Society Archives, Janney Family papers, 9 Jun 1875.

Janney (Derby), Frances. *Letter to parents John Jay Janney and Rebecca Smith Janney.*
        Columbus, OH: Ohio Historical Society Archives, Janney Family papers, 13 Feb 1876.

Jenness, Carrie L. "Dr. Mary J. Safford Blake." *Cottage Hearth.* 3: no. 5. Boston: Milliken and Spencer, May 1876. Courtesy Universtiy of Mississippi

Jolly, Ellen Ryan. *Nuns of the Battlefield.* Providence, RI: The Providence Visitor Press, 1977.

Johnson, Claudia D. and Johnson, Vernon. *The Social Impact of the Novel: A Reference Guide.* Westport, CT: Greenwood Press, 2002.

Jones, J. *Una and Her Paupers: Memorials of Agnes Elizabeth Jones.* New York: Routledge, 1872.

Journal of the Executive Proceedings of the Senate of the United States of America, from March 5, 1860, to March 3, 1871, Inclusive. 17. Washington, DC: GPO, 1901.

Kagin, Donald. *Private Gold Coins and Patterns of the United States.* New York: Arco, 1981.

Kaufman, Polly Welts. *Boston Women and City School Politics 1872-1905.* New York: Garland, 1994.

Kerner, Robert J. ed. "The Diary of Edward W. Crippin, Private 27th Illinois Volunteers, War of the Rebellion, August 7, 1861, to September 19, 1863."
        Transactions of the Illinois State Historical Society for the Year 1909. Springfield, IL: Illinois State Historical Society, 1909.

Khan, Yasmin Sabina. *Enlightening the World: The Creation of the Statue of Liberty.* Ithaca: Cornell University Press, 2010.

Kilgo, Dolores. *Tarpon Springs.* Charleston: Arcadia Publishing, 2002.

King, Moses. *The Harvard Register.* 2. Cambridge, MA: Moses King, 1880.

King, William Harvey. *History of Homeopathy and Its Institutions in America.* 3. New York: Lewis Publishing, 1905.

Kinglake, Alexander William. *The Invasion of the Crimea: Its Origin, and an Account of its Progress Down to the Death of Lord Raglan.*
        Leipzig: Bernhard Tauchnitz, 1863.

Kionka, T. K. *Key Command: Ulysses S. Grant's District of Cairo.* Columbia, MO: University of Missouri Press, 2006.

Kirschmann, Anne Taylor. *A Vital Force: Women in American Homeopathy.* New Brunswick, NJ: Rutgers University Press, 2004.

Kittridge, Herman E. *Ingersoll A Biographical Appreciation.* New York: Dresden Publishing Co, 1911.

Knox, John Jay, Rhodes, Bradford and Youngman, Elmer Haskell. *A History of Banking in the United States.* New York: Bradford Rhodes & Co, 1903.

Koerner, Gustav Philipp. *Memoirs of Gustav Koerner 1809-1896.* Cedar Rapids, IO: The Torch Press, 1909.

Koliopoulos, John S. and Veremis, Thanos M. *A Modern Greece: A History Since 1821.* West Sussex, United Kingdom: Wiley-Blackwell, 2010.

Lande, R. Gregory. *The Abraham Man: Madness, Malingering, and the Development of Medical Testimony.* New York: Algora, 2012.

Lander, James. " 'Herndon's Auction List' and Lincoln's Interest in Science." *Journal of the Abraham Lincoln Association.* 32: no. 2.
        Springfield, IL: Abraham Lincoln Association, Summer 2011.

Lander, James. *Lincoln and Darwin: Shared Visions of Race, Science, and Religion.* Carbondale, IL: Southern Illinois University Press, 2010.

Lankford, Nelson D. *An Irishman in Dixie: Thomas Conolly's Diary of the Fall of the Confederacy.* Columbia, SC: University of South Carolina Press, 1988.

Lansden, John McMurray. *A History of the City of Cairo, Illinois.* Chicago: R. R. Donnelley & Sons, 1910.

Lansden, John McMurray. "General Grant, Judge William H. Green and N. B. Thistlewood, of Cairo, Illinois."
        Journal of the Illinois State Historical Society. 8: no.3. Springfield, IL: Illinois State Historical Society, October 1915.

Larson, Orvin Prentiss. *American Infidel: Robert G. Ingersoll.* New York: Citadel Press, 1962.

Lasell College, Winslow Archives. http://library.lasell.edu/Archives.htm.

Leach, William. *True Love & Perfect Union: The Feminist Reform of Sex and Society.* New York: Basic Books, 1980.

"Lecture of Dr. Mary Safford Blake." *Boston Medical and Surgical Journal.* 102: no. 7. Boston: Houghton, 12 Feb 1880.

"Lecture Subjects: Professor Mary S. Blake." *Boston University Year Book.* 2. Boston: Houghton, 1875.

Leonard, John W., ed. *Marquis Who's Who in America 1903-1905.* Chicago: A. N. Marquis & Company, 1905.

Leonard, John W., ed. *Who's Who in Engineering A Biographical Dictionary of Contemporaries 1922-1923.* New York: John W. Leonard, 1922.

Letter. *American Journal of Homeopathic Materia Medica and Record of Medical Science.* 7: no. 53. Philadelphia: J. M. Stoddart & Co., 1874.

"Library Chat." *Cambridge Tribune.* 13: no. 37. Cambridge, MA: F. Stanhope Hill, 22 Nov 1890.

Lilienthal, Samuel, M. D. *Homeopathic Therapeutics.* 2. New York: Boericke & Tafel, 1879.

"List of Permanent Members." Transactions of the Illinois Homoeopathic Medical Association. Chicago: U.S. Medical Investigator Publishing Co, 1875.

"Literature Reviews." The Musical Herald. Boston: Musical Herald Co, May 1884.

Livermore, Mary A. "After the Battle of Fort Donelson." The Ladies Repository. 39: no. 5. Cincinnati: Methodist Episcopal Church, May 1868.

Livermore, Mary A. My Story of the War: A Woman's Narrative of Four Years Personal Experience. Hartford, CT: A. D. Worthington and Co, 1889.

Livermore, Mary A. The Story of My Life: Or, The Sunshine and the Shadow of Seventy Years. Hartford, CT: A. D. Worthington & Co, 1899.

Livingston, Luther Samuel and Rogers, Bruce. Franklin and His Press at Passy: An Account of the Books, Pamphlets, and Leaflets Printed There
    including the Long-Lost 'Bagatelles.' New York: The Grolier Club, 1914.

Lloyd, H. H. Lloyd's Battle History of the Great Rebellion, Complete. New York: H. H. Lloyd & Co, 1866.

"Local Brevities." Los Angeles Daily Herald. 4: no.102. Los Angeles: Herald Print Co, 23 Jul 1875.

"Local Brevities." Los Angeles Daily Herald. 4: no.108. Los Angeles: Herald Print Co, 29 Jul 1875.

"Local Matters: Tucson Public School." Arizona Citizen. 6: no. 39. Tucson, Arizona Territory: Wasson, 1 Jul 1876.

"Local Matters: Tucson Public School." Arizona Citizen. 6: no. 40. Tucson, Arizona Territory: Wasson, 8 Jul 1876.

"Local News." Cairo Evening Bulletin, Daily Edition. Cairo, IL: Oberly, 7 May 1869.

"Local News." The Daily Illini. 4: no. 1. Champaign, IL: Illinois Industrial University, Oct 1874. Courtesy University of Illinois Archives. 41/8/801.

Lockwood, Dr. Frank C. (Early Arizona Recollections) Statements made in conversations with J. S. Vosburgh, "Vosburgh Conversation"
    interview with John Vosburgh, October 1879, V959-7, Tucson: Arizona Historical Society Library Archives.

Logan, Mrs. John A. Reminiscences of a Soldier's Wife: An Autobiography. New York: Charles Scribner's Sons, 1916.

Logan, Mrs. John A. Thirty Years in Washington; or, Life and Scenes of Our National Capital. Hartford, CT: A. D. Worthington & Co, 1901.

"Lotta's Fountain." Art Inventories Catalog of Smithsonian American Art Museum, online:www.siris-artinventories.si.edu.

Lopez, Claude Anne. Mon Cher Papa: Franklin and the Ladies of Paris. New Haven: Yale University Press, 1990.

Lowell, Delmar R. The Historic Genealogy of the Lowells of America from 1639-1899. Rutland, VT: Tuttle, 1899.

Madsen, Peter and Plunz, Richard. The Urban Lifeworld: Formation Perception Representation. New York: Routledge, 2002.

Maghraoui, Driss, ed. "The mellah without walls Jewish Space in a Moroccan City, Tangier 1860-1912." Revisiting the Colonial Past in Morocco.
    New York: Routledge, 2013.

Maher, Teresa L. "Shawneetown Believes Restoration of Harbor Will Cause City to Boom." Illinois Catholic Historical Review (1918-1929). 9. Chicago:
    Chicago: The Illinois Catholic Historical Society, 1929.

Marckhoff, Fred. "Currency and Banking in Illinois Before 1865." Journal of the Illinois State Historical Society. 52: no. 3.
    Springfield, IL: Illinois State Historical Society, Autumn 1959.

"Marriage of Dr. Mary J. Safford." Cairo Daily Bulletin. Cairo, IL: Oberly, 1 Oct 1872.

"Marriage Records." "Illinois, Cook County, Marriages, 1871-1920." Springfield, IL: Illinois Department of Public Health Records, Division of Vital Records, #1030079.

"Marriages solemnized in 1884 and for which certificates have been filed." Annual Report of the Receipts and Expenditures Town of Hyde Park.
    Hyde Park, MA: Press of the Hyde Park Times, 1884.

"Married." Cairo Evening Bulletin, Daily Edition. Cairo, IL: Oberly & Co., 17 Aug 1869.

Marsh, George Perkins and Lucia Ducci. George P. Marsh Correspondence: Images of Italy, 1861-1881. Madison, NJ: Fairleigh Dickinson University Press, 2012.

Marshall-Cornwall, James. Grant as Military Commander. 1970. New York: Barnes & Noble Books, 1995.

Martin, C. Brenden. Tourism in the Mountain South: A Double-Edged Sword. Knoxville: University of Tennessee Press, 2007.

Massachusetts Death Index, 1901-1980. 70. Dorchester, MA: Registry of Vital Records and Statistics.

"Massachusetts Homoeopathic Hospital." Publications of the Massachusetts Homoeopathic Medical Society. 7. Boston: Homoeopathic Medical Society, Franklin Press, 1885.

Matile, Roger. "Was Dr. Conrad Will Really Worth His Salt?" Ledger-Sentinel. Oswego, IL: Farren, 22 Jun 2006.

Matteson, Frederick W. listing. Registers of Deaths of Volunteers, Compiled 1861-1865. Adjutant General's Office Records, 1780s-1917. Record group 94.
    Washington, DC: NARA.

McCaul, Edward B. To Retain Command of the Mississippi: The Civil War Naval Campaign for Memphis. Knoxville: University of Tennessee Press, 2014.

McClintock, James H. Arizona: Prehistoric—Aboriginal, Pioneer—Modern. 2. Chicago: S. J. Clarke, 1916.

McDowell, Katherine Sherwood Bonner. Dr. Anne Gowdy, ed. A Sherwood Bonner Sampler, 1869-1884. Knoxville: University of Tennessee Press, 2000.

McMullin, Thomas A., and Walker, David Allan. Biographical Directory of American Territorial Governors. Westport, CT: Meckler Publishing, 1984.

McParland, Robert. Charles Dickens' American Audience. Lanham, MD: Lexington Books, 2010.

McPherson, Edward. The Political History of the United States of America, During the Great Rebellion. 4th ed. Washington, DC: James J. Chapman, 1882.

McShane, Clay and Tarr, Joel A. The Horse in the City. Baltimore: The Johns Hopkins University Press, 2007.

"Medical View of the Chicago Fire." Homeopathic World. 6. London: Jarrold and Sons, 1 Dec 1871.

Meek, Fielding Bradford and Gabb, William More. Paleontology. 1. Sacramento: Legislature of California, 1864.

Member Listing. Transactions of the Forty-First Session of the American Institute of Homoeopathy. Philadelphia: AIH, 1889.

"Memorial of James Barnard Blake Late Mayor of the City of Worcester, Mass." Worcester, MA: Snow Brothers, 1871.

"Memorial to Carl Braun." The American Journal of Obstetrics and Diseases of Women and Children. 24: no. 6. New York: W. A. Townsend & Adams, Jun 1891.

Metropolitan Museum of Art. "19th Century America Paintings and Sculpture." Exhibit Catalog. New York: Metropolitan Museum of Art, 1970.

Michelet, Maren. Glimpses from Agnes Mathilde Wergeland's Life. Minneapolis, MN: Folkebladet Publishing, 1916.

Minutes of the Trustees of the Internal Improvement Fund of the State of Florida. 10. Tallahassee: J. Stuart Lewis, 1915.

"Miss Dr. Mary J. Safford." Cairo Daily Bulletin. Cairo, IL: Oberly, 18 Jul 1872.

Molloy, Johnny. The Land Between the Lakes National Recreation Area Handbook. Birmingham, AL: Menasha Ridge Press, 2003.

"Moral Education Association." Boston Post. Boston: Beals & Green, 2 Jun 1876.

Morris, Roy, Jr. *Lighting Out for the Territory: How Samuel Clemens Headed West and Became Mark Twain.* New York: Simon & Schuster, 2010.

Mountain, Carol. *Tarpon Springs.* Charleston: Arcadia Publishing, 2012.

"Murder by the Indians." *Sacramento Daily Union.* 3: no.404. Sacramento: E. G. Jefferis, 8 Jul 1852.

Musee Calvet @www.musee-calvert-avignon.com/.

Myrick, David F. and Angel, Myron. *Thompson & West's History of Nevada, 1881.* Oakland, CA: Thompson & West, 1881.

Napheys, George H. M.D. *Physical Life of Woman: Advice to the Maiden, Wife, and Mother.* Philadelphia: George Maclean, 1871.

Neely, Charles and Spargo, John Webster. *Tales and Songs of Southern Illinois. 1938.* Carbondale, IL: Southern Illinois University Press, 1998.

Newberry, J. S. "Events of 1862: The Spring Campaign." *Sanitary Commission No. 96: The U. S. Sanitary Commission in the Valley of the Mississippi, During the War of the Rebellion, 1861-1866.* Cleveland: Fairbanks, Benedict & Co., 1871.

New York Medical College for Women. Fifth Annual Announcement, 1867-1868. New York: Edward O. Jenkins, 1868.

New York Medical College for Women. Sixth Annual Announcement, 1868-1869. New York: Edward O. Jenkins, 1869.

New York Medical College for Women. Seventh Annual Announcement, 1869-1870. New York: Frances & Loutrel, 1869.

"New York Medical College for Women." *New York Times.* New York: Times Co, 24 Mar 1869.

"New York Medical College for Women-Note." *Woman's Advocate* 1: no. 4. New York: Tomlinson, Apr 1869.

News Item untitled. *Arizona Citizen.* 2: no. 12. Tucson, Arizona Territory: Wasson, 30 Dec 1871.

News Item, untitled. *Arizona Citizen.* 8: no. 43. Florence, Arizona Territory: Wasson, 2 Aug 1878.

News Item, untitled. *Arizona Citizen.* 9: no. 9. Florence, Arizona Territory: Wasson, 14 Dec 1878.

News Item, untitled. *Arizona Citizen.* 10: no. 1. Tucson, Arizona Territory: Wasson, 18 Oct 1879.

News Item, untitled. *Daily Alta California.* 30: no. 10407. San Francisco: Gilbert, 9 Oct 1878.

News Item, untitled. *Lowell Daily Citizen and News.* No. 6778. Lowell, MA: Knapp, 8 Mar 1878.

News Item, untitled. *Nunda News.* 16. Nunda, NY: Sanders 14 Apr 1883.

News Item, untitled. *Ottawa Free Trader.* 32: no. 30. Ottawa, IL: Osman & Hapeman, 2 Mar 1872.

News Item, untitled. *Tampa Tribune.* 11 Aug 1887. Online at: http://scholarcommons.usf.edu/cgi/viewcontent.cgi?article=3526&context=flstud_pub.

News Item, untitled. *TJ.* 1: no. 42. Tampa: Cooper, 5 Oct 1887. Online at: http://scholarcommons.usf.edu/cgi/viewcontent.cgi?article=3526&context=flstud_pub.

News Item, untitled. *The Index.* 9: no. 429. Boston: Index Association, 14 Mar 1878.

News Item, untitled. *The Index.* 9: no. 489. Boston: Index Association, 19 Dec 1878.

News Item, untitled, Dr. Mary J. Safford's request for information on offspring of consanguineous marriages for her study. *The Index.* 2. Boston: Free Religious Association, 28 Jul 1881.

News Item, untitled. *The Tarpon.* 1: no. 38. Tarpon Springs: Truax, 18 Aug 1887. Florida State Library.

News Item, untitled. *The Tarpon.* 1: no. 49. Tarpon Springs: Truax, 17 Nov 1887. Florida State Library.

News Item, untitled. *The Weekly Arizona Miner.* 18: no. 28. Prescott: Beach, 8 Jul 1881.

News Item, untitled. *Union Signal.* 17: no. 19. Chicago: Woman's National Christian Temperance Union, 10 May 1883. Frances Willard Memorial Library and Archives, Evanston, IL.

News Item, untitled. *Union Signal.* 17: no. 41. Chicago: Woman's National Christian Temperance Union, 25 Oct 1883. Frances Willard Memorial Library and Archives, Evanston, IL.

News Item, untitled. *West Hillsborough Times.* Clearwater, FL: A. C. Turner. 19 Aug, 1886.

Nightingale, Florence. *Florence Nightingale on Society and Politics, Philosophy, Science Education and Literature.* Waterloo, Ontario: Wilfrid Laurier University, 2003.

Ninth Census of the U.S. 1870, Boston, Ward 16, Suffolk, MA: NARA.

Ninth Census of the U.S. 1870, Worcester, Ward 8, Worcester, MA: NARA.

Nolan, Edward Henry. *The Liberators of Italy: or The Lives of General Garibaldi; Victor Emmanuel, King of Italy: Count Cavour, and Napoleon III, Emperor of the French.* London: J. S. Virtue, 1864.

"Notes and Comments." *The Index.* 5: no. 225. Boston: Index Association, 16 Apr 1874.

"Notes of the Sixty-First Regular Meeting, September 26, 1871." *Journal of the Gynaecological Society of Boston.* 6: no.1. Boston: James Campbell, Jan 1872.

"Notice." *Medical Investigator.* 9: no.107. Chicago: C.S. Halsey, Nov 1872.

"Notice." *New England Medical Gazette.* 9: no. 6. Boston: Otis Clapp & Son, Jun 1874.

"Notice." *Nunda News.* 25: no. 44. Nunda, NY: Sanders, 1 Nov 1884.

"Oak Park Unity Church Dedication." *New Covenant.* 25: no. 31. Chicago: Hanson, 8 Aug 1872.

Obituary, "Gorham Blake Buried." *San Francisco Call.* 83: no. 20. San Francisco: Shortridge, 20 Dec 1897.

Obituary, "Carl Rudolph Braun." *Medical Record.* 39. New York: W. Wood, 2 May 1891.

Obituary, "Dr. Arvilla Britton Haynes." *New England Medical Gazette.* 19: no. 2. Boston: Otis Clapp & Son, Feb 1884.

Obituary, "Dr. Mercy Jackson." *New England Medical Gazette.* 13: no. 1. Boston: Otis Clapp & Son, Jan 1878.

Obituary, "Soledad Safford Martin." *Arizona Citizen.* Tucson. 26 Mar 1931. Arizona Historical Society's newspaper articles scrapbook.

Obituary, "Soledad Safford Martin." *Arizona Historical Review.* 4. Tucson, AZ: University of Arizona, July 1931.

Obituary, "C. P. Putnam." *Harvard Alumni Bulletin.* Boston: Harvard Bulletin, Inc., 1913.

Obituary, "James Jackson Putnam." "News from the Classes." *The Harvard Graduates' Magazine.* 27. Boston: The Harvard Graduates' Magazine Association, 1918-1919.

Obituary, "Johann Ritter von Oppolzer." *Medical Times and Register.* 1. Philadelphia: Lippincott & Co., 1 Jun 1871.

Obituary, "Julia Safford." *Cairo City Weekly Gazette.* Cairo, IL: J. A. Hull, 6 Feb 1862.

Obituary, "Marguerite G. Safford." *New York Times.* New York: Times Co, 9 Jan 1880.

Obituary, Dr. Mary J. Safford. "Died in Florida." Newspaper clipping from unknown source, context suggestive of a Cairo paper.
    Safford Family ephemera, Cairo, IL, Public Library.
"Obituary for Dr. Mary J. Safford." Lasell Leaves. Auburndale, MA: Lasell Seminary, Feb 1892.
Obituary, "Dr. Mary J. Safford." New England Medical Gazette, 27, no. 1, Boston: Otis Clapp & Son, Jan 1892.
Obituary, Dr. Mary J. Safford. Report of the Women's Education and Industrial Union for the Year Ending May, 1892. Boston: WEIU, 1892.
Obituary, Dr. Mary J. Safford. "A Notable Family." Bennington Banner. Bennington, VT: Thomas J. Tiffany, 15 Jan 1892.
Obituary, Dr. Mary J. Safford. "Dr. Mary J. Safford." "Deaths Here and Elsewhere." Pittsburg Dispatch. Pittsburgh: Rook O'Neil & Co, 18 Dec 1891.
Obituary, Dr. Mary J. Safford. "Dr. Mary Safford's Career." The Inter Ocean. 20: no. 268. Chicago: Inter-Ocean, 17 Dec 1891.
Obituary, Dr. Mary J. Safford. Death notice. Cairo Citizen. Cairo, IL: Oberly, 19 Dec 1891.
Obituary, "Elizabeth Ingalls Sage." Tarpon Springs Leader. Tarpon Springs, FL: Tarpon Springs Pub Co, 28 Feb 1922.
Obituary, "Elizabeth B. Sammons." Blue Island Sun Standard. Blue Island, IL: John H. Volp, 9 Oct 1924.
    South Suburban Genealogical and Historical Society, Hazel Crest, IL.
Obituary, "W. E. D. Scott." "Notes and News." The Auk. 27: no. 4. Cambridge, MA: American Ornithologists' Union, Oct 1910.
Obituary, "Otto Spiegelberg." The Boston Medical and Surgical Journal. 105: no. 26. Boston: Houghton, Mifflin and Co, 29 Dec 1881.
Obituary, "Israel Tisdale Talbot." Transactions of the Fifty-sixth Session of the American Institute of Homoeopathy. New York: AIH, 1901.
Obituary, "Fidelia Jane Merrick Whitcomb." The Nunda News. 24: no.16. Nunda, NY: Sanders, 7 Apr 1888.
Obituary, Flora Payne-Whitney. "In Youth and Womanhood." New York Times, 6 Feb 1893. Online.
Obituary, "Lydia Safford Wilson." Cambridge Transcript. Cambridge, VT: Brush and Bourn, 13 Feb 1890. Anna Safford Memorabilia Book, Cairo Public Library.
"Of Interest to All Women." The Arrow. Ann Arbor: Pi Beta Phi Fraternity, 1892.
Owens, Dan. California Coiners and Assayers. New York: American Numismatic Society, 2000. Original is in the Francis P. Farquhar Collection,
    Bancroft Library, University of California, Berkeley.
Papers and Letters Presented at the First Woman's Congress of the Association for the Advancement of Woman. 1. New York: Mrs. Wm. Ballard, 1874.
Papers Read at the Fourth Congress of Women. Washington, DC: Association for the Advancement of Women, 1877.
Papers Read Before the Association for the Advancement of Woman 14th Women's Congress. Louisville, Kentucky, October 1886. Atlantic Highland, NJ: AAW, 1887.
Passenger Listing, Bark Kepler, from Sumatra, New York Evening Post. New York. 11 Dec 1850.
"Passenger Lists." Daily Alta California. 37: no. 12506. San Francisco: Gilbert & Co, 12 Jul 1884.
"Passengers Sailed." New York Times. New York: Times Co, 5 Nov 1876.
"Past Officers." Transactions of the American Institute of Homeopathy Sixty-Second Session. Cleveland: AIH Publication Committee, 1906.
Payne-Whitney, Flora. Letters #3852. Courtesy Division of Rare and Manuscript Collections, Carl A. Kroch Library,
    Cornell University, Ithaca, NY, Jan 1863-Nov 1864.
Pent, R. F. History of Tarpon Springs. St. Petersburg: Great Outdoors Publishing, 1964.
"Periscope." The Medical Investigator. 7: no. 4. Chicago: C. S. Halsey, Jan 1870.
Perrin, William Henry. History of Alexander, Union and Pulaski Counties, Illinois. Chicago: O. L. Baskin and Company Historical Publishers, 1883.
"Personal." New England Medical Gazette. 8: no. 1. Boston: Otis Clapp & Son, Jan 1873.
Phelps, Elizabeth Stuart. Letter to the Editor. New England Medical Gazette. 8: no. 1. Boston: Otis Clapp & Son, Jan 1872.
"Plat of the Subdivision of Dr. Mary J. Safford." Old Hillsborough County Deeds. Book K. Clearwater, FL: Pinellas County Clerk of the Circuit Court Office.
Pickard, John B. Letters of John Greenleaf Whittier. 1. Cambridge, MA: President and Fellows of Harvard College, 1975.
"Police Search for Portree Fossil Hunters." Oban Times & West Highland Times. Oban, Argyll, Scotland: Wyvex Media, 22 Nov 2011.
Powell, James Henry. William Denton, the Geologist and Radical: A Biographical Sketch. 4th ed. Boston: Colby & Rich, 1870.
Powers, Hiram. Hiram Powers Papers, 1819-1953. Washington, DC: Smithsonian Institution Archives of American Art.
"Pratt, Sarah Marinda Bates." The Joseph Smith Papers. Church Historian's Press online: josephsmithpapers.org.
"Preceptors." Boston University Year Book. 2. Boston: Houghton, 1875.
"Proceedings of the American Association for the Advancement of Science." AAAS: Twenty-First Meeting. Salem: Permanent Secretary, 1872.
"Proceedings of the American Association for the Advancement of Science." AAAS: Thirty-First Meeting. Salem: Permanent Secretary, 1882.
"Proceedings of the Twenty-Fifth Session of the American Institute of Homoeopathy." Transactions of the Twenty-Fifth Session of the American Institute of Homoeopathy.
    Philadelphia: Sherman & Co, 1872.
Publications of the Massachusetts Homoeopathic Medical Society 1884. 7. Boston: Committee on Publication, 1885.
Quinlan, Kieran. Strange Kin: Ireland and the American South. Baton Rouge, LA: Louisiana State University Press, 2005.
R. M. H. Letter. Weekly Arizona Star. Tucson: Hughes & Fay, 29 Jan 1880.
"Reading for Health." "Books and Authors." The Christian Union. 29: no. 6. New York: New York and Brooklyn Publishing Co, 7 Feb 1884.
"Real Estate Transactions." Daily Alta California. 37: no. 12516. San Francisco: Gilbert & Co, 23 Jul 1884.
Register of Former Students with an Account of the Alumni Association. Cambridge, MA: Massachusetts Institute of Technology, May 1915.
"Register of the Members of the Vieusseux," of the Il Libro dei Soci del Gabinetto Vieusseux Il Marzocco. 6. Dec 1862-Spring 1867, files 218 and 256.
Report extracted from the Mining Index. Gulf Coast Herald. 1: no 8. Tarpon Springs: Camp & Buckner, 26 Jul 1884.
    University of South Florida Special Collections Library, Tampa, FL.
"Report from the Committee on Commitment and Detention of the Insane." Proceedings of the National Conference of Charities and Correction at
    the Seventeenth Annual Session Held in Baltimore, MD, May 14-21, 1890. Boston: Geo. H. Ellis, Isabel C. Barrows, ed., 1890.
Reports Made to the General Assembly of Illinois, at the Twenty-Eighth Session Convened January 8, 1873. 3. Springfield, IL: State Journal Printing Office, 1874.
"Report of Regular Meeting, Monday, Oct. 20, 1873." Bulletin of the Essex Institute. 5: no. 10. Salem, MA: Salem Press, 1874.

"Report of the Illinois Homeopathic Medical Association." *Transactions of the Twenty-Fifth Session of the American Institute of Homeopathy.* Philadelphia: AIH, 1872.

Report of the International Council of Women Assembled by the National Woman Suffrage Association March 25 to April 1, 1888. Washington, DC: National Woman Suffrage Association, 1888.

Report of the Secretary of the Class of 1863 of Harvard College, June 1893 to June 1903. Cambridge, MA: John Wilson and Son, 1903.

"Report of the Social Affairs Committee for the Year Ending May 1892." *Report of the Women's Educational & Industrial Union for the Year Ending May 1892.* Boston: WEIU, 1892. Harvard University Library Open Collections Program, Women Working 1800-1930. WEIU (Boston, Mass), Reports of the WEIU 1892.

Report of the Women's Educational & Industrial Union for the Year Ending May 7, 1879. Boston: WEIU, 1879. Harvard University, Widener Library Collection Development Department.

Report of the Women's Educational & Industrial Union for the Year Ending May 3, 1881. Boston: WEIU, 1881. Harvard University, Widener Library Collection Development Department.

Report of the Women's Educational & Industrial Union for the Year Ending May 1, 1884. Boston: WEIU, 1879. Harvard University, Widener Library Collection Development Department.

Report of the Women's Education & Industrial Union for the Year Ending May 1894. Boston: WEIU, 1894. Harvard University, Widener Library Collection Development Department.

"Report on the Women's Congress." *Annual Report of the Association for the Advancement of Women.* Boston: Cochrane & Sampson, 1881.

"Resident Members." *Proceedings of the California Academy of Natural Sciences.* 2-1858-1862. San Francisco: Town & Bacon, 1863.

Reynolds, John. *The Pioneer History of Illinois.* Chicago: Fergus Printing Co, 1887.

Rhodes, Albert. *Jerusalem As It Is.* London: John Maxwell and Co, 1865.

Richardson, Albert Deane. *A Personal History of Ulysses S. Grant.* Hartford, CT: American Publishing Co, 1868.

Richardson, Albert Deane. *The Secret Service, the Field, the Dungeon, and the Escape.* Hartford, CT: American Publishing Co, 1864.

Richardson, Benjamin Ward, MD. *Hygeia: A City of Health.* London: MacMillan, 1876.

Richardson, John. *The Annals of London: A Year by Year Record of a Thousand Years of History.* Berkeley: University of California Press, 2000.

Ripley, Martha, MD. "Some Overlooked Causes of Disease in Children." *Transactions of the Forty-Fifth Session of the American Institute of Homoeopathy.* Philadelphia: Sherman, 1892.

Robinson, Sarah. *Genealogical History of the Families of Robinsons, Saffords, Harwoods, and Clarks.* Bennington, VT: 1837.

Rooks, Sandra W. and Mountain, Carol. *Tarpon Springs, Florida.* Charleston: Black America Series, Arcadia Publishing 2003.

Rummel, Edward. *The Illinois Hand-book of Information for the Year 1870.* Springfield, IL: Hudson, 1870.

Russler, Fern I. "A Museum's Life-Story." *Daily Illini.* 56: no. 131. Champaign-Urbana: University of Illinois, 13 Feb 1927.

Ryan, Jeffrey R. *Pandemic Influenza: Emergency Planning and Community Preparedness.* Boca Raton: CRC Press, 2009.

Safford, Alfred B. and Julia Massey, marriage announcement, Joliet Signal, last published 25 Apr 1854, http://files.usgwarchives.net/il/will/vitals/marriages/1849mar.txt.

Safford, Alfred B. and Anna Candee, marriage record. Alexander County, IL, Court Record Microfilms no. 0961420-0961425, 7 Apr 1863.

Safford, Anna. "Memorabilia Book." Assembled letters, obituaries and newspaper clippings relating to Safford family members, some items of unknown origin and date, in a handmade scrapbook. Cairo, IL, Public Library.

Safford, Anna E. "Letter to Mary Ann Bickerdyke." circa 1897. Topeka: Kansas State Historical Society Library and Archives.

APKS. *Sketch of the Life of Gov. A. P. K. Safford.* California Manuscripts, Bancroft Library, University of California, Berkeley, 1872.

APKS. "Last Will and Testament Safford, Anson P. K." Hernando County, Florida, Book A, 157, Book 1, 40-48. Citrus County Will Book Index, 15.

APKS. *Handwritten Biography of Margarita Safford.* Available through the courtesy of Dr. Frank Dunton and Mr. Charles Dunton, recipients of Margarita (daughter) Safford's belongings at her death.

APKS. "Letter to Sam Hughes." 31 Dec 1888. Tucson: Arizona Historical Society Charles R. Drake Papers.

APKS. To Sam Hughes in Arizona Territory. 16 Dec 1890. Arizona Daily Citizen. 19: no. 307. Tucson: Citizen Print & Publishing Co, 16 Dec 1890. Arizona Historical Society.

Safford, Dr. Mary. "Extracts from a Letter of Dr. Mary Safford, in Vienna, Austria." *The Medical Investigator.* 7 no. 5. Chicago: C. S. Halsey, Feb 1870.

Safford, Dr. Mary J. "Nervous Prostration." *The Union Signal.* 17: no. 20. Chicago: Woman's National Christian Temperance Union, 17 May 1883. Evanston, IL: Frances Willard Memorial Library and Archives.

Safford, Dr. Mary J. "Personal and News Items." *The New England Medical Gazette.* 18: no. 4. Boston: Otis Clapp & Son, Apr 1883.

Safford, Dr. Mary J. "Physiological Effects of Alcoholic Beverages." "Health Talks." 17: no. 10. Union Signal Chicago: Woman's National Christian Temperance Union, 8 Mar 1883.

Safford, Edward Stanley, *Saffords in America,* Library of Congress typescript, 1923.

Safford, Frank Alfred. "Death Notice." Arizona Citizen. 1: no. 48. Tucson: J. Wasson, 9 Sep 1871.

MJS. "A Visit to a Harem." *Woman's Advocate.* 1: no. 1. Philadelphia: William P. Tomlinson, Jan 1869.

MJS. "An Evening at a German Professor's." *The Woman's Advocate.* 1: no. 6. New York: William P. Tomlinson, Jun 1869.

MJS. "An Extraordinary Case of Constipation." *The New England Medical Gazette.* 19: no. 2. Boston: Otis Clapp & Son, Feb 1884.

MJS. "Artificial Alimentation." *The New England Medical Gazette.* 15: no. 4. Boston: Otis Clapp & Son, Apr 1880.

MJS. "Case of Ovariotomy By Prof. Freund, of Breslau, as submitted on behalf of Dr. A. L. Norris of East Cambridge, Massachusetts, at the January 2, 1872, meeting of the Gynecological Society of Boston." *Proceedings of the Gynaecological Society of Boston,* 7: no. 7. Boston: James Campbell, Jul 1872.

MJS. "Complete Inversion of the Uterus." *New England Medical Gazette.* 8: no. 5. Boston: Otis Clapp & Son, May 1873.

MJS. "Concerning European Medical Universities." *The Medical Investigator.* 9: no. 101. Chicago: C. S. Halsey, May 1872.

MJS. "Correspondence." *The Medical Investigator.* 7: no. 8. Chicago: C. S. Halsey, May 1870.

MJS. "Dear Brother." Boston, 18 Nov 1881. Available through the courtesy of Dr. Frank Dunton and Mr. Charles Dunton, recipients of Margarita (daughter)
        Safford's belongings at her death.
MJS. "European Correspondence-No. 3." New Covenant. 15: no. 48, Chicago: Livermore, 30 Sep 1862.
MJS. "European Correspondence." New Covenant. Chicago: Livermore, Damascus (Syria) 5 Oct 1863. From reprint in Humboldt Register.
        Unionville, Nevada Territory, 18 Jun 1864.
MJS. "European Correspondence." New Covenant. Chicago: Livermore, Beyroot and Damascus 28 Nov 1863. From reprint in Humboldt Register.
        Unionville, Nevada Territory, 11 Jun 1864.
MJS. "European Correspondence-No. 53: Letter from Miss Mary J. Safford, Antwerp July 8, 1864." New Covenant. 18: no. 1, Chicago: Livermore, 7 Jan 1864.
MJS and Allen, Mary E. Health and Strength for Girls. Boston: Lothrop, 1884.
MJS. "How a Daughter Was Educated." Herald of Health. 23: no. 5. New York: Wood and Holbrook, May 1874.
MJS. "How They Treat American Women Medical Students in Germany—A Lesson For Bellevue—A letter from Dr. Mary Safford."
        16 Tauenzien Strasse, Breslen, Germany, 30 Jul 1871. Herald of Health. 18: 3. New York: Wood and Holbrook, Sep 1871.
MJS. "Lacerated Cervix." New England Medical Gazette. 16: no. 10. Boston: Otis Clapp & Son, Oct 1881.
MJS. "Last Will and Testament." Signed and witnessed in Boston, Massachusetts, 20 Jun 1884. Proven in Suffolk County, MA, 11 Jan 1892.
        Tarpon Springs, FL: TSAHS Archives.
MJS. "Letter." Anti-Slavery Standard. 29: no. 50. New York: American Anti-Slavery Society, 17 Apr 1869.
MJS. "Letter from Austria." New Covenant. 24: no 5. Chicago: Hanson, 4 Feb 1871.
MJS. "Letter from Germany." New Covenant. 24: no. 21. Chicago: Hanson, 27 May 1871.
MJS. "Letter from Mary Safford." Vienna, 12 Jun 1870. The Herald of Health. 16: no. 3. New York: Wood & Holbrook, Sep 1870.
MJS. "Letter from Vienna." New England Medical Gazette. 6: no. 1. Boston: S. Whitney, MD, Jan 1871.
MJS. "Letter from Vienna—The Skoda Ovation." New England Medical Gazette. 6. Boston: S. Whitney, MD, May and June 1871.
MJS. "Letter to the Herald." Gulf Coast Herald. 1: no. 18. Tarpon Springs: Camp & Buckner, 1 Nov 1884.
MJS. "Ornament and Dress." Herald of Health. 21: no. 1, 3, 6. New York: Wood and Holbrook, Jan, Mar and Jun 1873.
MJS. "Protest Against Pepper. Soups and Their Value." Woman Suffrage Cookbook. Boston: Hattie A. Burr, 1886.
MJS. "Pruritis." The New England Medical Gazette. 8: no.5. Boston: Otis Clapp & Son, May 1873.
MJS. "Remembrances of Moscow." The Woman's Advocate. 1: no. 2. New York: William P. Tomlinson, Feb 1869.
MJS. "Sights in Vienna." The Revolution. 4: no. 8. Rochester, New York: Susan B. Anthony, 25 Aug 1870.
MJS. "Sure Test of Death." Brisbane Australia Courier. Brisbane, Australia, quoted in Boston Transcript 14 Jun 1873.
MJS. "The Effects of Stimulants and Narcotics Upon the Health and Morals of Women."
        Papers Read Before the Association for the Advancement of Women 14th Women's Congress. Atlantic Highlands: AAW, 1887.
MJS. The United States Cremation Company, Opinions on Cremation. New York: New York Cremation Society, 1889.
MJS. "To Clara Barton." 6 Mar 1870. Barton Papers. Library of Congress, Manuscript Division.
MJS. "To Dr. Mary Holywell Everett," 11 Mar 1881 Boston. Everett Family Papers. Chicago: Newberry Library.
MJS. "To Caroline Crane Marsh." 10 Apr 1867. George Perkins Marsh Collection. Burlington, VT: University of Vermont Library Special Collections.
MJS. "To George Perkins Marsh." 30 Dec 1865. George Perkins Marsh Collection. Burlington, VT: University of Vermont Library Special Collections.
MJS. "To Mr. & Mrs. George Perkins Marsh." 7 Oct 1869. George Perkins Marsh Collection. Burlington, VT: University of Vermont Library Special Collections.
MJS. "To George Perkins Marsh." 30 Oct 1869. George Perkins Marsh Collection. Burlington, VT: University of Vermont Library Special Collections.
MJS. "To Frank Moore." 28 Dec 1866 Cairo, Illinois. American Historical Manuscripts Collection-Safford, Mary Jane.
        New York: New York Historical Society Manuscripts.
MJS. "To James Jackson Putnam." 16 Apr 1871. Cambridge, Massachusetts: Harvard University, MS/c 4.2,
        Francis A. Countway Library of Medicine's Women in Medicine Collection.
MJS. "To Caroline Severance." 14 Jul 1876. Caroline M. Seymour Severance Collection. San Marino, CA: Huntington Library.
MJS. "To Caroline Severance." 14 Mar 1885. Caroline M. Seymour Severance Collection. San Marino, CA: Huntington Library.
MJS. Untitled item regarding her medical school graduation. Cairo Evening Bulletin. Cairo, IL: Oberly, 27 Mar 1869.
Safford, Miss. "Indications for Ovariotomy." Proceedings of the Gynaecological Society of Boston. 7: no. 7. Boston: James Campbell, Jul 1872.
Safford-Blake, Mary I. (sic). "Lac Defloratum." North American Journal of Homoeopathy. 4: no. 4. New York: Boericke & Tafel, May 1874.
MJSB. "A Glimpse of California." The Woman's Journal. 6: no. 38. Boston: 18 Sep 1875.
MJSB. "A New Dress for Women." Science of Health. New York: Samuel Robert Wells, 1 Mar 1875.
MJSB. "A Supposed Uterine Tumor." The United States Medical Investigator. 6: no. 5. Chicago: United States Medical Investigator Press, 1 Sep 1877.
MJSB. "A Visit to Cornell University." Woman's Journal. 5: no. 50. Boston: 12 Dec 1874.
MJSB. "A Visit to Dr. Harriet K. Hunt." Woman's Journal. 2. Boston: Julia Ward Howe, 23 Nov 1872.
MJSB. "Annie Conway Damer." Woman's Journal. 6: no. 17. Boston: 24 Apr 1875. Republished by American Antiquarian Society.
MJSB. "Boston News." The Medical Investigator. 11: no. 121. Chicago: C. S. Halsey, Jan 1874.
MJSB. "Circulate the Paper." Woman's Journal. 6: no. 39. Boston: 25 Sep1875.
MJSB. "Etiquette and Custom." The New Age. 1: no. 30. Boston: 27 May 1876.
MJSB. "Glastonbury Criticized." Woman's Journal. 5: no. 17. Boston: 25 Apr 1874.
MJSB. "Hopeful Things." Woman's Journal. 5: no. 48. Boston: 28 Nov 1874.
MJSB. "How the Mighty Have Fallen!" New Age. 1: no. 35. Boston: 1 Jul 1876.

MJSB. "Inversion of the Uterus." Transactions of the Twenty-Sixth Session of the American Institute of Homoeopathy Held in Cleveland, Ohio, June 3-6, 1873. Philadelphia: Sherman, 1873.

MJSB. "Prenatal Influence." Herald of Health. 25: no. 1. New York: Wood and Holbrook, Jan 1875.

MJSB. "Pre-Natal Influence, An Essay Read to the Second Radical Club, Boston, March 8, 1875, by Dr. Mary J. Safford-Blake." The Index. 6: no. 274. Boston: Index Association, 25 Mar 1875.

MJSB. "Reminiscences of German Hospitals." The New England Medical Gazette. 9: no.5. Boston: Otis Clapp & Son, May 1874.

MJSB. "The Etiology and Infectiousness of Puerperal Fever." Transactions of the Twenty-Seventh Session of the American Institute of Homoeopathy. Philadelphia: Sherman & Co, 1875.

MJSB. "The Ideal Sunday School." The Index. 8. Boston: Index Association, 23 Aug 1877.

MJSB. quoted on undergarment design in Science of Health (Mar 1875). The Evening Post. 74. New York: William C. Bryant & Co, 26 Feb 1875.

MJSB. "W. C. and L. L. A." Cairo Bulletin. 9: no. 116. Cairo, IL: Oberly, 13 May 1877.

MJSB. "What Ladies Should Wear." The Health Reformer. 9: no. 7. Battle Creek, MI: J. H. Kellogg, Jul 1874.

MJSB. "Women in Utah—Letter from Dr. Mary Safford-Blake" Woman's Journal. 6: no. 33. Boston: 14 Aug 1875.

Sage, Elizabeth Ingalls. Death Certificate. Florida Bureau of Vital Statistics File No. 1979.

Sajous, Charles E., M. D. ed. "Reasons Why Far-sighted Investors are Purchasing Lots in Tarpon Springs," Annual of the Universal Medical Sciences. 5. Philadelphia: F. A. Davis, 1891.

Sajous, Charles, M.D. Sajous' Analytical Cyclopaedia of Practical Medicine. 3rd revised ed. 4. Philadelphia: F. A. Davis Co, 1906.

Sammons, Elizabeth B. "Mary J. Safford, MD." To-Day. 1:6, Philadelphia: Bisbee & Whitcomb, Jun 1896.

Sargent, Mary Elizabeth Fiske, ed. Sketches and Reminiscences of the Radical Club of Chestnut Street, Boston. Boston: James R. Osgood and Co, 1880.

Sarti, Roland. Italy: A Reference Guide from the Renaissance to the Present. New York: Facts On File, 2004.

Schnur, James Anthony. "Springing into Action by the Bayou: The Boyer Family and Tarpon Springs During Florida's Gilded Age." Punta Pinal. 33. Seminole, FL: Pinellas County Historical Society, Fall 2006.

"School of All Sciences." Boston University Year Book. 2. Boston: Houghton, 1875.

Schweikart, Larry. A History of Banking in Arizona. Tucson: University of Arizona Press, 1982.

Scott, William Earl Dodge. The Story of a Bird Lover. New York: MacMillan, 1904. Reprint by Bibliolife.

Scrivener, Laurie and Barnes, J. Suzanne. A Biographical Dictionary of Women Healers. Westport, CT: Oryx Press, 2002.

Semmelweis, Ignaz. Carter, K. Codell, translator. The Etiology, Concept, and Prophylaxis of Childbed Fever. 1860. Madison, WI: University of Wisconsin Press, 1983.

Seventh Census of the U.S., 1850, Crete, Will County, IL. NARA.

Seventh Census of the U.S., 1850, Manchester, Hillsborough County, NH. NARA.

Seventh Census of the U.S., 1850, Newton, Middlesex, MA. NARA.

Sewell, Alfred L. The Great Calamity: Scenes, Incidents and Lessons of the Great Chicago Fire of the 8th and 9th of October 1871. Chicago: Alfred L. Sewell, 1871.

Shalley-Jensen, Michael. Encyclopedia of Contemporary American Social Issues. Santa Barbara: ABC-CLIO, LLC, 2011.

Sheahan, James Washington and Upton, George Putnam. The Great Conflagration. Chicago: Its Past Present and Future. Chicago: Union Publishing Co, 1871.

Shearer, Benjamin F. Home Front Heroes: A Biographical Dictionary of Americans During Wartime. 3. Westport, CT: Greenwood Press, 2007.

Shepheards Hotel History: www.shepheard-hotel.com/history.html.

Sheridan, Thomas E. Los Tucsonenses: The Mexican Community in Tucson, 1854-1941. Tucson, AZ: University of Arizona Press, 1986.

Sherman, Irwin W. The Malaria Genome Projects. London: Imperial College Press, 2012.

Shindler, Robert. From the Usher's Desk to the Tabernacle Pulpit: The Life and Labours of Pastor C. H. Spurgeon. London: Alabaster, Passmore and Sons, 1897.

Silcox, Harry C. A Place to Live and Work: The Henry Disston Saw Works and the Tacony Community of Philadelphia. University Park: Pennsylvania State University Press, 1994.

Simon, John Y., ed. The Papers of Ulysses S. Grant: April–September 1861. Carbondale, IL: Southern Illinois University Press, 1967.

Simon, John Y., ed. The Papers of Ulysses S. Grant: January 8-March 31, 1862. 1973. Carbondale, IL: Southern Illinois University Press, 1991.

Simon, John Y., ed. The Papers of Ulysses S. Grant: April 1-August 31, 1862. 1973. Carbondale, IL: Southern Illinois University Press, 1991.

Simon, John Y., ed. The Papers of Ulysses S. Grant, January 1-September 30,1867. 1973. Carbondale, IL: Southern Illinois University Press, 1991.

Simon, Linda. William James Remembered. Lincoln, NE: University of Nebraska Press, 1996.

"Sixth Annual Commencement of the Boston University School of Medicine." New England Medical Gazette. 14: no. 4. Boston: Otis Clapp & Son, April 1879.

Sixth Census of the U. S., 1840, Thorn Creek Precinct, Will County, IL. NARA.

"Sixty-eighth Regular (Annual) Meeting, January 2, 1872." Proceedings of the Gynaecological Society of Boston. 7: no.7. Boston: James Campbell, July 1872.

Skrabec, Quentin, R., Jr. The 100 Most Significant Events in American Business. Santa Barbara: ABC-CLIO, 2012.

S. L. Correspondence. The Medical Investigator. 7: no. 5. Chicago, C. S. Halsey, Feb 1870.

Smith, George Washington. A History of Southern Illinois. 1. Chicago: Lewis, 1912.

Smith, Stephen, M. D. and Sanborn, F. B. "State Legislation for the Insane." Proceedings of the National Conference of Charities and Correction at the Sixteenth Annual Session Held in San Francisco, Cal., September 11-18, 1889. Boston: Geo. H. Ellis, Isabel C. Barrows, ed., 1889.

Society of Homeopaths website: www.homeopathy-soh.org/research/research-and-the-society/provings/

Society for Psychical Research website: www.spr.ac.uk/page/history-society-psychical-research-parapsychology

Souvenir Nineteenth Annual Congress of the Association for the Advancement of Woman. Washington, DC: Todd Brothers, 1877.

Souvenir of Settlement and Progress Will County, Ill. Chicago: Chicago Directory Publishing Co, 1884.

Squier, Effie J. "Sojourner Truth, New York." The Christian at Work. New York: H. W. Adams, 28 Sep 1882.

"Special Notice." Real Estate Record and Builder's Guide. 28: no. 717. New York: Real Estate Record Association, 10 Dec 1881.

"Special Notices." Woman's Journal. 5: no. 10. Boston: Julia Ward Howe, 7 Mar 1874..

"Specimens of Silver from Nevada." Cairo Evening Bulletin, Daily Edition. Cairo, IL: Oberly, 11 Jun 1869.

Sprague, Julia A. "New England Women's Club." The Woman's Journal. 11. Boston: 26 Jun 1880.

Stahnisch, F. "Graefe, Friedrich Wilhelm Albrecht von (1828-1870)." Dictionary of Medical Biography. 2. Westport, CT: Greenwood Press, 2007.

"Standing Committee Members." "Committee on Climatology." Publications of the Massachusetts Homoeopathic Medical Society 1886. 9.
    Boston: Committee on Publication, 1887.

Stanton, Andrea L., Ramsamy, Edward, Seybolt, Peter J., Elliott, Carolyn M. Cultural Sociology of the Middle East, Asia, and Africa: An Encyclopedia. 1.
    Los Angeles: Sage Publications, 2012.

Stanton, Elizabeth Cady, Anthony, Susan B. and Gage, Matilda Joslyn, ed. History of Woman Suffrage. 3--1876-1885. Rochester, NY: Susan B. Anthony, 1886.

"State Banks of Issue in Illinois." The Bankers' Magazine. 57. New York: Bradford Rhodes & Co., Jul-Dec 1898.

"State Natural History." Prairie Farmer. 4. no. 2. Chicago: Union Agricultural Society, 14 Jul 1859.

Sterling, Albert Mack and Sterling, Edward Baker. The Sterling Genealogy. New York: Grafton Press, 1909.

Stern, Madeleine B. So Much in a Lifetime: The Story of Dr. Isabel Barrows. New York: Messner, 1964.

Stevens, William Wallace. Past and Present of Will County, Illinois. 1. Chicago: S. J. Clarke Publishing Co, 1907.

Stewart, William Morris and Brown, George Rothwell, ed. Reminiscences of Senator William M. Stewart, of Nevada. New York: Neale Publishing, 1908.

Stoughton, Gertrude. Tarpon Springs Florida—The Early Years. 2 ed. Tarpon Springs, FL: TSAHS, 1975.

Straub, W. L. History of Pinellas County, Florida. St. Augustine, FL: The Record Co, 1929.

Straus, Terry. Indians of the Chicago Area. Chicago: NAES College, 1989.

"Suburban Short Notes." Boston Post. Boston: Beals & Greene, 14 Nov 1879.

Sullivan, John, M.D. "The Roman Fever." The Medical Times and Gazette. no.1. London: J & A. Churchill, 12 Jan 1878.

Swanberg, W. A. Whitney Father, Whitney Heiress. New York: Charles Scribner's Sons, 1980.

Swift, Henry Walton. "Edward A. Hunting & Another, trustees, vs. Gladys Safford." Massachusetts Reports,
    Cases Argued and Determined in the Supreme Judicial Court of Massachusetts. 183. Boston: Little, Brown & Co, 1904.

Tangier American Legation Institute for Moroccan (TALIM) Studies director's blog @ www.talimblog.org/2012/03/consul-mcmaths-sentence-to-tangier.html.

"Tarpon Springs" and "Physicians." Florida State Gazetteer and Business Directory. New York: South Publishing Co., 1886.

"Tarpon Springs, Florida: The Gem of the Gulf Coast: Health, Pleasure & Comfort: Homes for All."
    Ann Arbor: University of Michigan, William L. Clements Library, 1884.

"Tarpon Topics." Gulf Coast Herald. 1: no. 15. Tarpon Springs: Camp and Buckner, 27 Sep 1884.

"Tarpon Topics." Gulf Coast Herald. 1: no. 18. Tarpon Springs: Camp and Buckner, 1 Nov 1884.

"Tarpon Topics." Gulf Coast Herald. 1: no. 20. Tarpon Springs: Camp and Buckner, 15 Nov 1884.

Taylor, Joshua C. The Fine Arts in America. Chicago: University of Chicago Press, 1979.

Tenth Report of the Board of Trustees of the Illinois Industrial University. Springfield, IL: H. W. Bokker, 1881.

Tenth Census of the U. S., 1880, Boston, Suffolk County, MA. NARA.

Tenth Census of the U. S., 1880, Wrentham, Norfolk County, MA. NARA.

"The American Froebel Union." Kindergarten Messenger. 1: no. 9. Cambridge, MA: Elizabeth P. Peabody, Sep 1877.

"The Boston Anniversaries." New York Daily Tribune. New York: Greely & McElrath, 1 Jun 1877.

"The Boston Directory." Boston: Sampson & Murdock, 1872.

"The Boston University." New England Medical Gazette. 8: no.2. Boston: Otis Clapp & Son, Feb 1873.

"The Committee on Medical Legislation." The Homoeopathic World. 16. London: Homoeopathic Publishing Co, 1 Oct 1881.

"The Consumptive Home." "Public Documents of Massachusetts." 3: no. 17. Appendix to the Secretary's Report. Boston: Secretary of the Commonwealth, 1874.

"The Dress Reform Lectures." New England Medical Gazette. 9: no.5. Boston: Otis Clapp & Son, May 1874.

"The Dress Reform Meeting in Boston." Frank Leslie's Illustrated Newspaper. 38: no. 977. New York: Frank Leslie, 20 Jun 1874.

"The Dress Reformers. How the Boston Women Propose to Regenerate Their Sex." New York Times. New York: Times Co, 15 Jun 1874.

"The Essex Institute." Bulletin of the Essex Institute. 5: no. 1. Salem, MA: Salem Press, Jan 1873.

"The Folly of Fashion." Terre Haute Daily Gazette. Terre Haute, IN: Hudson & Rose, 29 Feb 1872.

"The Hotels, Who are at Them, and Where They Came From." Ashville Daily Citizen. 7: no. 142. Asheville, NC: Cameron, Tuesday Evening Edition, 20 Oct 1891.

"The marriage record of Sammons, Walter W., and Pond, Elizabeth B." (1892) University of South Florida: Florida Studies Center Publications,
    Paper 1620 online: http://scholarcommons.usf.edu/flstud_pub/1620

"The Mining Wealth of Arizona." The Weekly Arizona Miner. 16: no. 39. Prescott: Beach, 18 Sep 1879.

The National Cyclopaedia of American Biography. 5. Entry for Richardson, Abby Sage. New York: James T. White & Co., 1891.

"The Prayer Gauge." New York World. New York: Manton, 22 Nov 1872.

The Richardson-McFarland Tragedy: Containing All the Letters and Other Interesting Facts and Documents Not Before Published. Philadelphia: Barclay & Co, 1870.

"The Utah Theocracy." The New York Herald. No. 14,879. New York: James Gordon Bennett, 18 May 1877.

"The Woman's Congress." The Unitarian Review and Religious Magazine," 14: no. 5. Boston: Office of the Unitarian Review, Nov 1880.

"The Women's Congress in Chicago." The Daily Graphic, 2nd ed. New York: Graphic Co, 21 Oct 1874.

"The Woman's Congress Chicago, October 15." New York Tribune. 34: no. 10. New York: New York Tribune, 16 Oct 1874.

Thomas, M. Louise. Centenary Voices or, A Part of the Work of the Women of the Universalist Church from its Centenary Year to the Present Time.
    Philadelphia: Women's Centenary Association, 1886.

"Tilghman's Sand Blast: Patented Oct. 8, 1870." Boston: Rand Avery & Co, 1874.

"Transactions of Societies: Society for Promoting the Welfare of the Insane." The Medico-legal Journal. 3. New York: Medical-legal Journal Association, 1885.

Transactions of the New England Cremation Society 1893. 2. Boston: New England Cremation Society, 1894.

Transactions of the Twenty-Sixth Session of the American Institute of Homoeopathy Held in Cleveland, Ohio, June 3-6, 1873. Philadelphia: Sherman, 1873.

"Transactions of the Twenty-Seventh Session of the American Institute of Homoeopathy, held at Niagara Falls, June 9th to 12th, 1874."
    Book review in The North American Journal of Homeopathy. 24 (new series, 6). New York: Boericke & Tafel, 1875.

Transactions of the World's Congress of Homeopathic Physicians and Surgeons. Philadelphia: AIH, 1894.

"Travels in the East." Sacramento Daily Union. 2: no. 26. Sacramento: E. G. Jefferis & Co, 22 Mar 1876.

Triebold, Carol and Monks, Phyllis. Crete Remembered. 1. Chicago: Solution Graphics, 2003.

Triebold, Carol and Monks, Phyllis. Crete Remembered. 2. Chicago: Solution Graphics, 2004.

Trollope, Anthony. North America. II Leipzig: Bernhard Tauchnitz, 1862.

Truax, George A. "A Tribute." The Truth. Tarpon Springs: George Truax, 12 Dec 1891.

Tselos, George D. and Wickey, Colleen. A Guide to Archives and Manuscript Collections in the History of Chemistry and Chemical Technology.
    Philadelphia: Center for History of Chemistry, 1987.

Tucker, Spencer C. The Civil War Naval Encyclopedia. Santa Barbara: ABC-CLIO, 2011.

Tuckerman, Henry Theodore. Book of the Artists: American Artist Life. New York: G. P. Putnam & Sons, 1867.

Turner, John G. Brigham Young: Pioneer Prophet. Cambridge: Harvard University Press, 2012.

Twelfth Census of the United States, 1900, Sycamore Township, DeKalb, IL, Waterman Hall School. NARA.

Ullman, Dana. The Homeopathic Revolution: Why Famous People and Cultural Heroes Choose Homeopathy. Berkeley, CA: North Atlantic Books, 2007.

"United States Ministers and Ambassadors to France." The World Almanac and Encyclopedia. New York: Press Publishing Company, 1911.

University Council, ed. Boston University Yearbook. 1. Boston: Houghton, 1874.

University of Chicago. "Second Annual Catalogue of the University of Chicago, Officers and Students for the Academic Year 1860-1861."
    Chicago: Church, Goodman & Cushing, 1861.

"University of Florida at Tarpon Springs." Newark, Delaware: University of Delaware Special Collections Library, Dr. Charles Sajous Papers (MS253), 29 May 1890.

Urquart, David. The Pillars of Hercules, Or, a Narrative of Travels in Spain and Morocco in 1848. 2. New York: Harper & Brothers, 1855.

U. S. Bureau of Education Bulletin. "History of Public School Education in Arizona." no. 17, Washington, DC: Government Printing Office, 1918.

U.S. Centers for Disease control website: www.cdc.gov/malaria/about/faqs.html "If I get malaria, will I have it for the rest of my life?"

U.S. National Library of Medicine at National Institutes of Health. "Wilhelm von Waldeyer-Hartz (1836-1921): an Anatomist Who Left His Mark."
    website: www.ncbi.nim.gov/pubmed/17072873

Usry, Glen and Keener, Craig S. Black Man's Religion, Can Christianity be Afrocentric? Downer's Grove, IL: InterVarsity Press, 1996.

Van Bibber, W. C., M. D. "Peninsular and Sub-Peninsular Air and Climates." Journal of the American Medical Association. 4: no. 20. Chicago:
    American Medical Association, 16 May 1885.

Van Tassel, David Dirck and Vacha, John. Beyond Bayonets: The Civil War in Northern Ohio. Kent, OH: Kent State University Press, 2006.

Van Wagoner, Richard A. "Sarah Pratt: The Shaping of an Apostate." Dialogue: A Journal of Mormon Thought. 19: no.2. Cambridge, MA: Dialogue Foundation, 1986.

LV. "A Gypsy Camp." TJ. 4: no. 14. Tampa: Cooper, 20 Mar 1890. LV's Tampa Guardian and Tampa Journal columns are available on microfilm as the Old Florida
    Newspapers collection at both Tampa's John M. Germany Public Library and the University of South Florida's Special Collections Library.

LV. "Correspondence--Our Tarpon Letter." TJ. 1: no. 15. Tampa: Cooper, 31 Mar 1887.

LV. "Lucie Vannevar's Letter." TWJ. 1: no. 9. Tampa: Cooper, 16 Feb 1888.

LV. "Lucie Vannevar's Letter." TWJ. 2: no. 14. Tampa: Cooper, 22 Mar 1888.

LV. "Lucie Vannevar's Letter." TWJ. 2: no. 27. Tampa: Cooper, 23 Jun 1888.

LV. "Lucie Vannevar's Letter." TWJ. 2: no. 28. Tampa: Cooper, 29 Jun 1888.

LV. "Lucie Vannevar's Letter." TWJ. 2: no. 49. Tampa: Cooper, 22 Nov 1888.

LV. "Lucie Vannevar's Letter." TWJ. 3: no. 6. Tampa: Cooper, 24 Jan 1889.

LV. "Lucie Vannevar's Letter." TJ. 3: no. 12. Tampa: Cooper, 7 Mar 1889.

LV. "Lucie Vannevar's Letter." TJ. 3: no. 21. Tampa: Cooper, 9 May 1889.

LV. "Lucie Vannevar's Letter—Her Impression of the State W.C. T. Convention." TJ. 4: no. 12. Tampa: Cooper, 6 Mar 1890.

LV. "Mrs. Vannevar's Party." TJ, West Coast Department. 4: no. 8. Tampa: Cooper, 20 Feb 1890.

LV. "Our Tarpon Letter." TJ. 1: no. 1. Tampa: Conoley, 29 Dec 1886.

LV. "Our Tarpon Letter." TJ. 1: no. 3. Tampa: Conoley, 13 Jan 1887.

LV. "Our Tarpon Letter." TJ. 1: no. 6. Tampa: Conoley, 2 Feb 1887.

LV. "Our Tarpon Letter." TJ. 1: no. 7. Tampa: Conoley, 9 Feb 1887.

LV. "Our Tarpon Letter." TJ. 1: no. 23. Tampa: Cooper, 26 May 1887.

LV. "Our Tarpon Letter." TJ. 1: no. 24. Tampa: Cooper, 2 Jun 1887.

LV. "Our Tarpon Letter." TJ. 1: no. 26. Tampa: Cooper, 16 Jun 1887.

LV. "Our Tarpon Letter." TJ. 1: no. 32. Tampa: Cooper, 28 Jul 1887.

LV. "Our Tarpon Letter." TWJ 1: no. 42. Tampa: Cooper, 6 Oct 1887.

LV. "Our Tarpon Letter." TJ. 2: no. 4. Tampa: Cooper, 12 Jan 1888.

LV. "Pine Crest Inn." TJ, West Coast Department. 4: no. 7. Tampa: Cooper, 30 Jan 1890.

LV. "Sensation at Tarpon Thirty Five Citizens Poisoned by Eating Ice Cream." TWJ. 2: no. 7. Tampa: Cooper, 9 Feb 1888.

LV. "Tampa As Seen by Tarpon Eyes, An Interesting Description of Our City." TWJ. 1: no. 39. Tampa: Cooper, 15 Sep 1887.

LV. "Tarpon News." TG. 12: no. 32. Tampa: Magbee, 24 Nov 1886.

LV. "The Fourth at Tarpon." TWJ. 2: no.30. Tampa: Cooper, 13 Jul 1888.

LV. "Three Days with Rose Cleveland." TJ, West Coast Department. 4: no. 2. Tampa: Cooper, 26 Dec 1889.

LV. "West Coast Department." TJ, West Coast Department. 4: no. 1. Tampa: Cooper, 19 Dec 1889.

"Virtual Tours—Historic Northampton Museum and Education Center." "Entrepreneurs and Philanthropists," Northampton, Massachusetts, area history:
    www.historic-northampton.org/virtual_tours/Markers/Markerpanels/entrepreneurs.html.

"Visitors' Guide to the Centennial Exhibition and Philadelphia." Philadelphia: Lippincott, 1876.

Volp, John H. The First Hundred Years 1835-1935: Historical Review of Blue Island, Illinois. 1938. Internet Archive, open library.

Wack, Henry Wellington. The Romance of Victor Hugo and Juliette Drouet. New York: G. P. Putnam's Sons, 1905.

Waggoner, Horace Q. "Shawneetown Bank Project Memoir." Springfield, IL: University of Illinois at Springfield,
    Norris L. Brooks Library, Archives/Special Collections interviews, 1978.

Wakefield, Eva Ingersoll. The Letters of Robert G. Ingersoll. New York: Philosophical Library, 1951.

Wall, John P., M.D. "The Yellow Fever in Tampa, Plant City, Manatee, and Palmetto." Annual Report of the Supervising Surgeon-General of the Marine
    -Hospital Service of the United States for the Fiscal Year 1889. Washington, DC: GPO, 1889.

Wallbridge, Gedney. Descendents of Henry Wallbridge Who Married Anna Amos December 25, 1688 at Preston, Connecticut. Litchfield, CT: Wallbridge, 1898.

Ware, Susan, ed. Forgotten Heroes: Inspiring American Portraits of Our Leading Historians. New York: The Free Press, 1998.

Warner, John Harley. Against the Spirit of System: The French Impulse in Nineteenth-Century American Medicine. Baltimore: John Hopkins University Press, 2003.

Wawro, Geoffrey. The Austro-Prussian War: Austria's War with Prussia and Italy in 1866. Cambridge, England: Cambridge University Press. 1996.

Weatherford, Doris. Real Women of Tampa and Hillsborough County from Prehistory to the Millennium. Tampa: University of Tampa Press, 2004.

Weatherford, Doris. They Dared to Dream: Florida Women Who Shaped History. Gainesville, FL: University Press of Florida, 2015.

Webb, Wanton, W. "Tarpon Springs." Webb's Historical Industrial and Biographical Florida, Part I. New York: W. S. Webb & Co, 1885.

Whitcomb, F. J. M., MD. "From the Land of Flowers: The Soil and Climate of Florida." Nunda News. 25: no. 3. Nunda, NY: Sanders, 19 Jan 1884.

Whitcomb, F. J. M., MD. "Our Florida Letter (Special Correspondence of the News)." Nunda News. 25: no. 2. Nunda, NY: Sanders, 12 Jan 1884.

Whitcomb, F. J. M., MD. "Our Florida Letter (Special Correspondence of the News)." Nunda News. 25: no. 7. Nunda, NY: Sanders, 16 Feb 1884.

Whitcomb, Merrick. Harvard College Secretary's Report, No. IV. Buffalo: Matthews, Northrup & Co Art Printing Works Office of the Buffalo Morning Express, 1890.

White, Mrs. Augusta Francella Payne and Holman, Mary Lovering. The Paynes of Hamilton: A Genealogical and Biographical Record. New York: Tobias Wright, 1912.

Whiting, Lilian. "Lilian Whiting's Pen." The Inter-Ocean. Chicago: Inter-Ocean, 25 Jun 1881.

Wiley, Edwin and Rines, Irving. Lectures on the Growth and Development of the United States. 4. New York: American Educational Alliance, 1916.

Willard, Frances E. Glimpses of Fifty Years, 1839-1889. Chicago: Woman's Temperance Publication Association, 1889.

Williams, Deborah. The Erie Canal. Woodstock, VT: The Countryman Press, 2009.

Williams, Wellington. Appleton's Southern and Western Travellers' Guide. New York: D. Appleton, 1853.

Willson, Francis Michael Glenn. The University of London, 1858-1900: The Politics of Senate and Convocation. Woodbridge, Suffolk, England: Boydell Press, 2004.

Wilson, Ella B. Ensor, ed. "Memorial Library Building, Cairo, Ill." Parson's Memorial and Historical Library Magazine. 1. St. Louis: Becktold, Jan 1885.

Wilson, James Grant and Fiske, John, ed. Appleton's Cyclopaedia of American Biography. 4. New York: D. Appleton, 1898.

Wilson, Lydia Safford. Letter to Niece Mary. Burlington, Vermont 15 Dec 1880. Through the courtesy of Dr. Frank Dunton and Mr. Charles Dunton,
    recipients of Margarita (daughter) Safford's belongings at her death.

Winslow, Donald J. Lasell: A History of the First Junior College for Women. Boston: Nimrod Press, 1987.

"Woman's Work." Buffalo Daily Courier. Buffalo, New York: Manchester, 21 Jun 1885.

"Women's Congress." Friends' Intelligencer. 31: no. 39. Philadelphia: An Association of Friends, 21 Nov 1874.

Woodlawn Cemetery Register of Interment #19175, Folio 235, Margaretta G. Safford. Bronx, New York City. Death 7 Jan 1880.

Woodruff, George H. and Hill, H. H. The History of Will County, Illinois. Chicago: William LeBaron Jr. and Co, 1878.

Woodward, Corodon Roswell. Recollections Reflections Collections of Seventy Years. Cairo, IL: C. R. Woodward, 1909.

Woolson, Abba Goold, ed. Dress Reform: A Series of Lectures Delivered in Boston, On Dress as it Affects the Health of Women. Boston: Roberts Brothers, 1874.

"World's Homeopathic Convention." United States Medical Investigator. 4. Chicago: United States Medical Investigator Press, 15 Sep 1876.

Young, Agatha. The Women and the Crisis, Women of the North in the Civil War. New York: McDowell, Obolensky, 1959.

Zeller, George. The Autobiography of George Zeller, MD 1858-1938. Peoria, IL: George A. Zeller Mental Health Center, undated but apparently from late 1930s.

Zweifel, P., "Occlusion of the Os Uteri." Archives of Gynaecology, translation by Mary J. Safford-Blake. New England Medical Gazette. 8: no. 10.
    Boston: Otis Clapp & Son, Oct 1873.

ACKNOWLEDGMENTS

The author thanks the following individuals and institutions while apologizing to those inadvertently neglected in the listing:

Ed and Jane Hoffman; Safford House Museum, Judy LeGath, Deborah Gammon; Carol and Wehlan Triebold, Crete, IL; Tarpon Springs Public Library and librarian Salvador Miranda; Hernando County Public Library; Monica Smith, Librarian, Cairo Public Library, IL; Mary Markey, Smithsonian Archives; Carolyn L. Clark, Librarian, Auburn Avenue Research Library on African-American Culture and History, Atlanta, GA; Scott Anderson and Tom Collins, Sharlot Hall Museum, Prescott, AZ; Dr. Ann Koblitz, AZ State University, Tempe; Cynthia Vickery and Brenda Wood, Shawneetown Library, IL; Lara Killian, Hyde Park Town Records, VT; Jack Eckert, Countway Library, Harvard University; Janet C. Olson, Northwestern University and Frances Willard House, Evanston, IL; Karen Maxville, U.S. Grant NHS; Dennis Taylor, U.S. Patent Office; Fred Holabird, Reno, NV; Fred Reed, Editor & Publisher *Paper Money* Magazine; Professor Virginia Hayssen, Smith College, Northampton, MA; Amy Crumpton, American Association for the Advancement of Science; Peter Reich, A'Llyn Ettien, Emily Beattie, and Dr. Julie Sandell, Boston University School of Medicine; Christa Jones, Chauncey Hall School, MA; Jill McCreary, AZ Historical Society, Tucson; Melanie Sturgeon and Nancy Sawyer, AZ State Archives; AZ Historical Foundation; Caroline Stoffel and others, American Antiquarian Society, Boston; Mario Ignacio Coppola-Joffroy, Antonio Coppola Bonorand and Michele Mahler, Soledad Safford's relations; Irene Axelrod, Peabody Essex Museum, Salem, MA; Eisha Prather Neely, Cornell University Division of Rare Manuscripts; Jeffery Flannery, Library of Congress, Manuscripts Division; Abraham Lincoln Presidential Library and Museum, Springfield, IL; Dr. Cynthia Patterson; Marilyn Negip, Librarian, Lasell College; Jinene Harvey, Unitarian/Universalist consultant; Earl Taylor, Dorchester Historical Society; Linda Morrison, Boston research; Joan Bates, NC research; Shirley Moravec, language consultant; Michael Coachman, photography; Debbie Scott, San Joaquin County Historical Society, Lodi, CA; Marcella Pertsas, FL Hospital-North Pinellas, Tarpon Springs; Wenxian Zhang, Rollins College Archives & Special Collections; Joan Schumaker, Pat Galbraith and Tom Cook, Nunda Historical Society, NY; Phyllis Kolianos, Sharon Sawyer and Tarpon Springs Area Historical Society; April Anderson and Ashley Pritts, IL State University, Bloomington, IL; Roxy Dunn, Linda Stahnke and Elizabeth Wohlgemuth, University of IL Archives; Amy Papola, Greentree Foundation; Caterina Del Vivo, Gabinetto Vieusseux, Florence, Italy; Sarah Dorpinghaus, University of KY Library, Lexington; Jay Stearns, IL researcher; Dr. Philip Abensur, Paris, France; Gerald Loftus, Tangier American Legation Institute for Moroccan Studies; Tiffany Cabrera, Historian, Policy Studies Division, U.S. Dept. of State; Cat Camp, University of South FL Library, Tampa; Dr. Patricia Likos Ricci, Elizabethtown College, PA; Doris Weatherford; Paula Everett, Mt. Greenwood Cemetery, Blue Island, IL; Mike Kaliski, Blue Island Historical Society, IL; Sally Costik and Molly Lindahl, Bradford Landmark Society, PA; Gina Giang and Laura Stalker, Huntington Library, San Marino, CA; Christophe LaBaune, archivist, College de France, Paris, France; Wm. L. Clements Library Librarians, University of MI, Ann Arbor; Sabina Beauchard, MA Historical Society, Boston; WI Historical Society personnel, Madison; Deborah Trehy, MD; Juliana Okulski Laitos, JD, initial manuscript review; Joseph Rivera, manuscript review/critic; Betty Hammock; Theodore A. Gantz.

ABOUT THE AUTHOR

Born in Evanston, Illinois, Elizabeth Grange Okulski
Coachman grew up outside Chicago before attending
Philadelphia's Moore College of Art and Rutgers University.
After two years in Okinawa, she returned to Philadelphia and
gained an MD at Temple University Medical School before
receiving pathology training in Florida. Practicing mainly in
western Florida she was also on the University of South Florida
Medical School's Clinical Staff. Upon retiring as Laboratory
Medical Director at Tarpon Springs' hospital, she returned
to her artistic roots as a printmaker and landscape painter.

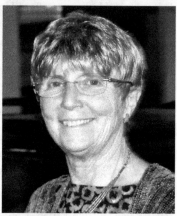

Elizabeth Coachman, MD

She and her husband Mike enjoy extensive travel throughout the US and Canada
but also relish their time at home on their Hernando County cattle ranch. Repeated
requests for her reenacting Dr. Mary Safford for Tarpon Springs' Safford House
Museum led to research that resulted in this book.

Printed in the USA
CPSIA information can be obtained
at www.ICGtesting.com
CBHW041128031023
1213CB00003B/5